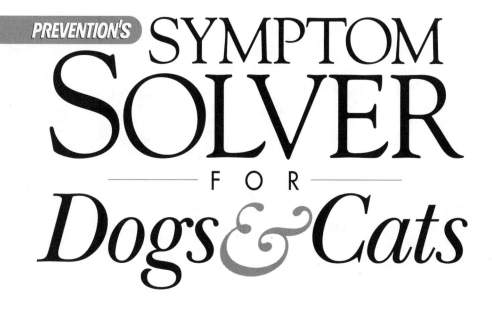

PREVENTION'S

SYMPTOM SOLVER

FOR

Dogs & Cats

PREVENTION'S SYMPTOM SOLVER

FOR

Dogs & Cats

From Arfs and Arthritis
to Whimpers and Worms,
An Owner's Cure Finder

Edited by Matthew Hoffman

Medical Advisor: Craig N. Carter, D.V.M., Ph.D., head of
epidemiology at the Texas Veterinary Medical Diagnostic
Laboratory at Texas A&M University

Rodale Press, Inc.
Emmaus, Pennsylvania

Library of Congress Cataloging-in-Publication Data

Prevention's symptom solver for dogs and cats : from arfs and arthritis to whimpers and worms : an owner's cure finder / edited by Matthew Hoffman.
    p.   cm.
  Includes index.
  ISBN 0–87596–523–7 hardcover
  1. Dogs—Diseases. 2. Cats—Diseases. 3. Symptoms in animals.
I. Hoffman, Matthew. II. Prevention for Pets. III. Prevention (Emmaus, Pa.)
IV. Title: Symptom solver for dogs and cats.
SF991.P74 1999
636.7'089—dc21   98–39964

Distributed to the book trade by St. Martin's Press

4 6 8 10 9 7 5 3   hardcover

OUR PURPOSE

We help you give your pets all the good health and loving care they deserve. In our books, you will find the latest information along with the wisdom and practical advice of the country's top veterinary experts. From behavior and training tips to improving quality of life, we will help you achieve the greatest reward of all—a lifetime of love and commitment.

PREVENTION PETS

Notice

This book is intended as a reference volume only, not as a medical manual. The information given here is designed to help you make informed decisions about your pet's health. It is not intended as a substitute for any treatment that may have been prescribed by your veterinarian. If you suspect that your pet has a medical problem, we urge you to seek competent medical help.

PREVENTION'S SYMPTOM SOLVER FOR DOGS AND CATS EDITORIAL STAFF

Editor: Matthew Hoffman

Senior Managing Editor: Edward Claflin

Contributing Writers: Betsy Bates; Lisa Bennett; Karen Commings; Robin DeMattia; Phil Goldberg; Joanne Howl, D.V.M.; Jill O. Kulig, V.M.D.; Lynn McGowen; Kristine Napier; Audrey Pavia; Fran Pennock Shaw; Kim Thornton; Margo Trott

Lead Researcher: Shea Zukowski

Editorial Researchers: Leah B. Flickinger, Nanci Kulig

Senior Copy Editor: Karen Neely

Cover Designer: Joanna Reinhart

Book Designers: David Q. Pryor, Joanna Reinhart

Associate Art Director: Charles Beasley

Cover Photographer: Dennis Mosner

Illustrator: Tim Phelps

Layout Designer: Faith Hague

Manufacturing Coordinators: Brenda Miller, Jodi Schaffer, Patrick T. Smith

Office Manager: Roberta Mulliner

Office Staff: Julie Kehs, Suzanne Lynch, Mary Lou Stephen

RODALE HEALTH AND FITNESS BOOKS

Vice President and Editorial Director: Debora T. Yost

Executive Editor: Neil Wertheimer

Design and Production Director: Michael Ward

Marketing Manager: Kris Siessmayer

Research Manager: Ann Gossy Yermish

Copy Manager: Lisa D. Andruscavage

Production Manager: Robert V. Anderson Jr.

Assistant Studio Manager: Thomas P. Aczel

Manufacturing Managers: Eileen F. Bauder, Mark Krahforst

Contents

Foreword

Veterinarians are often compared to pediatricians because our patients, like many of theirs, can't tell us what is wrong. It takes a lot of education and long hours before we learn to recognize most of the things that can make your little critter sick. Even then it is a tough job. We only see our patients once or twice a year. Sometimes it is difficult to tell if the way they are acting or feeling is normal for them. We just don't see them enough. And when we ask them what's wrong, well, who knows what they would say if they could talk?

This is where you, the owner, come in. One thing that I have learned over the years is how important it is to listen to what *you* think is wrong with your pet. Because of the strong bonds and incredibly intimate relationships you share with your furry companions, you are often better at recognizing a potential medical problem than your veterinarian is. When it comes to what your pet is feeling, you are an expert.

Of course, it is crucial for pet owners to learn the difference between those symptoms that are serious enough to warrant a veterinarian's attention and those that they can deal with at home. Many conditions can, in fact, be solved quickly and safely on your own.

Suppose your dog begins to choke on his dinner. If you recognize the symptom and know what to do, you can clear his windpipe with one simple Heimlich maneuver. Problem solved.

Or imagine that your cat is keeping one eye shut for no apparent reason. When you examine the eye, you may find a small foreign object inside, and so you safely flush it out with saline solution.

The information in this book will add an extra dimension to the care that you are able to give your pet at home. At the same time, it will send you straight to the phone on those important—sometimes critical—occasions when you need to see your vet.

The next time you are worried about your pet, turn to the book that is in your hands right now. It will help you both on your journey toward a healthier and happier life.

Craig N. Carter, D.V.M., Ph.D.
Head of epidemiology at the Texas Veterinary Medical Diagnostic Laboratory at Texas A&M University

Introduction

Dogs and cats are stoic creatures. They are very good at hiding their pain, and they can't say when they need some help. It is up to us to recognize their symptoms and signals—and to know how to help them get better.

A few years ago, I discovered the importance of "dognostics" firsthand. My dog, Max, is an elderly Airedale who normally smells a little musky. One day I came home from work and immediately noticed a strange, pungent odor in the room—quite different from Max's usual Airedalian aroma. He looked a little under the weather, too, so I called my vet. It turned out that Max had a mild skin infection that was causing the bad smell. I picked up a medicated shampoo at the pet store, and a few baths later, Max was his usual (if slightly smelly) self again.

I learned a valuable lesson that day—one I call the Max test. *Any change in a pet's usual behavior or appearance (or smell) is a warning sign.* When you know what is normal for your pet, you will also know when something is wrong. The problem, of course, is that while some symptoms are obvious—a limp, for example, or a cut paw—many are not. That is why this may be the most important pet-care book that you will ever own.

The editors at *Prevention for Pets* spent over a year interviewing more than 160 of the country's top veterinarians. Our goal was to discover every possible dog and cat symptom in order to help owners recognize—and treat—potential problems.

Maybe your cat is eating less than usual. Or your dog is going to the bathroom more often. The eyes are dilated. The coat looks dry. There are specks in the stool. These are just a few of the hundreds of symptoms that you will find in this book. And some of them are quite surprising.

We discovered that some of the symptoms we always worried about, such as a hot nose, aren't really problems at all. And some things we never thought about or even noticed are actually quite serious. Pets that suddenly develop sweet breath, for example, could have diabetes. A potbelly is common in humans, but in dogs or cats it could be a sign of internal diseases. Pets with dirty ears could have mites—or they could have a serious infection.

In this book, you will find more than 225 symptoms and clues—everything from appetite loss and aggression to eye changes, a dry nose, and tail limpness. In addition, every entry includes a special section called "What You Can Do," which provides practical, easy-to-follow instructions for helping your pet feel better and recover more quickly.

Some symptoms, of course, need a veterinarian's care. So we also included a section called "What Your Vet Will Do." You will discover the sorts of things that your vet will look for, the tests that will be run, and what the best medical treatments are. You will get fascinating, behind-the-scenes insights into veterinary care—insights that will help you understand your pet's health and make informed decisions.

The best medicine—for pets as well as people—is prevention. You will find everything you need to keep your pets healthy, from giving home exams to the best exercises for different breeds. Since even healthy pets will get sick from time to time, we have also provided a "nursing" guide. You will learn the best way to give a pill, how to take your pet's temperature, ways to relieve aches and pains, and how to keep your pet comfortable.

Dogs and cats are curious, adventuresome creatures who sometimes get into trouble, which is why knowing first-aid is so important. You will discover the best ways to stop bleeding. How to bandage a broken tail. How to give CPR. Techniques for moving an injured pet. How to save your pet from poisoning. And much more.

Finally, to make this book as practical as possible, we have also included more than 90 simple, easy-to-follow illustrations that show exactly what you need to do.

After reading this book, you may find yourself thinking like a "symptom detective." You will be alert to changes that you never noticed before. And your pets will soon get used to having you feel their paws, look inside their ears, and move their joints this way and that to make sure that everything is okay. You will feel confident knowing that if they ever do get sick or hurt, you will spot the problem quickly and will know exactly what to do.

Prevention's Symptom Solver for Dogs and Cats will help you give your pets the gift of good health—and nothing is better than that.

Matthew Hoffman

Matthew Hoffman
Editor, *Prevention for Pets*

Prevention: The Best Care

One of the first things we do when we bring a new pet home, after spreading newspapers on the floor or putting out the litter box, is browse through the Yellow Pages to find a veterinarian. It's a good place to start because your vet is the person that you'll call whenever you have questions or concerns—when your dog is limping for no apparent reason, for example, or your cat has been noshing on a plant that you're afraid may be poisonous.

But your vet only spends an hour or two a year with your pets. He can easily handle vaccinations, injuries, and illnesses, but he can't be there every day to notice the little changes in your pets' health and behavior that may turn into problems later on. Nor can he take your pets for walks or make sure that they are eating the right food. It's up to you to handle the daily care—all the little things that will keep your pets happy and healthy for the rest of their lives.

Like their owners, dogs and cats need to have good nutrition, daily exercise, a safe place to play, and regular grooming. The difference, of course, is that pets can't complain when they are tired and achy. They won't tell you when they have an eye discharge or a loss of hearing or that they are gaining weight. It's up to you to notice changes or symptoms. By watching your pets closely, you will know when trouble is brewing. In this chapter, you will also discover ways to keep them from getting sick in the first place.

Preventive care isn't expensive (it's a heck of a lot cheaper than veterinary care), and it doesn't take a lot of time. And the payoff is tremendous: a small amount of time for a lifetime of love.

HOME SAFETY

From your pet's point of view, your house is one big amusement park. There are chair legs to chew, curtains to climb, electrical cords to tug on, garbage to eat, slick floors to slide on, and any number of interesting potions, powders, and pills to lap up and swallow. When you first bring your pet home, you will be amazed at how much trouble he can get into in such a short time.

"Anything that a two-year-old child might put in his mouth or grab hold of, a puppy or kitten will undoubtedly do the same," says Peggy Rucker, D.V.M., a veterinarian in private practice in Lebanon, Virginia.

Every year, thousands of pets get hurt when their curiosity (and their appetites) lead them into dangerous territory. You don't want to stop dogs and cats from exploring, but you do want to keep them safe. Take a few minutes to see things the way they see them—from floor level. Get down on your hands and knees and explore the house, room by room. (Your pets will think this is all great fun, so you'll have plenty of company.) Look for things that they can reach, chew, or swallow, like string or sewing supplies, says Victoria Valdez, D.V.M., a veterinarian in private practice in Orange, California. Are there cabinets they can nose open or cleaning supplies in paw's reach? The more attractions you can identify— and either move or safely secure—the less likely your pets are to get hurt, she says.

Watch out for electricity. Electrical cords can seem like perfect chew toys—until your pet's sharp teeth penetrate the insulation and hit the wires inside. Dr. Valdez recommends

Which Plants Are Poison?

For dogs and cats, many houseplants and shrubs are as tasty as a fresh garden salad. But many of the same plants that tickle their tastebuds are also poisonous. Among the worst are poinsettias, philodendrons, and dieffenbachias. "There are alkaline chemicals in the leaves of poinsettias that cause gastrointestinal upset," says Robin Downing, D.V.M., a veterinarian in private practice in Windsor, Colorado. Here are a few other plants that you'll want to keep out of reach.

- Amaryllis
- Azalea
- Caladium
- Calla or arum lily
- Daffodil
- Delphinium
- Elephant's ear
- English holly
- Foxglove
- Ivy
- Jade plant
- Jerusalem cherry
- Morning glory
- Mums (pot and spider)
- Privet
- Wisteria

hiding electrical cords under carpets or behind furniture. Or tape them firmly to the floor.

Keep medicines out of reach. Even mild human medicines like acetaminophen can be extremely dangerous for dogs and cats. It's not enough to stash them on top of the bureau or in a partly closed drawer. Dogs and cats are intrepid explorers and will often find things you didn't expect them to. And a childproof cap won't slow down an inquisitive puppy for more than a minute or two, says Dr. Valdez. So be sure to keep medicines well out of reach or behind tightly closed doors.

Cover the windows. Young pets are attracted to open windows and balconies, but they don't fully grasp the concept of "down." Every year, a few unfortunate dogs and cats accidentally tumble from upper stories, causing injuries that vets refer to as high-rise syndrome. Take a few minutes to make sure that screens fit snugly and are in good repair. If you have a balcony, keep the door to it closed.

Shut the lids on appliances. You wouldn't think that the inside of a washing machine would hold much allure, but more than a few cats have dropped in to explore, then found themselves tumbling around with the wash. Vets recommend getting in the habit of closing appliances—including trash compactors and dishwashers—when they're not in use. It's also a good idea to check for visitors before hitting the "on" switch.

Cover the commode. "If you leave the toilet seat up, it looks like a chair from a kitten's point of view, and she's going to jump up," says Dr. Valdez. And the next thing you know, your cat's splashing around in an unsanitary place. For small cats particularly, it's not always easy to get out. "It's porcelain, so they can't get a foothold," she explains.

Do a car check. Cats love to curl up under the hoods of cars because heat from the engine keeps them pleasantly warm. You don't have to open the hood every time you go for a drive. Just rap it soundly with your hand—the noise will drive out guests before the gears and belts start turning, says Dr. Valdez.

Make the garage off-limits. Many chemicals that we use every day, like insecticides and antifreeze, are downright tasty—and deadly—to dogs and cats. "You'd be amazed at the things pets think are okay to put in their mouths, including lye and other chemicals," says Robin Downing, D.V.M., a veterinarian in private practice in Windsor, Colorado. It's essential to keep your pets away from danger zones and to keep chemicals off the floor and put away, she says.

Provide some traction. For puppies particularly, slick linoleum floors can be hard to negotiate. It's pretty cute when your roly-poly puppy goes slipping and sliding, but the lack of traction can actually damage his bones and joints. "A rug that won't slip will keep the young puppy from slipping and harming his hip socket, which is still being formed when he's young," says Jim Corbin, Ph.D., professor emeritus of animal nutrition at the University of Illinois in Urbana.

THE HOME EXAM

Most of us take our pets to the vet once or twice a year for shots and a checkup. While annual exams are essential, there are limits to what your vet can learn during a 30-minute visit. If your dog was a little achy a month ago but is fine on the day of the exam, your vet won't suspect that he is having hip problems or the beginnings of arthritis—unless you remember to tell him what was going on before. And you won't know yourself unless you have been keeping tabs on his health. This is why home exams are so important.

You don't need a white coat or a stethoscope to examine your pet. Really, all that's required is being alert for changes, says Dr. Downing. Maybe there is an eye discharge, a new bump on the skin, or tenderness in the abdomen or around the hips. Catching these and other problems early means that your pet is much less likely to get sick later on. "I teach my clients to smell the inside of the ear canal," she adds. "They can often notice an early ear infection—long before their pet is really scratching his ear and shaking his head—and get it treated before it gets serious."

Vets recommend doing a complete home exam at least once a month, says Priscilla Stockner, D.V.M., executive director of the Animal Center and Humane Society in Escondido, California. But you don't have to follow a formal plan. When you are giving him a bath, rubbing his belly, or playing in the yard, watch for *anything* that seems different. It probably isn't

Does the Nose Know?

Dogs and cats get fevers just as often as people do. But don't count on your pet's nose to be a reliable indicator. A warm nose doesn't mean he's sick, any more than a cool, wet nose means he's healthy.

"That's one of the oldest old wives' tales out there," says Robin Downing, D.V.M., a veterinarian in private practice in Windsor, Colorado. "I've seen pets with high temperatures that have cold, wet noses. I've also had owners bring a pet in because his nose was warm, but the pet was just fine. The temperature of the nose isn't a very reliable measure of an animal's wellness."

About all you can tell from the temperature of your pet's nose is where he has been spending his time, adds Peggy Rucker, D.V.M., a veterinarian in private practice in Lebanon, Virginia. "Your pet can come in from the outside, and his nose may feel cool, but he could still be running a fever," she says.

The only way to check your pet's temperature is the old-fashioned and never-popular way: by using a rectal thermometer.

anything serious—but if it is, you will have the advantage of catching it early. Here are the main things that you will want to watch for.

Do an infection inspection. Since the eyes, ears, and nose are always open to the elements, they are the places most likely to get infected. Signs of infection include a bad odor, redness, swelling, or a discharge, says Dr. Downing.

Check for mites. Ear mites are tiny parasites that can cause intense itching and, sometimes, infections in the ear canal. Look at the wax in your pet's ears. It should be light or dark yellow. If it's black or brown and gritty-looking, he probably has mites, and you will want to take care of them.

Monitor his weight. It's normal for pets to gain a little weight as they get older. If your dog or cat has suddenly put on a lot of weight—or if he has suddenly started to lose weight—you'll want to call your vet right away.

Look for lumps. Many dogs and cats will develop lumps under the skin. Some older pets, in fact, get so many lumps that they feel like furry beanbags. Unfortunately, there's no way to tell at home if a lump is harmless or not, so it's essential to call your vet if a new one develops. This is especially true of cats since they are more likely than dogs to develop cancerous lumps. "The four most dangerous words in the English language are 'Let's just watch it,'" says Dr. Downing.

EATING FOR HEALTH

Dogs and cats like to eat. Actually, they *love* to eat—everything from dry kibble to yesterday's steamed broccoli or leftover roast. They aren't thinking about their waistlines or cholesterol levels. They are just thinking about food—and when the next meal is going to be served.

What they don't think about—but we do—is whether or not what's going in their bowls is good for them. "Nutrition is an incredibly important part of wellness," Dr. Downing says. Pets that eat wholesome, nutritious foods are much less likely to be overweight. They are less likely to get diabetes and other digestive problems. A healthful diet may even reduce the risk of kidney stones, she says.

Choosing the right food can be tricky. The pet food aisle is often one of the biggest pieces of real estate in the supermarket, with dozens of brands and styles to choose from. Where do you begin?

Most vets recommend avoiding generic, "no-name" foods. Even though they are often half the cost of name-brand foods, they are not made with top-quality ingredients. "What I generally find with generics is that they are not very calorically dense, so you have to feed more of them to get the same amount of nutrition as you would from a national-brand food at a grocery store or a premium food," says Christine Wilford, D.V.M., a veterinarian in private practice in Seattle.

Are Vegetarian Diets a Good Choice?

The health concerns of people and pets are often similar, but when it comes to diet, the needs are entirely different. A vegetarian diet has been shown to be very healthful for people. Is the same true for pets?

For cats, the answer is an unequivocal no. Cats are known as obligate carnivores, which means that they need certain amino acids that they only can get from meat. Putting a cat on a vegetarian diet will make him ill and could be fatal, says Victoria Valdez, D.V.M., a veterinarian in private practice in Orange, California.

Dogs, on the other hand, are omnivores—they do quite well on a variety of foods, including a vegetarian diet. But it is essential to talk to your vet before putting your dog on a plant-based plan. Dogs need substantial amounts of protein as well as vitamin B_{12}, which can be difficult to get from plant foods alone. If you believe a vegetarian diet is the way to go, talk to your vet. She will recommend a diet that will provide all the nutrients that your pet needs.

There is nothing wrong with going to the other extreme and buying high-cost, premium foods, which are available from vets and pet supply stores. Premium foods are made from excellent ingredients, and vets sometimes recommend them for pets with special needs—those with urinary stones, for example, or those that are unusually active, like hunting dogs.

The advantage of premium foods is that they are very easy to digest. Many of them have a digestibility of more than 80 percent. "If you have a food that is only 50 percent digestible, that means that 50 percent of it is inert filler that is going to end up as poop in the yard or litter pan," she explains.

For most pets, however, premium foods won't make a big difference in their health, says Dr. Corbin. Unless your vet has suggested otherwise, you can't go wrong buying the less expensive, name-brand foods at the supermarket.

There is more to food than nutrition, of course. From your pet's point of view, taste is the most important thing. As long as you are buying a quality food, feel free to shop around until you find a brand or style of food that your pet likes best. Nutritionally, canned and dry foods are about the same, says John Hamil, D.V.M., a veterinarian in private practice in Laguna Beach, California. Given a choice, most dogs and cats prefer moist foods. Vets, on the other hand, lean toward dry. Kibble doesn't stick to the teeth the way moist foods do, and it scours the teeth when they eat, which can help prevent dental problems later on. And, of course, it's much less expensive.

LEAN FOR LIFE

Losing weight is never easy—for people or for pets. But when you are trying to keep your dog or cat healthy, there is no better place to begin than by keeping his weight in check. Overweight pets are at high risk for diabetes, a condition in which the body's insulin doesn't work as effectively as it should. They are also prone to hip dysplasia, arthritis, and other joint problems, says Dr. Wilford. In addition, vets have found that overweight pets don't live as long as their trimmer friends.

You don't have to buy exercise tapes or sign up with Weight Watchers to help your pet slim down. Giving him a little less food and a little more exercise will help restore him to a healthy weight. (Since weight gain may be a sign of medical problems, it's a good idea to check with your vet before starting a weight-loss plan.) Here is what vets advise.

Measure what goes in the bowl. Before changing your pet's diet, use a measuring cup to figure out how much you are actually giving him. Then cut the amount by no more than 25 percent. Most pets will lose weight this way, says Dr. Wilford. If your pet stays pudgy even on the leaner diet, Dr. Wilford suggests that you cut the amount of food again by up to 25 percent.

Of course, once your pet reaches his ideal weight, you will want to continue giving him smaller portions. This diet is safe for dogs and cats, says Dr. Wilford. But you have to be a little careful with cats since they will sometimes develop liver problems as they lose weight. If your cat seems to lose interest in food after being on the diet, check with your vet.

Keep track of treats. When you are trying to figure out how much your pets are eating, don't forget to include the little extras—the biscuits, fish snacks, or tasty table scraps. Treats are generally high in fat and calories and can sabotage the best-planned diet. Vets recommend cutting back on treats or replacing them with healthier snacks, like pieces of fruit or vegetables cut in bite-size pieces. Many pets like popcorn as well.

Forget the buffet. Some dogs and cats show admirable restraint at the dinner table, but most will eat whatever goes in the bowl. If you keep it full all the time, they will eat all the time. Vets recommend putting pets on strict eating schedules—feeding them once in the morning and again in the evening, for example. If for some reason your pet doesn't eat all of his food, pick it up after 15 to 20 minutes and put it away until the next meal. When your pets can't eat whenever they like, they will naturally start losing a little weight, says Dr. Valdez.

Tame their tummies. Dogs and cats don't like diets any more than people do, and you will probably see an increase in begging, whining, and mooching. To help them feel more satisfied, add a tablespoon or two of canned pumpkin to their food, says Craig N. Carter, D.V.M., Ph.D., head of epidemiology at the Texas Veterinary Medical Diagnostic Laboratory at Texas A&M University in College Station. It is high in fiber, low in calories, and filling—and most pets like the taste.

STAYING ACTIVE

No one expects their pet to be a feline Fonda or an Arnold *Schnauzer*negger. But giving your pet regular exercise is among the most powerful strategies for keeping him trim and healthy. Exercise keeps the heart and lungs working well. It strengthens muscles and ligaments so that they are better able to protect the joints. It even makes pets less likely to misbehave, says Geoffrey N. Clark, D.V.M., a veterinarian in Dover, New Hampshire, and editor of *Canine Sports Medicine Update*. "Many common vices, such as digging holes or chewing on furniture, are caused by boredom, especially when a dog or cat doesn't have an outlet for his energy," he says.

How much exercise does your pet need? Among dogs, energy dynamos tend to be terriers, herding breeds, and sporting hounds. They typically need an hour or more of vigorous exercise a day to stay happy and healthy. Dogs that are extra-large or extra-small tend to be more laid-back and can get by with one or two short workouts a day. Generally, all pets require at least 30 minutes of exercise a day: 15 minutes in the morning and 15 more in the evening, says Dr. Stockner.

If your pet hasn't been getting much exercise lately, take it slowly at first, Dr. Stockner advises. Take a couple of walks each day, preferably along a route without too many hills. Or play in the yard or the living room for a few minutes at a time. As he starts getting in better shape, you can increase the workout intensity—and explore other, more exciting ways of getting his paws moving.

For dogs, one of the best fitness plans is cross-training, in which they do a variety of activities such as swimming, walking, running, or chasing a ball.

Fun Ways to Exercise Your Cat

Unlike dogs, who jump with joy whenever you pick up the leash or open the door, cats aren't always eager to go for walks or to play games—unless it was their idea first. To help your cat stay in shape, you have to make exercise truly exciting from a feline's point of view. Here are a few things you may want to try, according to Robin Downing, D.V.M., a veterinarian in private practice in Windsor, Colorado.

- Get a tall scratching post, preferably one with "branches," that your cat can run up and down.
- Roll a table-tennis ball across the carpet. Sit back and enjoy the "pinball-machine effect."
- Wad up a piece of paper, tie a string to it, and drag it around. It won't take your cat long to launch an attack.
- Practice your fly-fishing by casting a line down the hall. Put a feathery fly (minus a hook) on the end of the line and watch your cat go wild.

"Swimming is particularly good for those breeds that will go in the water because it allows the use of most major muscle groups and it's easy on the joints," says Dr. Clark. It's important to supervise a dog in the water just as you would a child. That includes making sure he knows how to get out of the water and avoiding rivers and the ocean, where fast-moving currents can pose hidden dangers. And keep in mind that not every dog takes to water. So if he doesn't want to swim, don't force him—try some other exercise instead.

There is one exercise caution: Avoid doing hard exercise involving twists and turns on asphalt or cement. These surfaces are too slippery for furry feet to get a grip on, and the inevitable slipping and sliding is hard on their feet and joints. Instead, choose exercise on softer surfaces such as lawns or dirt paths.

LOOKING GOOD, FEELING GOOD

Whether you have a show-quality cat or a lovable dog of indeterminate origin, regular grooming will help him look his best. More important, grooming is a great way to find problems you might otherwise miss—fleas in the fur, for example, or small bumps on the skin. Vets have even found that regular grooming can help prevent a variety of health problems. Here is what they advise.

Brush them often. Brushing your dog or cat does more than keep the furniture clean. It also distributes natural oils over your pet's skin, which can help prevent rashes and infections. For cats, brushing is important because it reduces the amount of hair they swallow—and invariably cough up later on as a hair ball. Short-haired pets can be brushed once a week. For dogs and cats with longer fur, a daily brushing will help keep them healthy and looking good.

Go after mats. For pets with long fur, matting is a never-ending problem. The mats not only look scruffy but also trap moisture next to the skin, making it easier for bacteria or parasites to thrive, says Dr. Hamil.

Hair mats are tricky to remove because the skin underneath is often tender. If you can convince your pet to hold still, you can often work out mats using a brush and comb, says Virginia Parker Guidry, grooming columnist for *Dog Fancy* magazine. To make things easier, she recommends spraying the mat with a detangler spray, available in pet supply stores.

If the mat is too tight to remove or if it is right against the skin, you may have to clip it out with a pair of blunt-nosed scissors. Clip carefully so as not to nick the skin.

Do a "pet-acure." Just like human fingernails, your pet's nails are constantly growing. If you don't trim them regularly, they are more likely to crack or tear, says Dr. Valdez. (For a step-by-step guide to trimming nails, see Claws Won't Retract on page 245.)

Keep his teeth clean. Few of us are dedicated enough to brush our pets' teeth after every meal. But brushing them several times a week—or better yet, every day—will help keep them clean and bacteria-free. It's more than just cosmetic. Vets have found that the same bacteria in the mouth that cause gum disease can get into the bloodstream, possibly damaging the heart or other organs. (For more on caring for your pet's teeth, see Bad Breath on page 284.)

Don't forget the ears. The ears are naturally self-cleaning and don't require much care beyond regular inspections for ear mites. (To learn how to check for mites, see Dirty Ears on page 157.) But you can periodically swab out the outer portions of the ears with a dry cotton ball. Or your vet may recommend using a combination ear cleaner/disinfectant. Don't use cotton swabs to clean out the ear canal since this can push wax and debris in, Dr. Stocker warns.

Fighting Fleas

It's hard to believe that something so small can cause so much misery. Like little vampires, fleas are the scourge of dogs and cats everywhere—and their owners. Fleas are more than just itchy. They also transmit tapeworms, which can cause diarrhea or other intestinal problems. Controlling fleas is an important part of keeping your pet healthy, says John Hamil, D.V.M., a veterinarian in private practice in Laguna Beach, California.

Fighting fleas has always been a challenge, but veterinarians have recently found ways to make it a little bit easier. One strategy is to use an oral medication such as Program. Given monthly, this prescription drug stops fleas from reproducing on your pet. It doesn't affect dogs and cats, but it does cause the flea population to plunge.

Your vet may also recommend products that kill fleas directly when they are applied to the coat. Used in combination with an oral medication, they can help eliminate fleas for good, says Dr. Hamil.

The problem with fleas is that for every critter that's actually on your pet, there may be hundreds (or thousands) more in his bedding, in the yard, and around the house, says Christine Wilford, D.V.M., a veterinarian in private practice in Seattle. When you are ready to wage war on fleas, it is essential to clean the house thoroughly, especially in areas where your pet spends his time. Washing his bedding in hot water will help kill fleas as well as their eggs, stopping the flea cycle at the source, she says.

HOMEWARD BOUND

They are the size of a quarter and cost just a few dollars—and they could save your pet's life if he slips out the front door or jumps from the car. In fact, using identification tags is perhaps the most effective (and least expensive) way of keeping your pet safe, says Dr. Stockner.

Tags should have your name

and phone number. (With cats, some people go one step further and include a line that says, "If I'm outside, I'm lost.") Veterinarians advise against putting your pet's name on his tag because that could make it easier for thieves to lure him away.

For additional protection, you may want to ask your vet about tattoos or microchips. Tags often get lost, but tattoos are permanent. The same is true of microchips, which are implanted beneath the skin, usually between the shoulder blades. If your pet gets lost and doesn't have his tags, a veterinarian or animal shelter will still be able to identify him. Used together, tags, tattoos, and microchips will help ensure that a lost friend finds his way home again.

THE KINDEST CUT

Having your pet spayed or neutered does more than prevent unwanted litters. Veterinarians have found that these procedures are among the cheapest, most-effective strategies for preventing a number of serious health threats.

In males, neutering involves removing the testicles. This is important because in unneutered males the prostate gland typically enlarges with age, starting when a dog is six or seven years old. If the gland gets too large, it can begin pressing on the urethra, making it difficult to urinate. Unneutered males are also at risk for prostate infections, along with testicular cancer. Neutering your pet will completely eliminate the risk for all of these problems, says Dr. Rucker.

As a behavioral bonus, neutering males also makes them much less likely to roam or get in fights with other pets. They tend to bond more with their human owners as well. "An intact male cat's life span is about half that of a neutered cat's," adds Dr. Rucker.

When female pets are spayed, the uterus and ovaries are removed. This completely eliminates the risk of uterine infections and substantially reduces the risk for breast cancer, Dr. Rucker says.

Veterinarians recommend neutering pets when they are about six months old, although it can be done earlier or later. Generally, younger pets recover more quickly and are back to normal in a day or two, says W. Marvin Mackie, D.V.M., a veterinarian in private practice in the Los Angeles area.

WHEN TO SEE THE VET

One of the most important preventive strategies, and also the easiest, is to take your pet to the vet once or twice a year. Your vet will do many of the same things that you have been doing all year—checking your pet's ears and eyes, feeling the coat, and running his hands across the ribs to make sure the pet is not getting too portly. Your vet will also check some of the more subtle signs of health, like the size of your pet's lymph nodes, liver, and bladder. He may recommend blood tests to check your pet's kidney and liver functions.

The last part of the exam is the one dogs and cats like the least: getting their shots. Vaccinations aren't a lot of fun (although many pets don't even notice them), but they are essential for keeping your pet healthy—not just today, but for the rest of the year as well.

Caring for a Sick Pet

People spend a lot of time with their pets and can usually tell at glance when their animal companions are feeling down. Maybe your dog didn't sprint into the kitchen when kibble clattered into his bowl, or your cat totally ignored the sparrows twittering outside the window. Or perhaps your pet is moping around, so tired that his tail doesn't rise above half-mast.

It would be nice if dogs and cats were always healthy, but they are exposed to many of the same germs that people are. They catch colds, come down with the flu, and suffer through fevers and stomachaches. And it's usually no big deal. People don't rush to their doctors every time they get the sniffles; similarly, dogs and cats usually get better on their own without any help from the vet. "When you have a proper diagnosis and the situation is not critical, most pets will recover better at home in the comfort of familiar surroundings and faces," says Merry Crimi, D.V.M., a veterinarian in private practice in Milwaukie, Oregon.

In the meantime, of course, they can feel pretty lousy, which is why home care is so important. Taking care of your pet when he's sick will help him feel better and recover more quickly. More important, keeping tabs on his health is the best way to know when home care isn't enough and you need your veterinarian's help.

CHECKING YOUR PET'S TEMPERATURE

Until dogs and cats come equipped with digital readouts ("Help! I'm sick!"), there is no better way to check their health than with a ther-

When to Call for Help

Caring for pets is tricky because it is not always easy to tell whether or not they are seriously ill. Even though you can handle many health problems at home, some require a veterinarian's care. According to Craig N. Carter, D.V.M., Ph.D., head of epidemiology at the Texas Veterinary Medical Diagnostic Laboratory at Texas A&M University in College Station, here are some important warning signs to watch out for.

- Your pet is having trouble breathing or has a serious cough.
- He has been vomiting or has had diarrhea for more than 24 hours.
- Your dog hasn't eaten for two days. For cats, 24 hours is the limit.
- There is a lump anywhere on his body.
- His temperature is 103°F or higher.
- His abdomen appears to be tender or bloated.
- He is having seizures or appears disoriented or confused.

mometer, says Karen Mateyak, D.V.M., a veterinarian in private practice in Brooklyn, New York. Even if you have already taken your pet to the vet, checking his temperature periodically will let you know whether he is getting better or worse.

Unfortunately, you can't check your pet's temperature by slipping the thermometer under his tongue or by feeling his nose. You have to get more intimate than that and take his temperature the old-fashioned way, by using a rectal thermometer.

Start out by gathering the necessary supplies: a rectal thermometer, petroleum jelly, a bottle of alcohol, some cotton balls, and a friend who is willing to help. Shake down the thermometer and lightly coat it with petroleum jelly, says Dr. Mateyak. Then soak a cotton ball in the alcohol and set it aside. Now you are ready to begin.

While your helper holds your pet steady and lifts the tail, gently twirl the thermometer into the rectum about one to three inches. (For large dogs, you may have to insert it halfway to get an accurate reading.) Hold it in place for two minutes, then pull it out, wipe it clean with a dry cotton ball, and take the reading, says Dr. Mateyak. The normal temperature for dogs and cats is between 100.5° and 102.5°F. If your pet is half a degree (or more) above the normal range, he may have a fever, and you should call your vet. Use the alcohol-soaked cotton ball to clean the thermometer when you are done.

Fevers are rarely dangerous and will usually go away when the illness does, says Dr. Mateyak. But they can make your pet very uncomfortable for a few days. To lower the heat, your vet may recommend applying cool compresses to your pet's belly. Or, if your pet doesn't mind getting wet, your vet may recommend a cool bath to lower the fever. It is important, however, to check with your vet before using compresses or cool baths because in some cases cooling your pet off too quickly can cause problems.

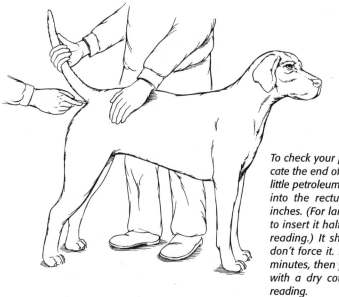

To check your pet's temperature, lubricate the end of the thermometer with a little petroleum jelly and gently insert it into the rectum about one to three inches. (For large dogs, you may have to insert it halfway to get an accurate reading.) It should slide in easily, so don't force it. Hold it in place for two minutes, then pull it out, wipe it clean with a dry cotton ball, and take the reading.

For some dogs, aspirin is a safe and effective way of lowering fever. The usual dose is about 10 milligrams of coated aspirin (like Ascriptin) for every 10 pounds of weight, given no more than twice a day, says Craig N. Carter, D.V.M., Ph.D., head of epidemiology at the Texas Veterinary Medical Diagnostic Laboratory at Texas A&M University in College Station. Aspirin can be dangerous for cats, however, and should never be used without a veterinarian's supervision. In fact, it's a good idea to check with your vet before giving any human medication to pets.

RESTFUL RECOVERY

You won't find your dog propped up in bed with an ice bag on his head or your cat curled up with a good book and a bottle of cough syrup, but pets need rest when they're sick just like people do. "They need to take some time off from the world," says Dr. Carter.

Pets know instinctively that rest is important and will do a lot of lying around when they are feeling ill. To encourage your pet to rest even more, it's a good idea to move his bed to a quiet part of the house—in a corner of the living room, for example, or next to your bed in the bedroom. To make his bed especially cozy, you can wrap a hot-water bottle in a towel and put in under his bedding.

If your pet doesn't have his own bed, you can cobble one together from a cardboard box. Be sure to get a box that's big enough for him to stretch out in, but not so big that it won't retain his body heat. Line the cardboard box with blankets to make it comfortable and cut down one side so that

Pets that are sick need a little privacy and comfort in which to recover. A cardboard box lined with a soft towel or blanket makes the perfect sickbed. It is a good idea to cut away one side so that your pet can get in and out more easily.

it's easy for him to get in and out. The more he rests, the quicker he is going to recover, says Dr. Carter.

Giving Medicines

If pets could talk, they would tell you that the worst part about being sick is—yuck—taking their medicine. You can't explain to them that the bad taste will last just a moment. As far as they're concerned, that nasty-tasting pill or liquid is the worst thing they have ever encountered, and they're going to do everything they can to keep it from going down.

Since persuasion won't work, you have to be a little sneaky. With dogs, this usually isn't too hard. Even when sick, they are often reluctant to pass up an appetizing treat, and you can hide a pill or capsule inside a tasty morsel—a chunk of cheese, for example, or a dollop of peanut butter. Most dogs will gobble it down, medicine and all, says Dr. Carter.

Cat aren't so easy to fool. Their sense of smell is incredibly sharp, and they will often turn up their whiskers and refuse to eat even when a seemingly odorless medication is concealed in their food. For recalcitrant cats (or reluctant dogs), the only solution is to give the medicine straight up.

Liquid medicines are easy to use, says Dr. Crimi. Before calling your pet, draw up the correct dose in a plastic eyedropper or needleless syringe. (Don't use a glass dropper because it could break in his mouth.) Open his mouth with one hand and use the other to slip the dropper toward the back half of the tongue. Squirt in the medicine slowly, but steadily. "Your pet will have no choice but to swallow it," she says.

Dogs will usually take liquid medicines without too much fuss, but cats, with their sharp teeth and claws, can be formidable patients. To protect your hands, you may want to wrap your cat in a towel, leaving just his head free. Better yet, enlist the help of a friend, Dr. Crimi says.

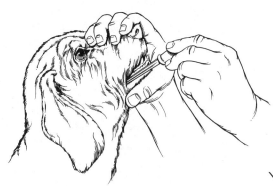

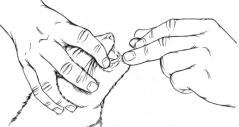

The way to get a cat to swallow a pill is to make it as difficult as possible for him to spit it out. Open your cat's jaw by gently squeezing the corners of his mouth with one hand. Holding the pill between your thumb and index finger, slip it as far back on the tongue as possible. When he closes his mouth, stroke his throat several times, which will stimulate the swallowing reflex. Don't hold his head up, or it will be difficult for him to swallow.

When giving liquid medicine, hold your pet's mouth slightly open and tilt his head upward at a 45-degree angle. Put the medicine dropper in the side of his mouth with the tip pointing backward. In this position, gravity will help the medicine go down. Don't use a glass dropper because it could break and splinter.

Using a towel and an extra pair of hands will make the process go much easier.

Some find pills more of a challenge than liquids—at least at first. When treating a pet, have a friend hold his body while you open his mouth with one hand and pop in the pill with the other. Put it as far back in the mouth as possible and hold his head upright until he swallows. Once the pill's inside, close his mouth and gently stroke his throat, which will encourage him to swallow. Blowing gently on his nose will also make him swallow, Dr. Crimi explains.

EYE AND EAR DROPS

If you think it's hard giving your pet pills, wait until it's time to put in eye or ear drops for quelling an infection, for example, or for treating ear mites. Dogs and cats hate the way drops feel, and by the time they are done shaking, twisting, and lunging, you'll consider yourself lucky if any of the medicine went where it was supposed to.

The trick to applying drops, besides moving quickly, is to keep a firm grip on your pet so that he can't twist away, says Dr. Carter. If your pet is both calm and small, you can probably do it by yourself. Most of the time, enlisting the help of a friend will make things go a lot more smoothly. When treating a cat, wrapping him in a towel first will save your hands a lot of scratches and bites, he adds.

To give eyedrops, raise the head slightly and hold the dropper directly over the eye. Use one hand to prop the eye open and the other to put in the drops. When giving eyedrops to a cat, it is a good idea to wrap him in a towel, leaving the head clear, to keep from getting scratched.

When giving ear drops, hold the dropper at the opening of the ear canal. When the drops go in, gently massage around the base of the ear to distribute the fluid.

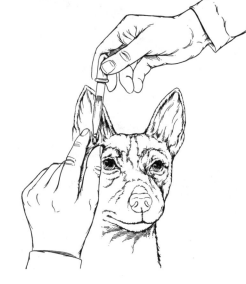

Eating for Health

Pets that are sick will often lose their appetites for a day or two. This is often a good thing. If they have been vomiting or having diarrhea, going without food will give their upset tummies time to recover.

With other types of illness, however, going without food means that they are missing out on essential nutrients they need to recover. "If you don't encourage them to take in small amounts of food and drink, they will become dehydrated quickly," says Dr. Carter.

Pets with colds or flu often lose their appetites simply because they are congested and can't smell their food. When they can't smell, they won't eat, Dr. Carter explains. An easy solution is to warm your pet's food slightly. "Warming food often releases the aroma, which can be helpful in stimulating the appetite," he says. When using dry foods, adding a little warm water will also release the appetizing smells.

If your pet still won't eat, you may want to tempt his tastebuds by adding a little broth or warm milk to his food. Or you can give him egg yolks, bits of meat, or strained baby food. These foods not only provide the calories and nutrition he needs to regain his strength, they also contain fluids, which will help keep his internal water supplies at healthy levels.

First-Aid: When Every Minute Counts

Dogs and cats are a lot like children—full of spontaneity and enthusiasm and a little short on common sense. The sight of a squirrel is enough to launch them into a high-speed chase—and the fact that a car is coming won't slow them down. They will venture onto glass-strewn sidewalks, leap onto hot stoves, or climb on tree limbs that won't support their weight. They will do everything, it seems, except think about the dangers that they are getting into. That's why knowing first-aid is so important.

"Knowing how to take quick, calm action can literally spell the difference between life and death," says Joseph Trueba, D.V.M., a veterinarian in Tucson, Arizona, who specializes in emergency care. You don't have to be a trained paramedic to handle most emergencies. But you do have to be prepared—emotionally and mentally—to do *something*. Even if your vet is only minutes away, knowing what to do in the moments right after an injury occurs can make all the difference.

Having a well-stocked first-aid kit is critical, says Dr. Trueba. You'll find everything you need in "Making a First-Aid Kit" on page 27. You also have to be prepared to stop bleeding, move your pet safely, or even do CPR. In the following pages, we will take a look at the basics of first-aid and show exactly what to do for some of the most common emergencies.

MUZZLING AN INJURED PET

It's hard to imagine your faithful companion lashing out at you with bared teeth or extended claws, especially when you are trying to help. But it happens all the time. "Once injured, any pet can become a ferocious biter or scratcher," warns Dr. Trueba. "Always protect yourself first, or you won't be able to help your pet."

Veterinarians recommend muzzling dogs and cats before performing first-aid. You can buy a ready-made muzzle at pet supply stores and keep

MUZZLING A CAT

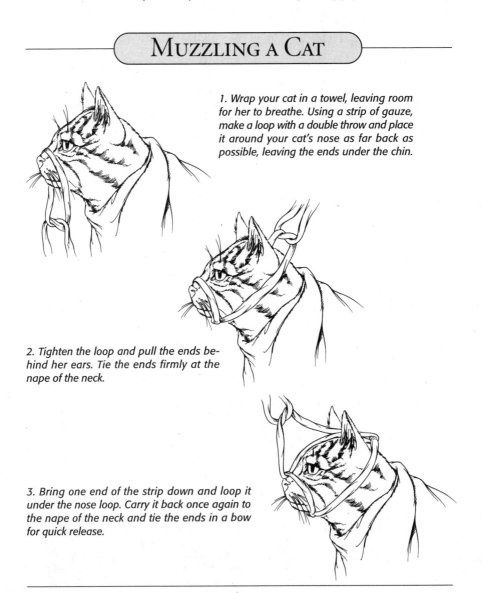

1. Wrap your cat in a towel, leaving room for her to breathe. Using a strip of gauze, make a loop with a double throw and place it around your cat's nose as far back as possible, leaving the ends under the chin.

2. Tighten the loop and pull the ends behind her ears. Tie the ends firmly at the nape of the neck.

3. Bring one end of the strip down and loop it under the nose loop. Carry it back once again to the nape of the neck and tie the ends in a bow for quick release.

it in your first-aid kit. Or you can make one on the spot by using a strip of gauze or even your pet's leash. Because of their longer snouts, dogs are a bit easier to muzzle than cats.

"While a muzzle generally provides sufficient restraint for a dog, you may have to further subdue your cat to avoid getting scratched," says Joan E. Antle, D.V.M., a veterinarian in private practice in Cleveland. She recommends wrapping your cat in a bath towel, leaving just enough room for her to breathe, before putting on the muzzle. Once her claws are under wraps, you will be able to get it on without too much fuss.

MUZZLING A DOG

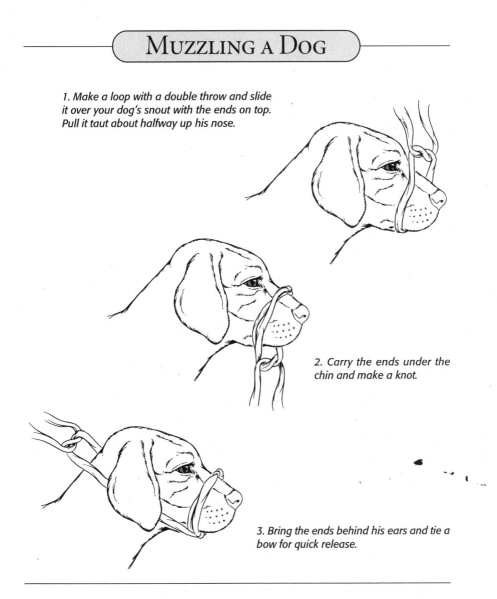

1. Make a loop with a double throw and slide it over your dog's snout with the ends on top. Pull it taut about halfway up his nose.

2. Carry the ends under the chin and make a knot.

3. Bring the ends behind his ears and tie a bow for quick release.

MOVING AN INJURED PET

If your dog or cat is seriously injured—having been hit by a car, for example—you are going to have to move her either to the side of the road or into the backseat of your car for the ride to the vet. Moving a pet with neck, back, or spinal cord injuries, however, can be as dangerous to your pet as the accident itself. It's essential to do it right.

To move your pet quickly, grasp her by the nape of the neck with one hand and by the back end with the other and drag her out of harm's way, advises Dr. Antle. You don't want to lift her off the ground because that can put dangerous pressure on the injured areas.

Time permitting, a pet with serious injuries should be immobilized before moving, says Dr. Antle. By moving her as one "unit," without allowing the spine or legs to move, you can help prevent further damage while you are getting your pet to the vet. It's easy to immobilize cats and small dogs—they can be lifted smoothly into a box or pet carrier. For large dogs, however, you are going to need a whole-body splint. Here are two approaches.

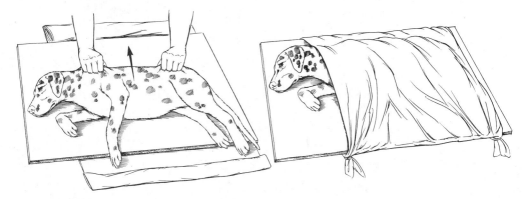

Being careful not to bend the spine, neck, or legs, drag your dog onto a firm surface like a piece of plywood with a sheet spread beneath it. Cover her with the sheet and tie her down by knotting the ends of the sheet around the board.

If you don't have a board handy, you can fashion a makeshift stretcher by taking a blanket or sheet and folding it in half. Drag your dog onto the blanket, then roll up the sides to take up the slack and form handles.

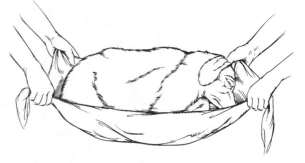

STOPPING BLEEDING

Most bleeding is caused by something minor—a piece of glass in a paw, for instance, or a spat with a neighborhood pet. "A little bit of blood can look like a lot because it spreads out quickly," says Dr. Antle. You can stop most bleeding by pressing on the area with a piece of gauze. (If blood soaks through the gauze, add some more. Don't remove the gauze because it may disturb clots that are trying to form.) Then it's just a matter of cleaning up the mess.

Bleeding that is unusually heavy or that doesn't stop within a few minutes needs more serious attention. Vets recommend keeping pressure on the wound by taping on a piece of gauze, for example, while also pushing down on one of your pet's pressure points (areas between the wound and the heart where a little finger pressure will partially collapse an artery, causing bleeding to slow). Regardless of the pressure point you use, be sure to relax the pressure for 1 or 2 seconds every 10 seconds. This permits some blood to get through, which will keep surrounding tissues healthy, Dr. Antle says. Wounds that are bleeding this heavily always require professional care, she adds, so get your pet to the vet as soon as possible.

YOUR PET'S PRESSURE POINTS

The easiest way to stop heavy bleeding is to put direct pressure on one of your pet's pressure points, areas where arteries lie near the surface of the skin. Pressing on a pressure point partially collapses the artery, causing less blood to get through. Be sure to relax the pressure for 1 or 2 seconds every 10 seconds. Here are the main pressure points.

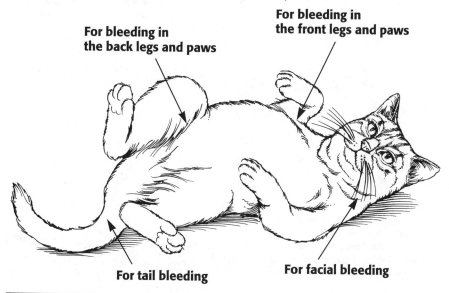

For bleeding in the back legs and paws

For bleeding in the front legs and paws

For tail bleeding

For facial bleeding

Using a Tourniquet Safely

For years, every first-aid manual recommended applying a tourniquet to stop bleeding. Today, most vets don't like them. Although tourniquets are very effective, unless they are used properly, they can make things worse by restricting blood flow to healthy tissues around the wound.

When you can't stop bleeding any other way, however, a tourniquet could save your pet's life. "Always use it as a last resort and only on a leg or tail," says Craig N. Carter, D.V.M., Ph.D., head of epidemiology at the Texas Veterinary Medical Diagnostic Laboratory at Texas A&M University in College Station. As soon as the tourniquet is in place, get your pet to the vet immediately, he adds. And be sure to loosen the tourniquet for a second or two every 10 seconds to keep the surrounding tissue healthy.

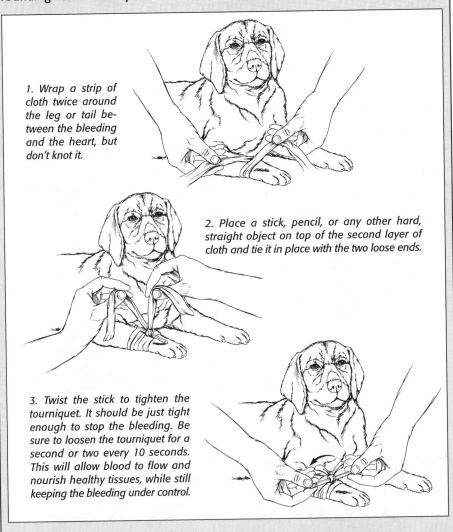

1. Wrap a strip of cloth twice around the leg or tail between the bleeding and the heart, but don't knot it.

2. Place a stick, pencil, or any other hard, straight object on top of the second layer of cloth and tie it in place with the two loose ends.

3. Twist the stick to tighten the tourniquet. It should be just tight enough to stop the bleeding. Be sure to loosen the tourniquet for a second or two every 10 seconds. This will allow blood to flow and nourish healthy tissues, while still keeping the bleeding under control.

Administering CPR

If your dog or cat has been in an accident, the heart and lungs may quit working. Once this happens, you only have anywhere from three to five minutes to restore the flow of oxygen to the brain to prevent permanent damage.

The best way to save your pet is with cardiopulmonary resuscitation, or CPR. "It's always worth trying CPR on your pet if he has stopped breathing and there is no immediate medical assistance," says Craig N. Carter, D.V.M., Ph.D., head of epidemiology at the Texas Veterinary Medical Diagnostic Laboratory at Texas A&M University in College Station. Even if you are en route to the vet, you (or a car passenger) should be prepared to do CPR until you get there. (To learn how to do it right, see "Performing CPR" on page 26.)

Bites

Dogs and cats are often braver than they should be. When an argument is brewing over territory, food, or the affections of the opposite sex, they will wade into battle, only to emerge with painful bites.

"Bites are often deep, and they are loaded with bacteria that can start an infection quickly," Dr. Antle says. "It's best to take your pet to the vet, who can clean the wound properly." Washing bite wounds at home often drives dirt and bacteria in deeper, making the injury worse.

One of the hidden dangers of bite wounds is simply their small size; they are not always easy to see. This means an infection may be quietly forming, getting worse every day. If you see an area that is red, swollen, or warm to the touch, call your vet right away. "Infected wounds need emergency veterinary care," says Dr. Antle. This is especially true if your pet has been spending time outdoors. Rabies isn't very common in dogs and cats, but it is common in skunks, raccoons, foxes, bats, and other wild animals. Your pet may need fast treatment.

Burns

Maybe your cat swiped some pizza off the counter, scalding her mouth and paws on the steaming mozzarella. Or perhaps your dog knocked a steaming cup of coffee from your hands. Or your puppy or kitten gnawed on a lamp cord and got a painful jolt—and an equally painful burn.

Thankfully, most burns aren't serious and can be treated at home the same way you would treat your own—by applying an ice cube or a cold pack or by flooding the area with cold water. "Applying cold stops a burn from penetrating into deeper tissues," explains Paul M. Gigliotti, D.V.M., a veterinarian in private practice in Mayfield Village, Ohio. "Apply the cold treatment for a full 20 minutes after the burn," he says.

PERFORMING CPR

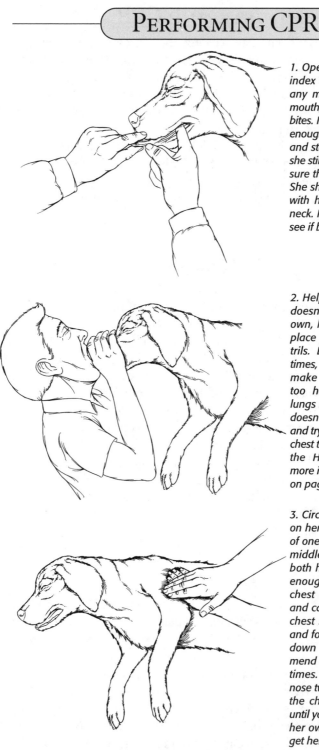

1. Open the airway: Using your index and middle finger, swipe any material out of your pet's mouth, being careful in case she bites. In some cases, this may be enough to clear a blocked airway and start her breathing again. If she still can't breathe, check to be sure that her neck isn't crimped. She should be lying on her side, with her head in line with the neck. Pull the tongue forward to see if breathing resumes.

2. Help her breathe: If your pet doesn't start breathing on her own, hold her mouth shut and place your mouth over the nostrils. Blow into the nose two times, using just enough force to make the chest rise. (Blowing too hard can overinflate the lungs in small pets.) If the chest doesn't rise, reposition the neck and try again. If you can't get the chest to rise, you may need to do the Heimlich maneuver. (For more information, see "Choking" on page 28.)

3. Circulate blood: Lay your pet on her right side. Place the heel of one hand over the ribs in the middle of the rib cage. Using both hands, press down, using enough force to compress the chest a ½ inch for small dogs and cats. For medium dogs, the chest should compress 1 inch; and for large dogs, it should go down 1½ inches. Vets recommend compressing the chest 15 times. Then breathe into the nose twice and start pressing on the chest again. Continue this until your pet starts breathing on her own again or until you can get her to the vet.

For most burns, applying cold is all you need to do. If the area is red and swollen, however, you should follow the cold treatment by applying an over-the-counter triple-antibiotic ointment twice a day, says Dr. Gigliotti. If the burn doesn't heal quickly or if it starts getting worse, call your vet right away.

Simple heat burns are usually the easiest to treat. Other types of burns, however, need more than a little bit of ice.

Chemical burns. These are caused by household cleaners or yard chemicals. "Flush the area with lots of water to wash away the chemical and stop further burns," says Dr. Gigliotti. Then take your pet to the vet immediately.

Electrical burns. A playful puppy or kitten will chew through almost anything, including electrical cords. This can cause a nasty burn around or inside the mouth. In more serious cases, electrical burns can damage lung tissue or even stop breathing entirely. Signs of lung injuries include coughing or difficulty breathing. Electrical burns are always an emergency that needs a veterinarian's care, says Dr. Gigliotti.

Making a First-Aid Kit

It would be nice if accidents unfolded slowly, giving us plenty of time to react. But that's not what happens. Emergencies occur in a flash, and you don't want to waste precious minutes searching for gauze pads or antibiotic ointments. Vets recommend always having a first-aid kit prepared and ready to go. Here's what to include.

- Your veterinarian's phone number
- The phone number to the closest emergency 24-hour clinic
- A first-aid manual, such as *Pet First-Aid*
- Antibacterial soap
- Antibiotic ointment
- Bandaging materials: two-inch stretchable and nonstretchable gauze rolls, gauze pads in a variety of sizes
- Blunt-tipped scissors
- Cotton balls
- Disposable rubber gloves
- Hydrogen peroxide (3 percent)
- Masking tape
- Needle-nose pliers
- Petroleum jelly
- Plastic, needleless syringe or turkey baster
- Rectal thermometer
- Saline solution (for an eyewash)
- Tweezers

CAR ACCIDENTS

Dogs and cats simply don't have street smarts. Whether they are lost and trying to get home or they have left the yard to chase another pet, they will often find themselves in the middle of the road—and they don't always look both ways first.

Getting hit by a car is always an emergency, even if your pet gets up afterward and walks away, says Dr. Carter. There could be brain damage, internal bleeding, or nerve injuries that won't show up right away. Getting your pet to the vet soon after an accident could save her life.

In the meantime, here's what you can do to help.

1. Muzzle your pet before trying to move her. It's the only way to get her to safety without getting hurt yourself. (For more information, see "Muzzling an Injured Pet" on page 20.)
2. Check for breathing by looking at the rise and fall of her chest. You should also check her pulse by feeling the inside of the leg near the groin. If there is no pulse or she isn't breathing, start CPR immediately. (For instructions on administering CPR, see "Performing CPR" on page 26.)
3. Stop bleeding by using a bandage, pushing on the pressure points, or, if necessary, applying a tourniquet. (For more information, see "Stopping Bleeding" on page 23.)
4. Cover her with a blanket or coat to prevent shock.
5. If you suspect a bone is broken, splint the area to keep it immobile. (For more on splinting, see "Fractures" on page 30.)
6. Get her to a vet immediately.

CHOKING

Cats are delicate eaters, but few dogs would earn top grades for gracious dining. They tend to gobble as much food as they can as quickly as they can. And the quicker they gobble and swallow, the more likely they are to start choking. This is especially true for older dogs, who sometimes lose control over their swallowing reflexes.

Choking usually doesn't last very long. A few good "acks" will often clear the windpipe of whatever is stuck inside. When the object doesn't come out, however, you need to act quickly. "Lacking enough oxygen,

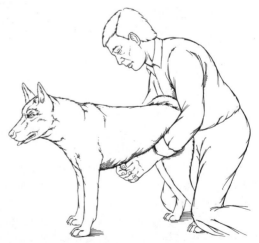

If your pet is standing, wrap your arms tightly around her belly under the rib cage. (For cats and smaller dogs, grab the sides with your hands.) Give your pet a quick, forceful squeeze, which will often pop the object right out. The smaller the pet, the more gently you should squeeze. If the object isn't dislodged with gentle force, slowly increase the force with each additional squeeze.

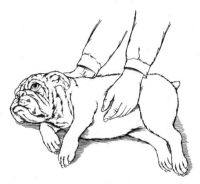

If your pet is lying on her side, feel for the last rib. For cats and small dogs, place one hand over the shoulder blades to keep them steady. With the other hand, push behind the last rib into the abdomen five times. For dogs over 40 pounds, lie down behind her and wrap your arms around her abdomen. Place one hand over your fist and press the abdomen five times, then check to see if the airway is clear. If not, try the abdominal press again.

your pet may faint," says Dr. Carter. This means that the brain isn't getting enough oxygen. In a way, fainting is good, he adds. When your dog faints, it is easier to reach inside her mouth and remove whatever is causing the choking.

If you are unable to remove the object by hand, you may need to do the Heimlich maneuver. By pressing on her sides below the ribs, you will cause the diaphragm to push forward, creating pressure inside the airways. This will often "blow" the object right out, Dr. Carter explains.

CUTS

Your pets don't wear shoes, and they tend to wander wherever they want. As a result, pets often get cuts—not only on the pads of their paws but also on their legs and backs. Taking care of cuts right away will help ensure that minor cuts stay that way. "Cleaning wounds helps prevent infection and speeds healing," says Beverly J. Scott, D.V.M., a veterinarian in private practice in Gilbert, Arizona.

Begin by trimming the fur around the cut, advises Dr. Scott. Wash the area thoroughly with warm water. Rinse it well, then pat it dry with gauze pads. (Don't use cotton balls to dry a wound because the fibers will get

When bandaging a cut on a paw, start at the toes and wrap gauze around the paw and the lower part of the leg. Cover the gauze with overlapping strips of cloth bandage tape, making sure that it isn't so tight that it cuts off circulation. If your pet is chewing at the dressing, put a sock over the foot and tape it in place.

stuck inside.) When the cut is clean, smear on some over-the-counter triple-antibiotic ointment several times a day.

Minor cuts usually don't need to be bandaged. In fact, they will heal a little faster when air is allowed to circulate. If your pet is licking or worrying the area, however, you are going to have to cover it up. It is also a good idea to bandage cuts on the feet because the pads contain a lot of blood vessels that bleed easily.

Most cuts don't need anything more than this, says Dr. Scott. But if the cut is deep, longer than a half-inch, or packed with dirt, it is going to need a thorough cleaning, and you should call your vet.

Drowning

Dogs and cats are capable swimmers, but they don't always take naturally to the water any more than some people do. They tire easily, and once they are in the water, it isn't always easy for them to get out. They can drown very quickly if you aren't there to bail them out, says Dr. Trueba.

Veterinarians recommend covering swimming pools when they are not in use or at least putting a fence around the pool area. If you have kittens in the house, don't forget to keep the lid to the toilet closed. Young cats may jump up and fall in. The slippery sides of the toilet bowl make it difficult for them to get back out.

If your pet has somehow gotten into water and is unconscious or choking, you will need to move very quickly. Here is what Dr. Trueba advises.

1. Put your arms around her belly below the ribs and lift her into the air so that her torso is lower than her hips. (For heavy dogs, heft them from the rear and leave the front feet on the ground.) Gently swing her back and forth to shake water from the lungs.
2. Lay your pet on her side with her head slightly lower than her body. (If you are not on a hill, elevate her body by putting a towel or pillow beneath her back haunches.) This will allow additional water to drain from the lungs.
3. Check her pulse and breathing. If she isn't breathing, perform CPR immediately. If possible, have someone else call the vet while you continue to do CPR. (See "Performing CPR" on page 26.)
4. Get her to the vet as soon as possible.

Fractures

When it comes to broken bones, pets are pretty smart and pretty lucky. Smart because Mother Nature teaches them to stay off an injured leg, especially a broken one. Lucky because they have "extra" legs; they can limp along pretty well on three legs.

FRACTURES ABOVE THE KNEE

Slide your pet onto a flat surface—a sturdy piece of cardboard, for example, or a small sheet of plywood—with the broken leg on the bottom. Tape the broken leg down with masking tape, then secure your pet's whole body to the board by covering her with a sheet or blanket and tying the ends together underneath the board. Then get her to the vet right away.

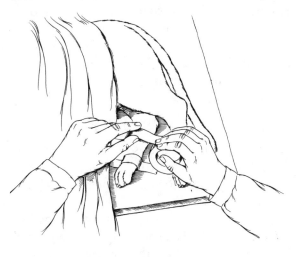

FRACTURES BELOW THE KNEE

Pad the leg with a towel to prevent chafing. Splint the leg using a pencil, a broken-off yard-stick, or even a rolled-up magazine. The splint should extend from above the elbow or knee down to the bottom of the paw. Wrap it in place with gauze strips or bandage tape. Don't make it too tight, which could cut off blood flow. Then get your pet to the vet.

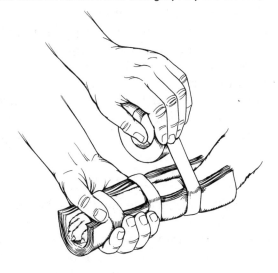

You will still need to see the vet if your pet has a fractured bone, of course. But unless the break is severe, it will probably be fairly easily to repair, says L. R. Danny Daniel, D.V.M., a veterinarian in private practice in Covington, Louisiana. There are two types of common leg fractures: those above the knee or elbow and those below. Those above the joints usually require orthopedic surgery to repair. Those below can often be stabilized with a splint alone. In either case, your pet will need to be kept quiet for six to eight weeks in order for the fracture to heal properly.

Before taking your pet to the vet, it is important to stabilize a broken bone to prevent further damage. To learn how to properly splint both types of fractures, see the illustrations on page 31.

HEATSTROKE

Heatstroke is an extremely serious condition in which a dog's or cat's internal temperature rises above 104°F, possibly causing damage to the brain or other organs. (Their normal temperature is between 100.5° and 102.5°F.) Short-faced breeds like pugs, boxers, and Persians, which have small airways, have an especially high risk of getting heatstroke. So do German shepherds, Old English sheepdogs, and other dogs with double coats, which retain a lot more heat than single coats.

"The leading cause of heatstroke in cats and dogs is leaving them in a parked car," says Lori A. Wise, D.V.M., a veterinarian in private practice in Wheat Ridge, Colorado. Pets that are elderly or overweight or those that get too much vigorous exercise on a hot day can also get overheated. Signs of heatstroke include heavy panting and drooling, glassy eyes, deep red gums, and excessive weakness.

Heatstroke is an emergency that must be treated by a vet, says Dr. Wise. In the meantime, you must act very quickly to bring the pet's temperature down. If possible, immerse her entire body in cool (not cold) water, either in the bathtub, a child's swimming pool, or a laundry sink. If you are unable to get her all the way in the water, soak her with a garden hose or cover her with wet towels. (Re-dip the towels in cool water every five minutes.) It is also a good idea to put her in front of a fan or the air conditioner, preferably in the car while you are on your way to the vet.

POISONING

Dogs and cats are always getting into things they shouldn't. Given half a chance, they will pick up stray pills, lick antifreeze off the floor, or roll in household chemicals, cleaners, and pesticides.

Poisoning is always an emergency that requires *fast* veterinary care, says Steve Hansen, D.V.M., vice president of the American Society for the Prevention of Cruelty to Animals' National Animal Poison Control

Purging the Poison

When your pet has swallowed poisons, vomiting is often the best way to get them out again. To induce vomiting, give a small amount of 3 percent hydrogen peroxide—about one teaspoon per 10 pounds of weight. Draw the liquid into a turkey baster or syringe and squirt it toward the back of your pet's mouth. Vomiting will usually occur within a few minutes. "If it doesn't work the first time, give the same amount in 15 to 20 minutes," advises Steve Hansen, D.V.M., vice president of the American Society for the Prevention of Cruelty to Animals' National Animal Poison Control Center in Urbana, Illinois. Don't use syrup of ipecac, however, because it can be toxic for dogs and cats.

Even though vomiting is recommend for some types of poisons, it can make things worse with others. Caustic substances like drain cleaner, for example, will do a "double burn"—once when your pet swallows them and again if she vomits them back up, Dr. Hansen adds.

The table lists some common poisons, along with advice regarding whether or not to induce vomiting. You should only induce vomiting if your pet is awake and alert. And, of course, you want to get her to the vet as quickly as you can.

Poison	Induce Vomiting
Antifreeze	Yes
Ant poison	Yes
Aspirin	Yes
Battery acid	No
Bleach	No
Drain cleaner	No
Fertilizer	No
Household cleaners	No
Insecticides	Yes
Medications (antihistamines, tranquilizers, barbiturates, amphetamines, heart pills, vitamins)	Yes
Paint thinner	No
Pesticides (water-based only)	Yes
Rodent poison	Yes
Sidewalk salt	No
Slug and snail bait	Yes
Turpentine	No
Weed killers (water-based only)	Yes
White glue or paste	No

Center in Urbana, Illinois. But unless you actually see your pet eating something she shouldn't, you won't know right away that she has been poisoned. Symptoms to watch for include difficulty breathing, depression, confusion, seizures, a slow or fast heartbeat, excessive salivation, burns around the mouth, or bleeding from the nose, mouth, or anus.

If you suspect that your pet has been poisoned, call your vet or the animal poison control center immediately. (It's a good idea to write down these numbers ahead of time and put them on the refrigerator or in your first-aid kit.) Have the container of the suspected substance in front of you so that you can explain to the experts exactly what she got into, says Dr. Hansen.

Porcupine Quills

Cats will rarely go head-to-head with a fully armed porcupine, but dogs don't always recognize the danger and wind up with a face full of quills for their efforts.

Porcupine quills can be extraordinarily painful. "The quills have multiple tiny barbs along their shafts," explains Dr. Trueba. The only way to get them out is to grip the quills with pliers as close to the skin as possible and work them out very slowly. The barbs really hang on, and most pets will have a hard time holding still. Most people take their punctured pets to the vet, who will often sedate or anesthetize them before removing the quills.

Once the quills are out, wash the area with warm, soapy water. Continue to keep the area clean for several days after the injury. "Check the wounds daily for four days, watching for signs of infection," says Dr. Trueba. If you see redness, swelling, or pus, get your pet to the vet right away.

Torn Nails

If you have ever snagged your fingernail on a sweater or torn it while working in the yard, you know how painful a torn nail can be. It is just as painful for dogs—and a lot more common because their nails are always out and on the ground. (Cats are able to retract their nails, so they rarely get this kind of injury.) A crack in the sidewalk or fibers in the carpet can trap long nails, causing a painful, bloody tear, says Dr. Antle.

Nails that are injured but not dangling usually aren't too serious, although they may bleed profusely, says Dr. Antle. The easiest remedy is to trim the ragged parts of the nail and clean the area well with warm, soapy water.

Nails that have been torn loose from the paw and are dangling are much more serious. "Removing an injured nail is excruciatingly painful, and your vet will need to numb the foot," says Dr. Antle. If you are unable to get to the vet, you can cut the nail yourself. She recommends sterilizing a pair of blunt-tipped scissors in alcohol and cutting the nail just above the tear. Then apply a local anesthetic like Orajel, which is used for teething babies. Bandage the foot for about 24 hours to keep your pet from licking the nail. Afterward, keep a close eye on the area to make sure that it doesn't get infected, she adds. If you see swelling or redness, get your pet to the vet right away.

Appetite
and Eating

In a perfect world, dogs and cats would always eat well, drink the proper amounts, and never munch on forbidden items like sweaters or the disagreeable snacks they find in the yard. But of course, dogs and cats, like humans, often have changes in their tastes or appetites. Sometimes they will eat themselves silly—or ignore food for days at a time. They will lap up water by the bowlful—or not take a drink all day. They will eat anything and everything that you put in their bowls, and then one day get extremely picky about what they will deign to eat. It is a challenge to know when everything is okay or if you need to be concerned.

Change in appetite is puzzling even for veterinarians because it can mean just about anything. At least a third of medical problems that affect dogs and cats can result in lost appetite, says Craig N. Carter, D.V.M., Ph.D., head of epidemiology at the Texas Veterinary Medical Diagnostic Laboratory at Texas A&M University in College Station. Between 50 and 60 disorders can cause excessive drinking.

Conditions that can cause appetite changes aren't always serious, he adds. Pets that have pulled a muscle or are having a flare-up of minor arthritis, for example, may lose their appetites simply because they are not feeling well. A stuffy nose can cause appetite to go on vacation. So can allergies or a temporary bout with the flu. Less often, appetite and eating changes really are caused by serious conditions, says Dr. Carter. Anything from diabetes to cancer to hormonal imbalances can cause pets to suddenly stop eating or, in some cases, to eat everything in sight.

Temporary changes in eating habits don't always mean that something is physically wrong. Dogs and cats will sometimes quit eating for a day or two when they are feeling stressed—because there's a lot of unusual activity in the house, or you have out-of-town guests that are making them nervous. In fact, any change in your pet's environment can cause a change in appetite. Even when these environmental changes are things you would never notice, such as the atmospheric changes that precede thunderstorms, your pets may be more sensitive to them than you realize.

Some appetite and eating changes don't have anything to do with what you put in the food bowl. Cats, for example, will sometimes develop a powerful taste for wool, cotton, or other fabrics. Veterinarians can't always tell why, but dogs and cats will sometimes eat nonfood items like soil or cardboard boxes. And dogs, given the chance, will often snack on droppings in the yard or litter box. These and other strange tastes don't always cause problems, but they do increase the risk for intestinal parasites or even blockages in the intestines, says Dr. Carter.

Since there are many reasons for changes in pets' appetites or tastes, it is worth paying attention to what they are—and aren't—eating. As a general rule, dogs and cats that are eating more or less than usual will return to their normal habits in a day or two and will be just fine. In fact, dogs can quit eating entirely for several days without suffering anything worse than occasional hunger pangs. For cats, however, going without food for more than a day can cause a serious liver disorder called hepatic lipodosis, which can be life-threatening if it isn't treated quickly. That's why a sudden loss of appetite can be a problem even when it doesn't last very long.

When your pets have a sudden change in appetite, it's fine to wait a day or two to see if they are going to get back to normal, says Dr. Carter. If they don't, there may be an underlying problem that needs looking into, and you will want to make an appointment to see your vet. In the meantime, here is some expert advice to help you understand your pets' puzzling behavior and to make sure that they get the nourishment they need.

See Your Vet If:

- Your pet has eaten antifreeze, houseplants, or other harmful substances.
- She has missing or broken teeth.
- Her teeth are gray or black.
- She has been vomiting for more than a day or is vomiting blood.
- She has had diarrhea or constipation for a day or more.
- You have noticed weight gain or weight loss.
- Your pet hasn't eaten for more than 24 hours.
- She is eating, drinking, or urinating much more than usual.
- Her abdomen is bloated or feels tight.
- She is drooling more than usual.
- There is a bulge in her throat.
- Your pet seems unusually tired and lethargic.
- She has sores on her gums or tongue.
- She seems to be having trouble chewing or swallowing.

SYMPTOM) APPETITE LOSS

Clues

- Your pet eats some foods but not others.
- She is anxious or depressed.
- Chewing seems painful.

Most dogs and cats are hearty eaters, and an untouched food bowl is unusual, to say the least. So you do the obvious thing and change the food, but your pet seems to find it about as appetizing as you do. This is a clear signal that something is wrong.

When pets are otherwise healthy, fasting for a meal or two isn't a problem, says Deborah C. Mallu, D.V.M., a holistic veterinarian in private practice in Sedona, Arizona. But when the abstinence persists, it is important to figure out why. This is especially true for cats since going without food for as little as a day or two can cause a liver disorder called hepatic lipodosis, which can make them extremely ill.

Loss of appetite may be caused by teeth and gum problems, such as periodontal disease or a fractured tooth, which can make chewing painful. It can also be caused by viral infections, like the flu, or even by everyday tummyaches caused, for example, by eating rotten leftovers from the trash. Constipation is another possibility since pets that aren't eliminating properly may stop eating, says Dr. Mallu.

If your pet persists in snubbing food, the underlying cause might be something more serious, such as a hormonal disorder or an illness affecting the kidneys, liver, or pancreas. Cancer often causes appetite loss. So does heart disease, which sometimes causes fluids to accumulate in the chest cavity, taking away a pet's appetite.

Pets that are anxious or depressed will often stop eating, says Karen L. Overall, V.M.D., Ph.D., head of the behavior clinic at the University of Pennsylvania School of Veterinary Medicine in Philadelphia. Even *your* moods can cause pets to quit eating. "Animals may go off food if they are emotionally connected to someone who is upset," she says. This occurs more often with dogs than with cats. "Cats can be sensitive to ups and downs in the household, but they usually don't stop eating because of it," she says. Dogs dislike being alone, and sometimes they will quit eating when their owners go away for a day or two.

And for dogs and cats, any change in the environment, such as moving to a new house or getting another pet, can cause them to temporarily lose interest in food. Even changes in the weather can cause appetites to flag. "When the temperature rises, the animal's metabolism slows down and the energy demands drop off," explains Craig N. Carter, D.V.M., Ph.D., head of epidemiology at the Texas Veterinary Medical Diagnostic Laboratory at Texas A&M University in College Station.

WHAT YOU CAN DO

Sometimes leftover food in the bowl only seems to be a sign of lost appetite. It is not unheard of for pets to be eating quite well, thank you—just not what you're feeding them. They might be feasting from the garbage or hunting prey instead, says Dr. Overall. "People will say, 'I leave dry cat food, but she never touches it.' Then they notice that a bunch of songbirds in the neighborhood have bitten the dust."

You may even discover that someone else in the family has been forking over tasty treats or leftovers, and your pet has abandoned her food for better offerings elsewhere.

If she is genuinely not eating, you need to figure out whether she has lost her appetite or simply developed a dislike for her usual food. Dr. Overall recommends putting different foods on the menu for a day or two. Most dogs and cats love chicken-flavored baby food. Cats are especially fond of tuna, sardines, and liverwurst. In addition, pet food companies such as Hill's Science Diet have created special formulas to whet pets' appetites. If your pet starts eating the new offerings with gusto, you will know that her appetite is doing just fine.

When dogs and cats have been feeling under the weather and not eating much, sometimes it is difficult to get them back to the food bowl. Here are a few additional tips to get them eating again.

- Most dogs and cats prefer canned food to dry. Mixing a little bit of canned food with their usual chow will often stimulate their appetites, especially if you warm the food first to make it smell more enticing, says Sandra Sawchuk, D.V.M., clinical instructor of small animal medicine at the University of Wisconsin School of Veterinary Medicine in Madison. Adding a little warm water to dry food will also make it more appealing, she adds.

- Pets may find home-cooked meals more palatable than packaged foods. Try giving them scrambled eggs or an omelet, suggests Dr. Mallu. Or feed them French toast cut up in chunks (but hold the syrup). She also recommends giving pets cooked grains, such as rice or oatmeal, with cooked vegetables and chunks of meat mixed in. Lightly braising the meat will bring out the flavor, she adds. Just be sure to let the food cool before giving it to your pet.

- Add some adventure to her meals. "These are predators whose ancestors spent most of their days solving the problem of how to get food, and we have put it in a bowl for them," says Patricia B. McConnell, Ph.D., assistant adjunct professor of zoology at the University of Wisconsin in Madison, a certified applied animal behaviorist, and author of *Beginning Family Dog Training*. To make mealtimes more exciting, she suggests tossing a handful of kibble across the grass so that your pet will have to forage a bit. "It's a way of making feeding more interesting by exercising the mind," she says. Exercising the body won't hurt her appetite either.

If you live in a multi-pet household, it's possible that there is rivalry between different pets for access to the food bowl. Some pets, in fact, will simply avoid their food rather than risk getting attacked. It won't hurt to try feeding your pets separately—in different places or at different times—for a day or two to see if things improve.

What Your Vet Will Do

You don't have to rush to the vet when your pet misses a meal or two. If her appetite doesn't come back, however, you are going to need professional advice. For dogs, three days is about the safe limit for going without food, says Dr. Carter. For cats, you should see your vet when they haven't eaten for more than a day, and you can't tempt them to eat with a change in diet. Of course, you will want to see your vet right away if there are also other symptoms, such as vomiting or diarrhea.

Your vet will begin by weighing your pet to see if she has lost weight. In addition, he will probably perform a number of tests, including blood work and possibly x-rays, to check for internal problems such as parasites, infections, or diabetes. Since there are literally hundreds of conditions that can cause lost appetite, don't be surprised if it takes a little time to figure out the problem. Once the underlying condition is taken care of, your pet's appetite will probably return very quickly.

See also Chapter 4: Finicky Eating; Chapter 14: Weight Loss

SYMPTOM

DRINKING FREQUENTLY

Clues

- Your pet's skin doesn't snap back into place when pulled.
- She is urinating frequently.

You discover that your pet is emptying the water bowl twice as often as usual, or she's making frequent trips to the toilet bowl to drink her fill. And she made a mess when she tried to lap up your glass of iced tea on the end table. What is giving your pet such a powerful thirst?

Veterinarians estimate that excessive drinking, also known as polydipsia, can be caused by roughly 67 different conditions in dogs and 56 in cats. But before you rush to your vet—or start drinking too much yourself—consider the possibilities.

In warm weather, dogs and cats naturally drink more water. They also drink more when they have been physically active or when they have been eating foods that are saltier than what they are used to. In some cases, they will drink more water simply because they are under stress— maybe you have visiting guests, for example, or have recently gotten another pet.

"If a dog or cat learns that you hover over them when they do something that you are worried about, they will keep doing it because they like the attention," says Karen L. Overall, V.M.D., Ph.D., head of the behavior clinic at the University of Pennsylvania School of Veterinary Medicine in Philadelphia.

Veterinarians worry about excessive drinking because there are a number of serious conditions that can cause it. Kidney failure is a possibility, especially in older animals that are urinating a lot, says Craig N. Carter, D.V.M., Ph.D., head of epidemiology at the Texas Veterinary Medical Diagnostic Laboratory at Texas A&M University in College Station. "When the kidneys can't regulate the water in the body, pets can't retain fluids, so they drink more and urinate it all out."

Diabetes is another condition that causes pets to urinate a lot and to crave more fluids, says Deborah C. Mallu, D.V.M., a holistic veterinarian in private practice in Sedona, Arizona. Other conditions that can cause pets to drink a lot include hormonal problems, such as having an overactive thyroid gland; urinary tract infections; and liver disease. Females that haven't been neutered will sometimes develop a uterine infection called pyometra. Also caused by hormonal problems, it can cause pets to drink huge amounts of water, she says.

WHAT YOU CAN DO

Unless you are in the habit of measuring your pet's drinking water, it is not always easy to tell if she is drinking more than usual or if the amount she is drinking is excessive. "Measure the amount of water she drinks for a few days," says Dean Gebroe, D.V.M., a veterinarian in private practice in Los Angeles. "Then call your vet and ask if that's too much."

To tell how much your pet is drinking, use a measuring cup to fill the water bowl. After 24 hours, measure the remaining water. To get an accurate measure, make sure that she doesn't have access to toilets or other sources of water, he adds.

Since a pet with medical problems may be dehydrated even when she is drinking a lot, you need to check the body's fluid levels right away. Try this tip from Dr. Carter. Lift the skin on her back and let go. "The skin should return to its normal position quickly. If it creeps back slowly or not at all, your pet might be severely dehydrated and should see a veterinarian," he says. In the meantime, let her keep drinking until you can get her to your vet.

Diabetes is another condition that requires a veterinarian's help. In some cases, however, it can be controlled by making simple changes in your pet's diet, such as feeding her several smaller meals instead of one big one or helping her lose weight if she is overweight.

If it turns out that your pet is drinking a normal amount of water, but it is still more than she used to drink, she is probably just nervous or under stress. Providing a change of pace—a bit more play and exercise, for example—might be a welcome diversion, says Dr. Mallu.

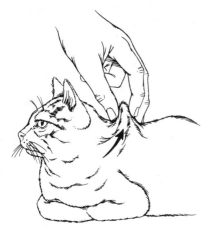

Dehydration is always an emergency, so you need to know what to look for. Here's one simple test. Gently pull up on the skin above the shoulder blades, then let go.

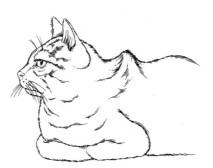

If your pet is getting enough water, the skin will return quickly to its normal position. If it doesn't, as illustrated here, call your vet immediately.

WHAT YOUR VET WILL DO

Since drinking too much is often a sign of physical problems, your vet will recommend bringing your pet in for a checkup—the sooner the better. Once you are there, he will probably begin by collecting a urine sample to test for diabetes and other internal problems.

You can help by bringing a urine sample with you, Dr. Gebroe adds. "With dogs, you can take them outside and slip a plastic bowl underneath while they urinate," he says. For cats, your vet will give you a pack of plastic beads that go in an empty litter box. The beads feel like litter to your cat, but they don't absorb the urine. After she uses the box, you can pour the urine into a jar or plastic bag and take it to your vet. If you don't bring in your own urine sample, your vet may need to use a needle to withdraw urine directly from the bladder, Dr. Gebroe explains.

If it turns out that your pet has diabetes, she may need insulin—along with oral medications or changes in her diet—to keep it under control. Hormonal problems can often be controlled with medications, although in some cases, surgery may be necessary to remove all or part of a gland. And for urinary tract infections, oral antibiotics are usually necessary.

Your vet will also want to know what medications your pet is already taking. "Certain medications, especially drugs in the steroid family, can make animals drink and urinate more," says Sandra Sawchuk, D.V.M., clinical instructor of small animal medicine at the University of Wisconsin School of Veterinary Medicine in Madison. Even drugs as simple as ear drops, if they contain steroids, may cause pets to drink more, she adds.

Finally, some cats with kidney failure need intravenous fluids in order to stay hydrated. The treatments are often done at the veterinarian's office, but they can also be given at home once your vet shows you how.

EATING GRASS

Clues

- Your pet is vomiting or has diarrhea.
- He has worms or other parasites.
- His abdomen feels tender or bloated.

Dogs and cats developed as hunters, which is why they have strong teeth and stomachs designed to digest high-protein foods. Meat is really their ideal meal. From time to time, however, most pets will act more like cows than carnivores, munching grass and watching the world go by.

No one knows for sure why dogs and cats crave the occasional salad. It may be because their hunting ancestors developed a taste—and a need—for greens when they ate the stomachs of their grass-eating prey. But some vets suspect that eating grass plays more of a medicinal role—that dogs and cats eat grass as a way of relieving digestive problems. When pets are vomiting or have diarrhea, it is not uncommon to see them on the lawn munching away, says Robert Washabau, V.M.D., Ph.D., associate professor and section chief of medicine at the University of Pennsylvania School of Veterinary Medicine in Philadelphia.

One possible cause of grass eating is a condition called pancreatic insufficiency, in which the pancreas doesn't produce all the enzymes needed for proper digestion. Eating grass may help settle pets' stomachs while providing a few additional nutrients.

Another possible cause of grass eating is parasites. Pets with hookworms or roundworms, for example, often feel sick to their stomachs, and the grass may act as nature's Pepto-Bismol.

While eating small amounts of grass may settle your pet's stomach, eating too much can make things worse, says Carol A. Tice, D.V.M., a veterinarian in private practice in Cary, North Carolina. Mature blades of grass have sharp, barbed edges that can irritate the soft lining of the stomach, which is probably why many pets throw up a few minutes after indulging in a grassy meal. Worse, grass is a natural haven for intestinal parasites, the same critters that may be upsetting your pet's stomach in the first place.

WHAT YOU CAN DO

"If your pet wants to graze, it's fine to just let him enjoy himself," says Dr. Washabau. Rather than letting cats eat in the dirty outdoors, however, some people plant indoor grass gardens. (These petite gardens won't work for dogs.) All you have to do is fill a shallow, wide clay pot with soil, sprinkle on some pesticide-free ryegrass or oat seeds, and keep the pot moist and warm. In about three weeks, you will have three-inch shoots that are perfect for grazing.

Of course, if your pet has diarrhea, is vomiting, or generally seems under the weather, the grass eating is probably a warning sign, and you will want to call your vet.

What Your Vet Will Do

When you make an appointment to see your vet, she will probably ask that you bring in a fresh stool sample since that's the easiest way to test for parasites, says Elvira L. Hall, D.V.M., a veterinarian in private practice in Odenton, Maryland. Your pet will also be given a blood test to check for things such as internal infections or problems with the pancreas. If your pet's abdomen is swollen or tender, he may be given an x-ray to check for intestinal obstructions.

Since intestinal parasites are a common cause of eating grass, there is a good chance that your vet will send you home with a liquid worming medication such as pyrantel pamoate. Pancreatic problems are more serious, of course. If it turns out that your pet isn't making enough digestive enzymes, he may need daily supplements, which will help him digest his food properly again.

EATING LITTER

Clues

- Your cat is on a vegetarian diet.
- Your pet has pale or white gums.

Cats are well-known for being fussy eaters, always demanding the freshest, tastiest foods. But occasionally a cat will go to the other extreme and begin snacking in the most unappetizing of places, the litter box.

Eating litter isn't necessarily dangerous, although cats that take more than a small nibble may get obstructions in their intestinal tracts. The real problem isn't the litter lunch itself but the underlying condition that is causing them to take up the habit.

"A cat that suddenly starts eating litter is almost always sick," says Jane Brunt, D.V.M., a veterinarian in private practice in Towson, Maryland. For example, cats with anemia, a condition in which the body doesn't have enough red blood cells, will sometimes eat litter. Vets aren't sure why they do it, but it may be nature's way of getting more iron into their systems. Cats with kidney disease or feline leukemia will also eat litter on occasion, she says.

"Cats with poor diets, especially those given vegetarian diets, may crave nutrients," adds Carol A. Tice, D.V.M., a veterinarian in private practice in Cary, North Carolina. The clay used to make litter is rich in minerals and may act as a natural supplement. Cats that keep eating litter, however, may actually lose nutrients because the clay will leach out more minerals like iron, zinc, and potassium than it puts back in.

It doesn't happen often, but sometimes cats will develop unusual compulsions, in which a normal habit, such as licking litter off their fur after using the litter box, becomes an uncontrollable urge, says Elizabeth Shull, D.V.M., a veterinary behaviorist and neurologist at the University of Tennessee College of Veterinary Medicine in Knoxville. This type of compulsion is thought to be caused by chemical imbalances in the brain, she explains.

WHAT YOU CAN DO

Even when the box is perfectly clean, eating litter is a disturbing habit, to say the least. "I know of a few perfectly healthy cats that take an occasional litter snack," adds Dr. Tice. "I only worry when it's a new problem or if the cat is eating a lot of litter."

Since anemia is the most common cause of litter eating, it is worth taking a minute to do this quick check: Look at your pet's gums. They should be a bright pink. If they appear pale pink or even white, he almost certainly has anemia. Some cats with mild anemia may have normal-looking gums, so this isn't a foolproof test, Dr. Brunt adds.

If your cat gets a clean bill of health from the vet, you may want to experiment a bit at home to see if you can stop the habit. "Try switching foods," recommends Dr. Tice. If your cat is eating a grocery-store brand, try switching to a premium brand, such as Iams or Science Diet. If you have been giving him a vegetarian diet—and most vets agree that vegetarian diets can be dangerous for cats—add some meat or canned food to the menu. This will help ensure that he is getting all the nutrients he needs. But be prepared to be patient: Even if the litter eating is caused by a nutritional shortfall, it may be a month or more before he gives up the habit, Dr. Tice says.

Of course, your cat can't eat what he doesn't have, so you may want to replace the clay litter—both the clumping and the coarse types—with a less "appetizing" litter that is paper-based. "I like one called Yesterday's News," says Dr. Tice. It's available from your vet or pet supply stores.

Cats with a compulsion to eat litter can get quite ill, both physically and emotionally, unless they get professional help. One thing that you can do yourself, however, is to try to keep your cat occupied. Spend some time each day tossing a ball or encourage him to chase a string across the floor. The more time you spend together and the more energy he burns in play, the less likely he will be to focus all his attention on the litter, says Dr. Shull.

WHAT YOUR VET WILL DO

To check for anemia, your vet will need to count your pet's red blood cells. This is often done with a simple blood test called PCV, which stands for "packed cell volume." It only requires a few drops of blood, and you will have results within a few minutes.

A slower, but more complete blood test is called a CBC-plus panel. This is actually a series of blood tests that will show signs of infection, low mineral levels, or other whole-body problems. Your vet may want to check for such things as feline leukemia or thyroid problems as well.

Cats that have eaten a lot of litter will sometimes develop bowel obstructions. So if your cat is a little tender or swollen around the abdomen, your vet will want to take x-rays to check for problems in the stomach or intestines. X-rays can also reveal whether there are signs of cancer or kidney failure, which can also lead to litter eating.

Pets with nutritional deficiencies can often be treated with supplements or simply a higher-quality food. Cats with anemia, of course, need to be treated for whatever is causing the number of red blood cells to decline. Often this is nothing more serious than hookworms or other parasites, and your vet will give medications to get rid of them.

Cats with a compulsion to eat litter are often given mood-changing drugs, which help make the brain's chemistry more normal. This commonly relieves the problem, says Dr. Shull.

EATING OBJECTS

Clues

- Your pet is hungry all the time.
- He is restless or nervous.
- He seems obsessed with sweaters or other objects.

No matter what you put in their food bowls, some dogs and cats will "supplement" their diets with rocks, jewelry, plastics, and just about anything else they can wrap their lips around. This can be serious because even though most small objects will pass right through the digestive tract, some may lodge inside, causing a dangerous obstruction. String, a favorite of cats, is surprisingly dangerous because it can literally tie up the intestine. Pennies are just as bad because coins minted in 1983 or later are mostly zinc, not copper. When zinc comes into contact with stomach acid, it can dissolve and cause severe poisoning.

Young pets, puppies in particular, tend to swallow things because they are naturally curious and use their mouths to explore, says Elizabeth Shull, D.V.M., a veterinary behaviorist and neurologist at the University of Tennessee College of Veterinary Medicine in Knoxville. Kittens are less likely than puppies to swallow objects deliberately, but they may accidentally swallow things that they are playing with, says Vance Case, D.V.M., a veterinarian in private practice in Sunbury, Pennsylvania. Sewing needles, string, fishhooks, and Christmas tree tinsel are common and *dangerous* objects of choice, he adds.

Most pets stop swallowing foreign objects by the time they are a year old. But some dogs and cats develop physical or emotional problems that send them in search of inedible objects. These cravings, known as pica, can leave your pet with a belly full of indigestible trash, says Dr. Shull.

Some pets with pica are always hungry even though they are getting plenty of food, says Robert Washabau, V.M.D., Ph.D., associate professor and section chief of medicine at the University of Pennsylvania School of Veterinary Medicine in Philadelphia. Pets with inflammatory bowel disease, for example, may eat all their food but not be able to absorb all the nutrients. They feel hungry all the time and may turn to objects in order to fill the void.

Hormonal problems can also cause odd eating habits. Pets that produce too much thyroid hormone can develop a very fast metabolism—too fast to be supplied by the amount of calories they are taking in. So they look elsewhere for satisfaction.

It isn't very common, but some pets actually feel a compulsion to eat foreign objects, Dr. Shull adds. Vets aren't sure what causes these unhealthy and uncontrollable urges, but they suspect they are caused by an imbalance of chemicals in the brain.

Finally, some cats develop a taste for fabrics, a condition called wool chewing. They will spend hours chewing and sucking on sweaters, socks, or blankets. This condition isn't serious, but cats that take up the habit can destroy a closetful of sweaters in no time.

WHAT YOU CAN DO

Even though it is normal for young pets to occasionally chew and swallow objects they shouldn't, it is never safe. It is worth taking a few minutes each day to pick up any tempting items, whether they are pennies on the floor or panty hose in the laundry basket, says Dr. Case.

Older pets that suddenly turn their attention to inedible objects probably have problems with their diets or digestion, says Dr. Washabau. If your pet isn't getting enough calories—either because you are not feeding him enough or he is having trouble digesting his food—you may want to pour a little more kibble in the bowl. If that doesn't help, switching foods may be an option. Pets foods provide nutrients in different forms. Some use rice, for example, while others depend on corn.

Every pet is unique, and a food that satisfies one dog or cat may leave another feeling hungry, says Dr. Case. If your pet is still eating the wrong things, you should call your vet right away.

It's not always easy to discourage cats from chewing sweaters, woolen sheets, or other toothsome fabrics. Some experts believe that cats that aren't getting enough fiber in their diets will naturally turn to material replacements, says Dr. Case. In fact, giving cats lettuce to munch on will sometimes cause them to lose interest in material. Another remedy you may want to try is Vetasyl, a fiber-filled capsule that you can get from your vet.

Even if your pet doesn't make a habit of eating objects, doing it even once can be a problem if the object doesn't come out again. If you see your pet swallow something that he shouldn't, like a small stone, switch him immediately to a high-fiber food, says Dr. Case. This will help coat the object in the intestine so that it slides out more easily. If it doesn't come out in a week, you should play it safe and call your vet. Don't wait that long if your pet swallows something that is potentially dangerous, like a battery, or if he is acting mopey or seems to have a stomachache, he adds. Call your vet immediately.

WHAT YOUR VET WILL DO

Your vet won't waste a lot of time discussing the issue if your pet has swallowed something harmful. He will want to get the object out right away, and the quickest way to do that is often with an emetic, a drug that causes vomiting.

Vomiting will bring up things like pennies without any problem, but it doesn't work for sharp objects like needles, which can do additional damage on the way back up. Your vet may decide to fish the objects out with a procedure called endoscopy, in which a long tube, lit with fiber optics, is slid down your pet's mouth and into his stomach. The procedure is very safe and your vet may be able to remove the object through the tube without resorting to surgery.

Inedibles that have been in the digestive tract for hours or days aren't so easy to dislodge. Your vet may need to do x-rays to see exactly what the object is, where it is located, and whether it can easily be removed. Some objects can be left inside until nature takes its course. But others, like batteries, are too dangerous to leave inside, and your pet may need surgery to get them out.

Pets that consistently swallow what they shouldn't invariably have an underlying medical or behavioral problem. Your vet will probably take blood samples to check for such things as thyroid or pancreatic disease, diabetes, or other whole-body problems. If nothing appears to be wrong physically, your vet will attack the problem from another perspective. Pets that won't leave objects alone can sometimes be trained to ignore them. They can also be given medications such as fluoxetine (Prozac), which change the brain's chemistry and can help keep eating compulsions under control, says Dr. Shull.

See also Chapter 4: Eating Stool, Wool Chewing

SYMPTOM) EATING STOOL

Clues

- **Your pet is having diarrhea or other digestive problems.**
- **He doesn't seem to have enough to do.**
- **He is also showing dominant behavior, like fighting.**

Dogs are well-known for their adventuresome appetites, but sometimes they go too far—grazing in the litter box, for example, or having "lunch" on the lawn.

Distasteful as it is to humans, eating stool is normal for dogs. (Cats, on the other hand, never do it.) New mothers, for example, will eat the stool of puppies, presumably to keep the nest clean. Puppies, in turn, will sample whatever they come across, including stool. "Human babies explore with their hands, and puppies explore with their mouths," says Sandra Sawchuk, D.V.M., clinical instructor of small animal medicine at the University of Wisconsin School of Veterinary Medicine in Madison.

Nearly every dog will occasionally sample stool, but some have a real craving for it, including their own, and will eat it every chance they get. This may be caused by nutritional deficiencies, possibly due to a lack of certain enzymes in the digestive tract, says Karen L. Overall, V.M.D., Ph.D., head of the behavior clinic at the University of Pennsylvania School of Veterinary Medicine in Philadelphia. When a dog eats his own stool, he is giving the partially digested food another run through his digestive tract, where more nutrients will be absorbed.

In some cases, dogs will eat stool merely because they don't have enough to do. Or they will do it because it is a way of getting your attention. They will also eat stool as a way of establishing their dominance over other pets by removing their scent markers. (Pets that are wrangling for dominance will sometimes pick fights as well.) And in rare cases, eating stool may be caused by a condition called obsessive-compulsive disorder, in which dogs repeatedly do certain things simply because they are emotionally unable to stop.

WHAT YOU CAN DO

Eating stool usually isn't a health threat, although some dogs may develop dental disease from bacteria lodging between their teeth. Most of the time it is a social disease: People don't like watching their dogs do it, and they certainly don't like smelling their breath later.

The easiest solution is to close the drive-up window. Put the cat's litter box out of reach, says Deborah C. Mallu, D.V.M., a holistic veterinarian in private practice in Sedona, Arizona. Clean the yard whenever your pet makes a pit stop. You may not be able to change his tastes, but you can make the foraging more difficult.

Some vets recommend taking a more aggressive approach. Rather than cleaning stools from the yard, give them a generous sprinkling of hot-pepper powder or hot-pepper sauce. Most dogs don't like hot, spicy foods. When your dog takes a bite, he will get an unwelcome surprise—and he may decide that stools simply don't taste the way they used to and give them up, says Dr. Sawchuk.

Vets and pet supply stores sell a product called For-Bid, which is added to a pet's food. Although it has little taste of its own, it becomes very bitter once it travels through the digestive tract, giving stools a taste dogs dislike. Vets advise adding it to your dog's food every day for three days. Some dogs will quickly learn to avoid stools, while others may take longer to get the hint.

If you don't want to give your dog chemicals, canned spinach has a similar effect, adds Kathalyn Johnson, D.V.M., clinical associate in companion animal behavior at Texas A&M University College of Veterinary Medicine in College Station. The usual strategy is to mix a quarter-cup of canned spinach in your dog's food every day, or until he stops snacking in the yard.

Adding more fiber to your dog's diet can also help, says Dr. Johnson. "We're not sure why some dogs respond to this," she says. It may be that fiber changes the consistency of the stool, making it less palatable to dogs.

You can buy high-fiber foods such as Hill's Prescription Diet W/D from your veterinarian. Or you can add a teaspoon or two of Metamucil, which is very high in fiber, to your pet's food every day until he stops eating stool, says Dr. Johnson. Canned pumpkin is also high in fiber, she adds, and dogs love the taste. You can mix between one tablespoon and a quarter-cup in your dog's food every day. Once he quits eating stool, you can put the pumpkin back on the shelf.

It's not always easy to train dogs to leave stools alone, but it can be done with a technique that vets call startle and redirect.

The next time your dog is nosing around for a snack, loudly clap your hands. This will startle him and get his attention, says Patricia B. McConnell, Ph.D., assistant adjunct professor of zoology at the University of Wisconsin in Madison, a certified applied animal behaviorist, and author of *Beginning Family Dog Training*.

Once he is paying attention to you, redirect his attention to something he enjoys, like playing catch or running around the yard. Eventually, he will get the idea that *not* eating stool is even more fun than eating it.

Since dogs that don't have enough to do will sometimes eat stool as a way of passing the time, it is a good idea to keep them active, says Dr. Overall. Play some catch or go for a quick walk. The more energy he burns up having fun, the less likely he is to go foraging later.

WHAT YOUR VET WILL DO

The very thought of it may upset your stomach, but most dogs can snack on stool their entire lives and never be sick a day. Others, however, may have underlying physical problems that are causing the habit. If your dog is vomiting, having diarrhea, or is losing weight as well as eating stool, he may have digestive problems and needs to see a vet.

Your vet will probably begin by feeling your dog's belly to see if organs inside are swollen. This may be a sign that undigested food is accumulating in the colon. She may also recommend blood tests to make sure that the liver and kidneys are working properly and to check the body's levels of trypsin and amylase, enzymes that are needed for digestion. These enzymes are available in supplement form from your vet, so a deficiency isn't always a serious problem.

If your vet suspects that your dog has obsessive-compulsive disorder, she will probably recommend that you take him to a professional who specializes in behavioral problems. In addition, the vet may recommend giving your pet anti-anxiety medications such as fluoxetine (Prozac), which will calm your dog down and make him less likely to fixate on his bad habits. Some dogs take the medication for life, but others are able to give it up after a reconditioning or training program, says Dr. Overall.

FINICKY EATING

Clues

- Your pet eats from one kind of bowl (made of ceramic or glass) but not another (made of metal or plastic).
- He lost his appetite suddenly.
- Your pet has lost weight.
- He eats human food but not pet food.

Sophisticated people who turn up their noses at certain foods are referred to admiringly as discerning eaters. Choosy dogs and cats, however, go by the less flattering term *finicky eaters.* For their frustrated owners, finding a menu to tempt the finicky diner can truly be a challenge.

The dictionary defines *finicky* two ways. First, it can mean picky, choosy, or difficult to please. Its second meaning? "Insisting capriciously on getting just what one wants." The second definition probably describes what your pet is doing—manipulating your emotions until you deliver whatever his tastebuds demand.

"Finicky eating is almost always caused by humans," says Karen L. Overall, V.M.D., Ph.D., head of the behavior clinic at the University of Pennsylvania School of Veterinary Medicine in Philadelphia. Owners love to make their pets happy, and an easy way to do it is by giving them what they like. And what they like may be steak rather than kibble or canned tuna fish instead of canned pet food. Eventually, they get the message: "Aha! If I hold out long enough, they'll give me the good stuff."

Finicky eating can also be caused by giving your pet a monotonous diet. Suppose, for example, that your dog has been eating one kind of kibble all his life, and one day he gets to sample another, tastier food. His kibble is going to seem awfully dull by comparison, and finicky eating may be the result.

Cats are even fussier in their tastes than dogs because cats notice the texture and shape of their food as well as its flavor. "We've found that if cats are fed a restricted diet from the time they are young, they get very finicky," says Dr. Overall. "If a cat has been fed only dry food, it's hard to switch to the wet kind, or even to a dry food with a different shape."

Finicky eating may also be caused by an unpleasant experience. "If an animal gets ill and associates the illness with a particular food, he may not eat that food again," says Dr. Overall.

While every pet has his likes and dislikes, some are so finicky that they will hold out for hours or even days until they get exactly what they want. This is not only frustrating for owners, but potentially dangerous for pets, especially cats. Cats that don't eat for a long time may develop a liver disorder called hepatic lipidosis, which can be extremely serious. If your cat refuses to eat for a day or two, it is a good idea to give him something that satisfies his choosy palate. Then call your vet for advice.

WHAT YOU CAN DO

Finicky eating isn't always a problem, as long as your pet is eating some food. In fact, if he is healthy and maintaining a normal weight, it really doesn't matter if he picks at his food, says Kathryn E. Michel, D.V.M., clinical assistant professor of nutrition at the University of Pennsylvania School of Veterinary Medicine. "What we may consider finicky eating may actually be appropriate for that animal," she says.

The problem with finicky eaters, of course, is that they often drive their owners crazy with whines, meows, or relentless mooching. To regain your peace of mind, here are a few things that you may want to try.

- Stop giving them human food. Once pets get a taste of tasty table scraps, they are often reluctant to return to their usual chow. At the very least, give them human food only when it is mixed in with the food you want them to be eating, says Dean Gebroe, D.V.M., a veterinarian in private practice in Los Angeles. While human food in moderation is okay, you don't want to get to the point where your pet only wants to eat what's on your plate, he says.

  In addition, don't put up with their begging. "Put their food down for 10 to 20 minutes, and if they don't eat, pick it up," Dr. Gebroe adds. "They may miss a couple of meals, but ultimately they will get the message." Dogs generally adjust quickly, but cats sometimes hold out for a long time—so long, in fact, that they will make themselves sick. If your cat's hunger strike lasts more than a day, call your vet for advice.

- Make sure that their food smells good, not necessarily to you but to them. "Odor is a big factor," says Dr. Michel. "Try to choose smellier foods, such as fish, for cats." For dogs, beef and liver are favorite choices. Warming the food slightly will release more of its aroma.

- Many pets prefer moist food over the dry stuff. This doesn't mean that you have to give your fussy eaters top-of-the-line canned food. Simply adding a little warm water to dry food or mixing in a little bit of wet food with a big serving of kibble may get them eating.

- Dogs are social animals, and sometimes they are reluctant to eat on their own. "They see the other members of the household as their pack, and one thing packs do is eat together," says Dr. Michel. You may want to try feeding your dog at the same time you eat with your family. You don't have to put his bowl right next to the table. Putting it in the next room but in sight of the table where you are eating may encourage him to eat with gusto again.

- While dogs enjoy taking their meals with company, cats often prefer a little bit of privacy. Moving their food into a quiet, out-of-the-way place may encourage them to eat, says Deborah C. Mallu, D.V.M., a holistic veterinarian in private practice in Sedona, Arizona.

- Some pets develop an intense dislike for plastic or metal food bowls, which may impart an unpleasant flavor to their food. Try using glass or ceramic instead, suggests Dr. Mallu. For small pets, use a flat dish instead of a deep bowl since they may dislike getting their whiskers bent when they stick their faces into the bowl.
- Some people have successfully stopped finicky eating simply by giving their pets a little less food and then acting indifferent when their pets turn up their whiskers. "The idea is to give them some food but not so much that they are satiated," says Patricia B. McConnell, Ph.D., assistant adjunct professor of zoology at the University of Wisconsin in Madison, a certified applied animal behaviorist, and author of *Beginning Family Dog Training*. When the finicky eaters realize that they can't push you around, they are more likely to grab what you give them, she says.

Once it starts, finicky eating can be very hard to stop. In most cases, however, it is easy to prevent. "Preferences are formed quite early in life," says Sandra Sawchuk, D.V.M., clinical instructor of small animal medicine at the University of Wisconsin School of Veterinary Medicine in Madison. "If you expose a pet to a variety of food flavors, shapes, sizes, and textures at a young age, he will tend to be more adventuresome later in life."

There is a big difference between pets that are hard to please and those that have abruptly lost their appetites, adds Craig N. Carter, D.V.M., Ph.D., head of epidemiology at the Texas Veterinary Medical Diagnostic Laboratory at Texas A&M University in College Station. Pets frequently lose their appetites when they are ill, so it is important to call your vet if your pet suddenly stops eating, he says.

WHAT YOUR VET WILL DO

If your pet isn't eating and is also losing weight, your vet will want to do a thorough checkup to see what's going on. She will begin by weighing your pet and by giving his body a good going-over with her fingers. If there is a bit of padding between the skin and the rib cage and his muscle mass is normal, he is at a healthy weight. If the ribs are especially prominent, however, he may be losing too much weight.

To find out if there is an internal problem causing your pet to lose his appetite, your vet will probably recommend doing blood tests to check for such things as infections and hormonal or intestinal problems. Once the underlying problem has been taken care of, your pet's appetite will quickly return to normal.

See also Chapter 4: Appetite Loss; Chapter 14: Weight Loss

SYMPTOM) OVEREATING

Clues

- Your pet gobbles everything in sight.
- He eats a lot but is losing weight.
- Your pet is taking steroids.

If you are perplexed because your pooch is getting a paunch or your feline is no longer streamlined, consider their ancestors. Dogs and cats were originally predators that ate whatever they could when they could. It made sense because they were never sure when their next meal was coming along.

Pets today, of course, "hunt" by stalking their food bowls, but they are genetically programmed to eat in the same way that their ancestors did—by stuffing themselves at every opportunity.

Overeating and the resulting weight gain usually occur because we, their owners, find it difficult to resist their pleading eyes and give them more food than they really need, says Craig N. Carter, D.V.M., Ph.D., head of epidemiology at the Texas Veterinary Medical Diagnostic Laboratory at Texas A&M University in College Station.

Overeating tends to be more of a problem when there is more than one pet in the family. Dogs and cats hate the idea that someone else is going to eat their food, so they may gobble as much as they can as fast as they can. In addition, dogs and cats, like people, will sometimes eat too much when they are depressed or anxious, says Deborah C. Mallu, D.V.M., a holistic veterinarian in private practice in Sedona, Arizona.

In rare cases, pets will eat and eat because they are emotionally incapable of stopping, a condition that vets call obsessive-compulsive disorder, says Karen L. Overall, V.M.D., Ph.D., head of the behavior clinic at the University of Pennsylvania School of Veterinary Medicine in Philadelphia.

There are a number of medical problems that cause dogs and cats to start eating more, Dr. Carter adds. Pets with Cushing's disease, for example, in which the adrenal glands produce too much cortisol (a steroid hormone), crave more food because the excess cortisol breaks down muscle and other tissue. This drains the body of necessary protein, and pets often eat more in order to replace it. An overactive thyroid gland, or hyperthyroidism, can also cause overeating, says Dean Gebroe, D.V.M., a veterinarian in private practice in Los Angeles. "You'll see your pet begin to overeat, yet maintain the same weight," he explains. "But as the disease progresses, he will start to lose weight."

Other physical problems that can cause overeating include parasites, diabetes, pancreatitis (an infection of the pancreas), or tumors in the pituitary gland. In addition, pets that are taking steroids, which are sometimes used after injuries, will sometimes eat everything in sight.

Overeating is always cause for concern—not only because it may be a sign of other, underlying problems but also because it is often followed by weight gain, which can be extremely unhealthy, says John E. Bauer, D.V.M., Ph.D., professor of clinical nutrition at Texas A&M University College of Veterinary Medicine in College Station. "The incidence of orthopedic problems in obese pets is incredible," he says, "and the cost of repairing ruptured ligaments is high."

WHAT YOU CAN DO

Most dogs and cats simply love spending time at the trough. The only solution may be to cut back on the amount you are feeding him or, at the very least, not to leave food out all the time. Vets usually advise feeding pets twice a day. If they don't eat all their food in half an hour or so, put the food away until it is time for the next meal.

If you are unsure whether your pet is overeating, here is a simple test: Rub your hand across his ribs. "You should feel your fingers slightly fall in the gaps between the ribs." says Dr. Bauer. If you can't feel the ribs, it's time to cut back on the amount you are feeding him, he says.

To help your voracious pet eat less and lose weight, cut back the amount you feed him by about 25 percent, says C. A. Tony Buffington, D.V.M., Ph.D., professor of veterinary clinical sciences at the Ohio State University Veterinary Hospital in Columbus. If he hasn't lost any weight in about two weeks, reduce the serving sizes a little more. Continue doing this until you can just feel the ribs through the coat, which will mean he is at a healthy weight.

Since overeating sometimes is a sign that pets don't have enough to do, you may want to keep your pet more active, says Dr. Overall. Taking regular walks and having more playtimes are excellent ways to get his mind off his food bowl.

Some vets recommend making the pet work a little harder for his grub. For example, put his kibble beneath an upside-down plastic flowerpot so that he has to knock over the pot to get to the tasty treat. Or spread his food over a large cookie sheet so that he has to eat it one nugget at a time. "Puzzles can make all the difference in the world to a dog or cat that's wolfing down food and immediately looking for more," says Dr. Overall.

If you don't mind spending a few dollars, a fun gadget to look for is the Buster Cube. It has hidden compartments inside where you can stash a little food. Your pet will have to manipulate the toy just so in order to open the doors that let him get to the food.

Food puzzles aren't just entertaining, adds Sandra Sawchuk, D.V.M., clinical instructor of small animal medicine at the University of Wisconsin School of Veterinary Medicine in Madison. Pets often eat so quickly that their brains don't get the "full" message until they have gobbled more than

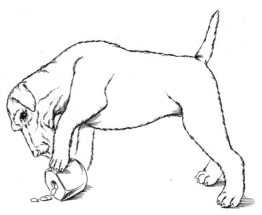

One way to curtail your dog's noshing and entertain him at the same time is with a Buster Cube. This is a fun toy with a hidden compartment that holds up to a cup of food. Your dog will have to work for each bite, and he will have a great time doing it.

they really need. Food puzzles cause pets to eat more slowly, so they are more likely to eat less, she says.

"Dry food tends to be eaten slower than canned food," Dr. Sawchuk adds. In addition, it's a good idea to feed your pets separately—in different places or at different times. Once they understand that no one is going to elbow in on their dinner, they are less likely to gobble it all down.

Since mealtimes are typically fun times, pets often gather around the food bowl simply because they are in the mood for extra attention. Instead of reaching for the food, do something else with them, suggests Dr. Mallu. "Pick up a brush and brush them or get a toy and play with them."

What Your Vet Will Do

It is not always easy for vets to tell if pets are truly eating too much. Before going into the office, it is a good idea to write down exactly how much you are feeding your pet and whether he has been gaining any weight. Is he eating more than usual? Is he drinking more water? Has he been vomiting or having diarrhea? "The best client is the one who comes in and whips out a piece of paper," says Dr. Gebroe.

Since parasites may cause pets to overeat, it is a good idea to take in a recent stool sample—one that is less than 24 hours old. In addition, your vet will check for hormonal problems, such as an overactive thyroid gland. Hormonal conditions can be serious without treatment, but they are usually easy to control with medications or, in some cases, with surgery.

When your pet's overeating has caused him to put on a few pounds, your vet will probably recommend that you begin a long-term weight-loss plan, says Dr. Bauer. A customized plan is especially important for cats since unsupervised dieting can result in liver problems that can be even more serious than the overeating was.

See also Chapter 14: Weight Gain

WOOL CHEWING

Clues

- Your cat is teething.
- She usually eats wet food.

First, she chewed your ratty old scarf. Then she took bites from your new angora sweater. Now she is showing interest in your Lycra tights. What's turning your otherwise normal cat into a material girl?

"We don't really understand it," says Karen L. Overall, V.M.D., Ph.D., head of the behavior clinic at the University of Pennsylvania School of Veterinary Medicine in Philadelphia, "but cats that chew wool seem to be born, not made."

Actually, the term *wool chewing* isn't entirely accurate since cats that take up the habit will go after other materials as well. They don't always chew the material either: Some prefer to suck and knead it, as though it were as tasty as mother's milk.

Vets suspect that certain cats, especially Burmese, Siamese, and Himalayans, simply have a genetic tendency to practice wool chewing. In some cases, it may be a way of easing teething pain or even of passing the time. In addition, cats that were weaned too early from their mothers may be more likely to turn their affections from the maternal to the material.

Wool chewing isn't likely to cause problems for cats (dogs don't practice the habit), although they conceivably could swallow indigestible material that could cause an intestinal blockage, says Debra Horwitz, D.V.M., a veterinary behaviorist in private practice in St. Louis. The main threat is to your clothes and furnishings.

WHAT YOU CAN DO

Since some cats have a natural urge to be oral, one of the easiest solutions is to give them more appropriate things to chew, says Kathalyn Johnson, D.V.M., clinical associate in companion animal behavior at Texas A&M University College of Veterinary Medicine in College Station. If your cat usually eats wet food, for example, feeding her dry kibble will give her jaws more of a workout and possibly satisfy the urge to chew. Or give your cat a bone. Sterilized bones are available at pet supply stores, and your cat will enjoy giving them a good going-over, particularly if she is also having teething pain.

If your cat insists on putting her teeth to work on fabrics, try giving her toys covered with fake sheepskin, says Patricia B. McConnell, Ph.D., assistant adjunct professor of zoology at the University of Wisconsin in Madison, a certified applied animal behaviorist, and author of *Beginning Family Dog Training*. "They are actually made for dogs, but a lot of cats really like them," she says. Watch her closely, however, and take the toy away if she is swallowing the fibers.

Cats take to training less readily than dogs, but there are ways to discourage your cat from dispatching your garments. When you see her sneaking up on your angora sweater, for example, stomp your foot or toss a shoe in her direction. The object isn't to hit or terrify her, but to redirect her attention, says Dr. Overall. Once her mind is off the sweater, tell her she is a good cat and give her an acceptable substitute to chew on, she suggests. Eventually, she will get the idea that crime doesn't pay.

Of course, you won't always be around when your cat has a view to chew. That's when booby traps come in handy. Dr. Johnson recommends putting hot-pepper flakes on the object of your cat's affections. Once she takes an unpleasant mouthful, your kitty may decide to be more careful of what she chews in the future.

Since cats tend to chew when they don't have other things to do, you can protect your wardrobe simply by having more fun together. For example, spend a half-hour dragging a piece of string or tossing a stuffed mouse. "Tired animals are well-behaved," says Dr. Overall. "They have less energy for obnoxious behavior."

Whatever remedies you try, be sure to start them as soon as you notice the behavior, adds Dr. McConnell. "If you wait too long, they can literally get addicted to the behavior."

WHAT YOUR VET WILL DO

Since wool chewing isn't likely to be dangerous, some owners simply put up with it—after hiding their best clothes, of course. But if you are tired of finding gaping holes in your linen or sweaters, your vet may have a solution.

It doesn't work for all cats, but giving anti-anxiety or antidepressant medications, such as asclomipramine (Anafranil), may be helpful in some cases. In addition, your vet may recommend that you see a specialist in behavior problems. "After you get them on medication, they might be more amenable to behavioral approaches," says Dr. Overall.

COMMON APPETITE AND EATING CONDITIONS

Cancer. As with any disease that affects the whole body, cancer will often stifle a dog's or cat's interest in eating. This is particularly true when the cancer affects the stomach, intestine, or any other part of the digestive tract.

"A common scenario with an older dog or cat that suddenly stops eating is an invasive cancer somewhere in the gastrointestinal tract, usually in the intestine," says Karen L. Overall, V.M.D., Ph.D., head of the behavior clinic at the University of Pennsylvania School of Veterinary Medicine in Philadelphia.

As with cancer in humans, there are many treatments available, from chemotherapy to radiation to surgery. And since it is essential for pets with cancer to eat properly in order to keep up their strength and keep the immune system working well, it is important to call your vet immediately if your pet's appetite seems to be dropping.

Cushing's disease. This is a condition in which the pituitary gland produces excessive amounts of the hormone ACTH, causing the body to produce high levels of cortisol and other steroids. When cortisol levels rise, so does your pet's interest in eating and drinking. Cushing's disease, which is often caused by a tumor on the pituitary gland, affects mainly middle-aged, purebred dogs. One of the main symptoms is an increase in appetite. It can also cause your pet's coat to get dry and thin. The usual treatment for Cushing's disease is to give medications (usually for life) that decrease the body's ability to make cortisol.

Dental disease. Sometimes eating can literally be a pain. If your pet is chewing in a funny way (gingerly or on one side of her mouth), has bad breath, or has gums that are inflamed or bleeding, chances are that she has dental problems.

Unlike humans, dogs and cats don't get cavities. But they do get other tooth and gum problems that can take away their appetites. Dental problems are quite common, affecting more than 80 percent of dogs and cats after the age of three. The most common dental problem is periodontal disease, in which bacteria-laden plaque on the teeth erodes gum tissue and possibly causes the teeth to loosen.

To prevent periodontal disease, vets recommend brushing your pet's teeth every day. It is also a good idea to give her dry food and crunchy snacks since these will help scour the teeth clean. In addition, some vets recommend giving the teeth a professional cleaning once a year to prevent plaque from accumulating.

Diabetes. Diabetes is a condition in which either the pancreas doesn't produce enough insulin or the body is unable to take full advantage of the insulin that is produced. Insulin is a hormone needed to transport glucose (blood sugar) and fats into the body's cells. When glucose and fats don't get inside cells, they stay in the bloodstream, damaging tissues throughout the body. Pets with diabetes will often drink enormous amounts of water—the body's attempt to dilute the sugar- and fat-rich blood before it does harm.

"There is all this sugar in the blood, but the cells are starving," adds Dean Gebroe, D.V.M., a veterinarian in private practice in Los Angeles. Pets with diabetes eat and drink with all their might, but without insulin, the cells are unable to take in the energy-giving glucose.

Some pets with diabetes will require daily shots of insulin to lower blood sugar levels. In many cases, however, this condition can be controlled or even eliminated by simple lifestyle changes—by helping overweight pets lose weight, for example, or by making changes in exercise and eating habits.

Hyperthyroidism. Pets with overactive (hyper) thyroid glands are hungry all the time, yet thin as a rail. They drink a lot, sleep less than they used to, and tend to be agitated and fidgety. "The thyroid is kind of like the gas pedal of the body," explains Sandra Sawchuk, D.V.M., clinical instructor of small animal medicine at the University of Wisconsin School of Veterinary Medicine in Madison. "It regulates metabolism. If it's producing too much hormone, it's like revving the engine constantly."

In cats, hyperthyroidism can be treated with medications that slow the metabolism to normal levels. Vets may also recommend treatments with radioactive iodine, which destroys abnormal thyroid tissue while keeping the gland intact. Radioactive iodine is usually the preferred option, says Dr. Gebroe, but also the most expensive. In dogs, surgery is usually needed to remove the overactive gland because it could contain a malignant cancer. "Because more than half of thyroid tumors in dogs are malignant, surgery will probably be required to help prevent the spread of the cancer to other organs," says Craig N. Carter, D.V.M., Ph.D., head of epidemiology at the Texas Veterinary Medical Diagnostic Laboratory at Texas A&M University in College Station. "The malignant form of thyroid cancer is much less common in cats, but it can occur and may also require surgery."

Hypothyroidism. Pets with underactive (hypo) thyroid glands don't produce enough of this important hormone to keep their metabolism running at healthy levels. As a result, their appetite drops, yet they gain weight. They may be sluggish and tired as well.

While hypothyroidism is very rare in cats, it is one of the most common hormonal conditions in dogs. In most cases, it is easily treated by giving pets thyroid hormone supplements, which replenish the body's natural supply.

Intestinal obstruction. When your pet develops a taste for inedible items, like pocket watches or rings, replacing your possessions may be the least of your concerns. Swallowing objects can cause an intestinal obstruction, resulting in a loss of appetite, constipation, nausea, abdominal pain, or vomiting. Intestinal obstructions can be life-threatening, so it is essential to see your vet immediately if you even suspect this is the problem.

Your vet can identify intestinal obstructions with an x-ray. In most cases, however, surgery is the only way to remove swallowed objects and relieve the blockage.

Kidney disease. In older pets particularly, kidney disease is a common cause of lost appetite. "If the kidney is not functioning properly, it can't filter all the toxins out of the blood," says Dr. Gebroe. "Toxins will accumulate, and your pet will lose her appetite."

In addition to lost appetite, symptoms of kidney problems include drinking a lot, weight loss, and possibly vomiting.

Kidney disease is serious, and your pet will probably need intravenous fluids to help flush the blood and keep her healthy. In addition, she will probably be given a special diet, along with medications, to help the kidneys work properly again.

Behavior

Nonstop barking. "Surprises" in the houseplants. Sofa backs ripped repairless. You know your pets don't mean to be so mean, but why are they acting this way?

Before you can understand why dogs and cats misbehave, you have to try to see the world from their point of view. Dogs and cats don't do "bad" things deliberately to annoy their human owners. In most cases, they are simply doing what comes naturally, like sharpening their claws or growling or fighting with other pets. In the days when dogs and cats lived in the wild, these and other activities weren't bad at all. They were part of their normal behavior and played valuable roles in day-to-day life. Cats scratched to keep their claws sharp and reading for hunting—an essential task in the days when food didn't come in a bowl. Dogs growled to warn off intruders. And dogs and cats would occasionally fight—or, more often, pretend that they were going to—to defend territory, establish hierarchies, and protect their young.

What's natural in the wild, of course, isn't always acceptable in your living room or while taking a walk. But dogs and cats follow instinct much more than people do, and it is not always easy to stop them from doing the same things that their ancestors did. In fact, the trick to solving most behavior problems isn't to stop the behavior entirely, but to make sure it is expressed in more appropriate ways, says Wayne Hunthausen, D.V.M., a veterinarian in private practice in Westwood, Kansas, who specializes in behavior problems. You may not be able to reduce your cat's urge to scratch, for example, but you can give him a more acceptable place to do it. You can't change a dog's dominant personality, but you can teach him to be submissive when he is dealing with members of the family or other humans. With a combination of patience, repetition, and clear direction, most behavior problems aren't that difficult to stop, he says.

The most important thing to remember is that misbehavior often occurs when something is happening in your pet's environment that's causing him to act in certain ways. It is up to you to provide an abundance of human understanding and care. Some dogs and cats, like people, experience stress and boredom that can lead to a wide range of behavior problems. While the problems aren't necessarily difficult to resolve, says Dr. Hunthausen, you can't even begin to do so until you have an inkling of why your dog or cat is doing the things he does.

It is not always easy for humans to have a pet's perspective of the world. But once you begin to see things the way your pets do, you will not only understand why they do things, but you will have a much better sense of how to improve their behavior. A dog, for example, will sometimes misbehave by grabbing your slippers and happily running around the house when you try to get them back simply because he wants more attention. Once you understand this, you will realize that spending a few extra minutes a day with your dog may be all it takes to stop his urge to grab and run.

Even though behavior problems can usually be solved, it is natural for owners to get angry or frustrated. In fact, behavior problems are among the most common reasons that people take their pets to the vet or, in extreme cases, put them up for adoption, says Dr. Hunthausen.

One of the best things that owners can do, he adds, is help prevent behavior problems from getting started. A pet often misbehaves because his owner thinks that a behavior is amusing, at least at first, and encourages it. Then later on, the owner wants the behavior to stop, but the pet didn't get the message at the beginning—and that's when problems begin.

In the following pages, you will learn about a variety of common problems—everything from barking and chewing to scratching and spraying—and discover what you can do to keep those problems under control.

See Your Vet If:

- Your pet has begun growling at or biting people.
- He gets panicky in certain situations, such as during thunderstorms.
- He has started pressing his head against walls.
- Your pet is having accidents in the house.
- He is overly possessive of food or toys.
- You can't stop him from barking or meowing.
- Your pet's voice has changed.
- He gets obsessed with odd behaviors, like chasing his tail or biting his feet.
- He urinates when people approach.
- Your pet seems depressed or lethargic.
- He is constantly biting, scratching, or licking himself.
- He often stands with his legs wide apart or at an awkward angle.
- His back arches even when he is not frightened.
- He appears to be having seizures.

AGGRESSION

Clues

• Your pet hesitates to take orders.
• He growls during play.
• He hisses for no reason.

It's fun to trade growls with your puppy when he is pulling a rope or to encourage cat attacks with a piece of string attached to a stuffed mouse. But when play aggression turns serious—and it is directed against you, your family, or your friends—it stops being fun and starts being a little bit scary.

Even a small dog can deliver a painful bite, and large dogs can do serious damage. Cats aren't as dangerous as their canine counterparts simply because they are smaller. Even so, cat bites and scratches often cause infections. That is why any form of aggression in dogs or cats must be dealt with immediately and firmly, says Wayne Hunthausen, D.V.M., a veterinarian in private practice in Westwood, Kansas, who specializes in behavior problems.

A dog's tendency to go on the offensive is influenced to a certain extent by his genetic makeup. Breeds such as Chow Chows, Rottweilers, and mastiffs have been bred to be aggressive. This doesn't mean that these dogs are automatically a threat to humans. What it does mean, says Dr. Hunthausen, is that they need careful training to keep their natural tendencies in check.

Regardless of the breed, pushy behavior such as biting, growling, or ignoring commands is a dog's way of saying that he is in charge. And the longer he gets away with it, the pushier he will become, says Dr. Hunthausen. This is because dogs live in natural hierarchies. If their owners don't tell them what to do, such as where to eat or to stay away from the door, dogs will naturally assume the leadership role. And that means they will start pushing you around.

Dogs that are frightened will frequently show flashes of temper, Dr. Hunthausen adds. Jealousy can also be a problem. In families with new babies, for instance, dogs will sometimes snap or growl because the newcomer is taking away some of their attention.

Dogs have surprisingly long memories, and if your pet had an unpleasant experience in the past, such as being abused by a previous owner, he may be snappish toward a person who reminds him of the bad old days. This may explain what happens when a normally peaceful dog shows a flash of anger at someone he just met—someone who, like his former abusive owner, for instance, wears a baseball cap.

Owners sometimes teach their dogs to be aggressive by playing rough games like tug-of-war and then rewarding them when they show spirit. Eventually, the dog learns that growling and other signs of play belligerence make his master happy. The problem, of course, is that dogs may get confused about the rules and get temperamental at the worst possible time—like when your toddler grabs his tail.

Cats are less likely than dogs to get into, well, cat fights with you. They do like to play, however, and sometimes this means honing their hunting skills by attacking your ankles or nipping your feet under the dinner table.

A cat can also be short-tempered when a well-meaning owner attempts to pet him and he isn't in the mood for affection. When you reach out too suddenly, he will sometimes react with a flash of teeth or claws. He may also show a similar reaction if you have been stroking him for a while, and something else becomes of interest.

A common form of aggression in cats, and the most dangerous, is called redirected anger. If your cat is upset because he has just been chased by an angry dog, for instance, it can take him hours to calm down. In the meantime, he may take out his anger or fear on you, explains Dr. Hunthausen.

Although aggression is usually considered a training or behavior problem, it can also be caused by physical problems, says Barbara Simpson, D.V.M., Ph.D., a veterinarian in private practice in Southern Pines, North Carolina, who specializes in animal behavior. Pets in pain—because of arthritis, for example—will often be short-tempered, she says. In addition, some older pets may be confused or disoriented, and this can also lead to displays of bad temper.

WHAT YOU CAN DO

"The most important thing to do with aggression is to nip it in the bud immediately," says Dr. Hunthausen. "This is a dangerous behavior, and you want to get it under control before it is too developed."

With dogs, you have to make sure they understand that you are the boss and that your commands are the law. If you tell your pet to get off the bed, he should get off immediately and not act like he is doing you a favor. If you let him get away with "attitude," Dr. Hunthausen says, he will start acting like he is in charge, and this invariably leads to additional problems.

What do you do when your commands don't work? The best strategy is to immediately withhold the two things your dog loves most—treats and affection. Dogs are social animals, and a few hours without your attention can seem like days to them. When he learns that his bad behavior leads to being ignored, he may decide that it is simply not worth it to act that way and will come around.

When he starts asking for your affection, make him work for it, Dr. Hunthausen advises. Give him a command like "Sit" or "Heel." When he obeys, reward him with a treat and a lot of love. Repeating this several times a day will help him remember that you are the one in charge and that he will be rewarded for obeying.

One of the best ways to keep your dog friendly is to expose him to a wide range of people and situations when he is still young. The more positive experiences he has, the less likely he will be frightened and snappish later on. This is why vets recommend taking your dog to obedience school—the earlier the better. Not only will you get good instruction, but your dog will learn to make friends with other people as well as other dogs, which will make him more easygoing later on.

Cats, though often more mild-mannered than dogs can be harder to train once problems begin. In most cases, Dr. Simpson says, cat aggression is simply caused by boredom. Giving your cat a little more attention and helping him burn off energy will make him less likely to vent his emotions in negative ways. "Young cats, especially, have a real need for social play," she says. "When you get home, spend 10 minutes really playing with him."

To discourage your cat from nipping or biting, Dr. Hunthausen recommends keeping a squirt gun nearby for a few days. When your cat does his usual, claws-out charge, give him a quick spray. He will soon learn that his misbehavior brings unexpected—and unpleasant—surprises, and he will look for other, more peaceful ways to get your attention.

What Your Vet Will Do

All aggression is potentially dangerous and should be taken seriously. Vets usually advise getting professional help as soon as it appears. For one thing, your vet knows how to deal with difficult pets without getting hurt. More important, your pet's moods may be a reflection of physical problems, so he will need a thorough checkup, just to be safe.

Since arthritis is a common problem associated with aggression, your vet will probably take x-rays to check the joints for unusual wear and tear. She will also do blood tests to see if your pet has an internal illness that is making him cranky.

Male pets that haven't been neutered are likely to be more temperamental than their fixed friends, Dr. Simpson adds. "In general, neutering has little effect on pets' personalities. If anything, they tend to become more people-oriented, and that's a plus," she says.

When the problem behavior doesn't go away, your vet may recommend giving your pet anti-anxiety medications such as diazepam (Valium) and fluoxetine (Prozac) to keep him calm. Given in small amounts, the drugs will have little effect on your pet's personality but can substantially reduce the aggressive behavior, Dr. Simpson says.

See also Chapter 5: Biting, Fighting, Growling, Hissing

BARKING

Clues

- Your dog barks when nothing is happening.
- The barking is rhythmic and monotonous.
- He barks only when you are gone.

Your dog's days are filled with excitement, from sirens and cats outside to the much-anticipated arrival of the mail carrier. With so much going on, he naturally wants to give his opinion, so he barks.

Some dogs, of course, have much more to say than others. They bark at everything and at all hours of the day and night. You would swear that they are trying to get a "barkalaureate" in public speaking.

It's tempting to respond to a dog's relentless barking with an irritable bark of your own. But it is important to figure out what he is trying to say. Dogs bark for all kinds of reasons, and understanding what's behind it will help you discover ways to turn down the volume, says Sandi Driscoll, owner of the Academy of Dog Obedience in Los Angeles.

Some breeds are naturally inclined to be barkers. Terriers and beagles, for example, were originally bred for hunting, and their vigilant barking alerted owners to the presence of game, says Wayne Hunthausen, D.V.M., a veterinarian in private practice in Westwood, Kansas, who specializes in behavior problems.

Dogs naturally bark as a way of sounding alarms. It is their way of telling approaching people (or pets), "This is my territory, buster, so you better back off!" They also bark when they are nervous or frightened. Some dogs are terrified about being left alone, a condition that vets call separation anxiety. When you leave for the day, they may vent their anxiety with nearly nonstop barking, Driscoll says.

Some dogs, unfortunately, don't need an excuse to let loose with resounding *woofs*. Dogs that spend their days alone, for example, often get bored and will bark as a way of filling the time, Driscoll says. This kind of barking is easy to recognize because the dog will actually sound bored—rhythmic, monotonous, and not very alert, she explains.

WHAT YOU CAN DO

Unless your dog is driving you or your neighbors crazy, barking really isn't something to worry about. "Sometimes I want my dogs to bark. I trust them as watchdogs," says Michael Moore, D.V.M., associate professor of specialty medicine at Washington State University College of Veterinary Medicine in Pullman.

Of course, there is a big difference between a helpful "there's someone here" bark and the kind that goes on all day. When your dog is barking simply as a form of recreation, you need to find ways to restore the peace.

One of the best ways to quell recreational barking is to help your dog have a more interesting life. The busier he is, the less likely he will be to entertain himself by making noise. Regular exercise is a great way to take his mind off his voice; exercise has a calming effect on dogs just as it does on people, Dr. Hunthausen says. At a minimum, vets say, you should take your dog for a vigorous walk before you leave for work in the morning and again when you get home at night. Some people ask neighborhood children or even professional pet-sitters to drop by in the middle of the day. Once he has burned off some of his energy, he will be more likely to be quiet.

A simple change of pace will also help keep him entertained. If he usually barks when you leave him inside all day, try keeping him in the yard now and then—as long as it is fenced, suggests William C. Beggs, D.V.M., a veterinarian in private practice in Colorado Springs, Colorado. If he is a vociferous outdoor barker, on the other hand, leave him inside a few days a week.

Getting a second dog will often help keep the barker quiet, says Dr. Moore. Dogs together are more likely to stay entertained than a dog alone, he says. And don't worry that the noisemaker will teach the other dog to bark. In most cases, barking is part of a dog's personality and not something he learns from other dogs.

Many small breeds of dogs have a natural tendency to get overexcited. You may be able to quiet their barks by keeping them in a less-stimulating environment, such as inside a comfortable crate or in a quiet room in the house, suggests Driscoll. The point isn't to punish them for barking, but simply to make it easier for them to relax. Most dogs don't mind spending time in enclosed places, as long as they get plenty of exercise and love the rest of the time.

If you are home when your dog starts barking, you may want to remind him that his loud opinions simply aren't appreciated. The next time he lets loose with a bark, quickly tell him, "Quiet." Don't yell, but be firm and no-nonsense. When he looks surprised and stops barking, praise him warmly for his good behavior, says Driscoll. Doing this consistently will help him understand that being quiet—or at least following your orders—will provide better rewards than merely making noise.

In addition, you may want to ask your vet about training collars like the Gentle Leader. When your dog starts barking, pulling the lead causes straps on the collar to gently press his mouth closed for the few seconds that you apply pressure.

Dogs that bark because they are anxious about being left alone won't respond well to scolding, Driscoll adds. In fact, your displeasure may

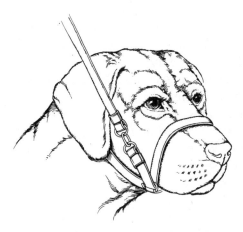

One way to curb unwanted barking is to use a training collar that closes your dog's mouth when you apply pressure. Each time you close his mouth, remind him to be quiet. Eventually, he will learn the command and will be more likely to keep his opinions to himself.

cause additional barking because they will be even more nervous than they were before. What these dogs need to understand is that your leaving the house doesn't mean that you are leaving for good.

To get them more comfortable with the idea of being alone, Driscoll recommends that you "practice" leaving. In other words, act like you are about to leave the house by grabbing your car keys, for instance, but don't go anywhere. Instead, sit down by the door and spend a little time with your dog. This will get him used to the idea that your leaving doesn't have to be scary. To make the training even more effective, put out some of his favorite toys just before you leave. When he learns that his alone times will also be fun times, he will be less likely to bark up the walls.

Once your dog becomes more at ease with being alone, take his training one step further by actually leaving the house. Again, put out some of his favorite toys or a chewy snack. Leave the house, spending a few minutes in the yard or taking a walk. Then come right back. This training may take a few weeks, but once he understands that your absences aren't forever, he will be more comfortable spending time on his own.

WHAT YOUR VET WILL DO

Barking isn't always an easy habit to change. Many vets specialize in behavior problems and will help you plan a strategy to keep your dog quiet.

As part of a training program, vets sometimes recommend giving dogs anti-anxiety medications, which will help keep them calm and quiet while they learn their new lessons. In addition, your vet may recommend that you use a training device called a shock collar. Available in some pet supply stores, they deliver a small, harmless shock to your dog's neck every time he barks. Some collars even have built-in warning systems: They vibrate with the first bark and deliver a shock with the second. This system gives your dog a few seconds to change his mind about speaking.

The collars aren't perfect, Dr. Moore adds. For one thing, *any* bark may signal the shock, even when the bark is coming from the dog next door. In addition, some dogs react negatively to the shocks and may get aggressive. That's why it is important to use the collars (and other training aids) with the guidance of a veterinarian or trainer.

For dogs that simply won't quit barking, vets sometimes recommend a surgical procedure called a ventriculocordectomy, in which some of the vocal folds are removed from a dog's voice box. Your dog will still be able to speak, but it will be more of a hoarse squeak than a loud bark. The operation can be somewhat tricky, Dr. Moore adds, and it is usually used only as a last resort.

See also Chapter 5: Crying and Whining, Fear of Being Alone

BITING

Clues

- Your pet plays aggressively or "mouths" your hand.
- Your cat's tail is swishing back and forth.
- Your dog's fur stands on end and his ears point forward.

Puppies and kittens experience the world through their mouths. Whatever fits goes in. And that may include your fingers and toes. Or your nose. Or any other part of your body that happens to be in nipping range.

Young pets don't mean any harm, of course, and their affectionate mouthings can't do real damage. But what's cute in young pets can be terrifying in older pets. Millions of people are bitten by dogs every year. And once a pet starts biting, he is likely to keep doing it unless you find ways to make him stop.

In dogs, biting is usually a display of dominance—their way of defending their territory and their status in the family. If another pet approaches their food, for instance, dogs will sometimes bite to prove that they are top dogs, says Wayne Hunthausen, D.V.M., a veterinarian in private practice in Westwood, Kansas, who specializes in behavior problems. In addition, some dogs will bite when they are startled or frightened. This is particularly true of dogs that have had abusive owners in the past, he says.

Cats are less likely than dogs to launch serious attacks. In fact, many cat bites are accidental—they were play-hunting, for example, and got a little carried away when your ankles came within reach. A cat may also bite when he wants to be left alone, such as during a petting, when he suddenly decides that he has had enough. Although cats are less likely than dogs to be seriously aggressive, even a minor cat bite can be dangerous because the wounds frequently get infected. It is essential to wash the wound with antibacterial soap and water and to check with your doctor to see if you need further treatment, which may include a tetanus shot.

Perhaps the most common cause of cat bites is what vets call redirected anger. When your cat is under stress after being chased by a dog, for example, he is likely to lash out at anything that comes close, including your ankle or hand.

Both dogs and cats may bite when they are in pain from a medical problem such as arthritis, adds Barbara Simpson, D.V.M., Ph.D., a veterinarian in private practice in Southern Pines, North Carolina, who specializes in animal behavior.

WHAT YOU CAN DO

Though dogs and cats are naturally inclined to use their teeth, it is up to you to make sure that they use them in an acceptable fashion. The next time your dog gets a little nippy, quickly offer him a chew toy. "This is a way to teach him to keep his mouth focused on toys instead of you," says Dr. Hunthausen.

Dogs are very respectful of their leaders. With puppies as well as grown dogs, it is essential to let them know that you are the boss and that you won't tolerate biting. The next time he bites, simply leave the room and ignore him for a while, says Dr. Hunthausen. When he starts craving your attention again, give him a command, like "Sit" or "Heel." When he obeys, reward him with a lot of love and perhaps a treat. Eventually, he will learn that biting has unpleasant consequences and that obeying has very pleasant rewards.

Another strategy is to keep your dog on a short lead with a training collar even when he is in the house. When he attempts to bite or even to "mouth" your hand, tell him, "No!" If he stops immediately, give him plenty of praise. If he continues biting, give a sharp pull on the lead and, again, praise him when he quits.

Some dogs are naturally aggressive, particularly toward other dogs. You can't change a dog's personality, but you can prevent problems when two dogs happen to meet.

- Watch the signs. "Look for growling, erect hair, ears directed forward, and any sign of teeth," says Dr. Hunthausen. These are signs that a fight is about to begin, and you will want to get away from the situation before an actual bite occurs.
- Distract him. Another way to prevent fights and bites when you see trouble coming is to make a sudden turn or to speed up or slow down your walk. This will make him pay attention to you and forget about the other dog.

It can take patience to train a cat not to bite. What you can do is change his mind before he makes the move. Dr. Hunthausen recommends that you keep a squirt gun nearby. If your cat begins an attack, give him a quick spritz. Nearly all cats hate water, and this will cause your cat to quickly retreat—and if you do it often enough, he will gradually get the idea to back off.

When squirting a cat, don't look him in the eye. Instead, pretend that the squirt of water had nothing to do with you. "You want to be as covert a possible so that he doesn't associate the punishment with you," Dr. Hunthausen explains.

Most cats adore human contact, but only on their terms. They will often scratch and bite when they are tired of being petted, he adds. Keep an eye on his tail: When it starts lashing back and forth, that's the signal that it is time to move your hand and let him be.

WHAT YOUR VET WILL DO

Biting and aggression can be extremely dangerous in cats as well as dogs. It is a good idea to call your vet if you even suspect that it is getting out of hand.

Since pets get cranky and short-tempered when they are sick, your vet will begin by checking for medical problems that cause pain, such as arthritis, which can bring on sudden displays of temper, says Dr. Simpson. You can expect your vet to take x-rays and perhaps do a blood test to check for internal problems. The treatment, of course, will depend on what the problem is. For pets with arthritis, anti-inflammatory medications will help relieve the pain, which, in turn, will make them less likely to bite, she says.

Intact males are much more likely to bite than their neutered friends, Dr. Simpson says. Neutering has little effect on a pet's overall personality, but it will make him less aggressive. Your vet will let you know if this is something that you should be considering.

Most of the time, of course, biting has more to do with personality or training or temporary emotional upsets than with anything that is physically wrong. Your vet will help you plan a training program for keeping the misbehavior under control. In addition, she may recommend giving your pet diazepam (Valium) or similar medications to keep him calm while he is learning his new ways.

See also Chapter 5: Aggression, Growling, Hissing

SYMPTOM # CHEWING OBJECTS

Clues

- Your pet is acting bored or anxious.
- He often chews when home alone.
- Your pet is teething.

Chewing the stuffing out of a pillow or gnawing wallpaper off the wall may not sound like fun to you, but it's a real party for pets, especially puppies and kittens, who put their teeth to work at every opportunity. When they are done with one item, they will move on to the next, and you're left paying for the repairs.

Kittens that are teething usually prefer gnawing on soft clothes, while puppies will chew just about anything, from a throw rug to the living-room chair, says Kathalyn Johnson, D.V.M., clinical associate in companion animal behavior at Texas A&M University College of Veterinary Medicine in College Station.

Some adult pets, unfortunately, retain the urge to be oral. This usually occurs because they are confused about what is acceptable to chew and what isn't, says Dr. Johnson. "It's not the chewing itself that's bad," she adds, "it's the chewing on furniture that is."

Dogs and cats with extra time on their paws often look for things to do, and chewing is always a favorite choice. It isn't as good as a walk or a game of chase-the-mouse, but it is better than nothing. "When dogs or cats get too little social interaction or inadequate exercise, they may begin chewing," says Dr. Johnson.

Less often, emotional problems such as separation anxiety cause stress and insecurity, and pets cope by chewing. This can happen in cats, but it is much more common in dogs.

WHAT YOU CAN DO

The combination of boundless energy and aching teeth means that puppies and kittens simply have to chew. The only way to protect your furnishings is to give the pets equally satisfying things on which to exercise their teeth, says Dr. Johnson. For kittens, toys covered with lamb's wool are always a good choice. Puppies will gladly chew almost anything, from rope toys to rubber bones. Don't give them discarded personal belongings, however. A puppy that enjoys a cast-off shoe today will eventually snack on your new Italian loafers—and then look surprised when your hair stands on end.

"Encourage your pet to use the toys you give him by playing with him and praising him when he shows interest in them," Dr. Johnson adds. That way, he will know which toys have your stamp of approval, and he will be more likely to leave other things alone. If you do catch him chewing something that he shouldn't, don't get upset, she says. Instead, tell him, "No!" and take it away. Then replace it with something that you would like him to chew and lavish him with attention when he goes after it. He will figure things out from there.

Cats aren't as easy to train as dogs. About all you can do when you catch your cat chewing is to startle him—by clapping your hands, for example, or by giving him a spritz from a water bottle, says Wayne Hunthausen, D.V.M., a veterinarian in private practice in Westwood, Kansas, who specializes in behavior problems. If you do this often enough, he will start to associate the forbidden object with the unexpected and unpleasant surprise, and he will gradually turn his attention elsewhere.

You can't be home all the time, of course. To protect things when you are gone, vets recommend putting pet repellents—a product called bitter apple can be very effective—on areas where your pet has been chewing. You may even want to try putting a little hot-pepper sauce on items that you want your pet to leave alone. (Test a small area first to make sure that it won't stain.) Giving pets more exercise is a great way to stop chewing. Tired pets are less likely to be mischievous pets, says Dr. Johnson.

What Your Vet Will Do

Although chewing is normal for youngsters, there is really no reason for older pets to be destroying your possessions. If it is happening regularly, don't try to solve it on your own, says Dr. Johnson. You are probably going to need help from a professional.

In some cases, chewing is caused by a condition called obsessive-compulsive behavior, in which pets have an overpowering emotional urge to do it. More often, chewing in adults is a sign of serious boredom or stress. Your pet may need more exercise and personal attention—and, in some cases, anti-anxiety medications from a veterinarian—to get it under control.

CHEWING SKIN, COAT, OR TAIL

Clues

- Your pet is focusing on his ears and rear.
- The chewing occurs late at night.
- Your cat's belly is bare.
- Your pet is biting at his feet and legs.

You have bought every chew toy you can find, but your pet seems more interested in licking and biting his own skin. He does it for what seems like hours at a time—usually after midnight when you are trying to get some sleep. What's going on?

Dogs and cats sometimes develop allergies to pollen, fleas, or even foods that make them itchy. Since they are a lot more limber than people, they can easily use their teeth, along with their paws and claws, to deliver a soothing scratch.

Fleas are a common cause of biting and scratching. For pets that are sensitive, just one or two bites are enough to cause problems, says Donna Angarano, D.V.M., professor of small animal surgery and medicine at Auburn University College of Veterinary Medicine in Auburn, Alabama. "Dogs predominantly get fleas over their rumps, on their tails, and on the backs of their legs," she says. Cats get them in the same areas as well as on the belly. In fact, cats may develop what vets call bald belly syndrome, in which they lick and chew their bellies until all the fur is gone.

You can make some guesses about what your pet is allergic to by paying attention to where he scratches.

- Dogs that are allergic to pollen, mold, or dust, for example, will often bite at their feet and legs. They may have itchy ears and weepy eyes as well, says Dr. Angarano. Terriers, retrievers, and Dalmatians are particularly susceptible to these types of allergies.
- Cats that are allergic to pollen or mold will usually scratch at their faces or ears, although in some cases they will chew their whole bodies. "Cats can be intensely itchy," Dr. Angarano says. "They will go to town in one spot until it becomes very red and inflamed."
- Although food allergies can cause itching almost anywhere on the body, pets with food allergies often chew or scratch at their ears and back end, Dr. Angarano adds. "We call this 'ears and rears,'" she explains.

If your pet is biting and licking at his tail, it could be because glands at the base of the tail are inflamed and tender. This occurs more often in males, which is why vets refer to it as stud tail.

Itchiness isn't the only condition that causes pets to bite their skin.

Some pets suffer from a serious condition called obsessive-compulsive disorder. Like people who are obsessive about washing their hands, for example, pets may be obsessive about biting at their skin. They will lick and chew an area until it gets raw and sore, says Jacque Schultz, director of companion animal services for the American Society for the Prevention of Cruelty to Animals, headquartered in New York City. This is particularly common in pets with high energy levels that don't get enough exercise or attention. They are easily bored and frustrated and will chew themselves merely to occupy the time, Schultz says.

What You Can Do

Since allergies are very common in dogs and cats, it is worth looking into. To identify food allergies, try giving him a balanced diet with none of the ingredients in his usual food. (Ingredients that cause problems for many pets include soy, beef, wheat, and dairy.) Your vet will help you plan a proper diet. If the itching and biting diminish in a few weeks to a few months, you may have identified the problem, explains Dr. Angarano.

Dogs and cats may be sensitive to household chemicals as well, Schultz adds. Even common products like rug shampoos, laundry detergents, and some cat-box litters may contain chemicals that cause some pets to bite themselves raw. In some cases, just changing brands will eliminate the problems.

"When pets are slurping on their paws or thumping the floors at 4:00 A.M., it is usually because house dust is a problem," Dr. Angarano says. Late-night scratching is common because that's when dogs and many cats have been inside—and in contact with whatever is bothering them—the longest.

Vacuuming thoroughly and often, particularly in areas where your pet spends a lot of time, can be very helpful. "Get under the bed and couch because that's where dust mite concentrations are higher," Dr. Angarano says. It's also helpful to cover the area where your pet sleeps with a washable sheet. This makes it easy to remove potential allergens before they accumulate to itch-and-chew levels. "Having sheets on everything makes it look like no one lives in your house, but it can make a pet with allergies feel better," she says.

If you suspect that your pet has stud tail—the surrounding skin will get oily, sore, and inflamed—vets recommend cleaning the area with an antibacterial cleanser, such as Betadine, then applying a light dusting of cornstarch to absorb the irritating secretions. You may also want to apply a little over-the-counter hydrocortisone, which will help reduce inflammation.

Fleas, of course, are the bane of every pet owner, and they can be a challenge to get rid of. Brushing your pet frequently, washing his bedding, and using flea powder or sprays will help keep their numbers down and reduce the chewing. But since a pet with allergies will react even after a bite or two, this can be a difficult problem to solve. "If the chewing doesn't stop, go to your veterinarian," Schultz advises.

If you suspect that your pet is simply bored, the solution may be as easy as taking him out for walks once or twice a day. Giving him plenty of attention and play will help take his mind off his skin, says Schultz. This is especially important for young dogs because they have a lot of energy. The more tired you can make him, the less likely he is to chew at his coat.

WHAT YOUR VET WILL DO

It's usually not difficult to treat the problems that cause pets to lick and bite their coats. But first, your vet has to find out exactly what the problem is. Your vet will get a pretty good idea just by seeing where your pet is doing the chewing. In addition, he may recommend a series of skin tests to test for allergies.

If you are having trouble controlling the fleas on your pet's hide, your vet may prescribe oral medications that fight them from the inside out, says Dr. Angarano. Drugs such as Program stop fleas by interrupting their ability to reproduce. Other products, such as Advantage and Frontline, are applied directly to the coat and last about a month.

If your pet has obsessive-compulsive disorder—that is, he is emotionally incapable of leaving his skin alone—your vet may prescribe an anti-anxiety medication such as fluoxetine (Prozac). This and similar drugs change the chemistry inside the brain, making pets calmer and less likely to focus on their skin and coats.

See also Chapter 5: Grooming Excessively; Chapter 7: Scratching and Shaking

SYMPTOM # CRYING AND WHINING

Clues

- Your pet doesn't respond to loud noises.
- There have been changes in your routine.
- He seems achy or stiff.
- He started crying only recently.

When Lassie whined, Timmy always knew why. "What? Someone fell down the well five miles past the creek? Let's go save him!"

In real life, you often have no idea why your pets are whining. All you know for sure is that you won't get any peace until you figure out what, exactly, they are trying to say. The messages are usually pretty simple. Pets often whine when they are trying to tell you something important, such as "I need to go out," "It's supper time," or "Scratch my head."

Because dogs and cats are very sensitive to high-pitched sounds, whines and cries sometimes mean that they hear something you can't—the power of an electric motor, for example, or the distant challenge from a pet outdoors, says Malcolm Riordan, D.V.M., a veterinarian in private practice in Santa Barbara, California.

Anything that upsets your pet's routine can result in frequent and noisy complaining, adds Dr. Riordan. Bringing a new baby into the family, packing for a trip, or even cleaning the house will make some pets anxious and whiny. And because pets crave human company, leaving them alone will often set their mouths in motion, at least until after you leave, when they will usually settle down.

Some dogs and cats, especially German shepherds and Siamese, are known for whining and crying. You can encourage them to be quiet, but they will always be somewhat noisier than other breeds, says Dr. Riordan.

When your normally quiet pet has suddenly started crying or whining, there could be a physical problem that is making him uncomfortable. Anything from earaches to urinary tract problems can cause pets to cry and whine. Among older pets, neurological problems such as senility are common causes of whining, as is a loss of hearing. Deaf pets will sometimes spend their days crying or whining—not even realizing that they are making those sad, plaintive sounds.

WHAT YOU CAN DO

In order to get any peace, you will have to figure out what your pet is trying to tell you or if he is making noise merely to hear himself talk. For starters, run your hands over his entire body, including the head and feet, to see if he is sore and tender. You can even do a quick hearing check by making noise when his back is turned and looking for his reaction to the sound. If you suspect that there is a physical problem, you will want to make an appointment to see your vet, says Wayne Hunthausen, D.V.M., a veterinarian in private practice in Westwood, Kansas, who specializes in animal behavior.

It is not always easy, even for vets, to figure out what is making pets whine and cry, explains Dr. Hunthausen. One way to find out is to keep a "crying and whining" diary for several days. In the diary, jot down everything that seems to be happening when your pet's vocal cords go to work. Does he cry and whine only at mealtimes? Is he more persistent later in the day (perhaps when people outside are walking their pets)? Does he make the most noise on weekends (when lawn mowers are running)? As you accumulate more and more information, you may eventually see patterns that can provide valuable clues to what the problem is.

Figuring out what your pet is trying to say is only part of the problem. The harder part is making him stop. This is particularly true for pets that are begging for attention. When they don't get what they are looking for, they ask again . . . and again. Giving them the attention isn't the solution since that will prove to them that whining works.

What you can do, however, is make it rewarding for them *not* to cry, says Dr. Hunthausen. He recommends giving your pet an abundance of attention—along with treats and plenty of strokes—only during his quiet, nonwhining moments. If you do this consistently, he will eventually learn that he doesn't have to cry and whine to get the attention he craves.

It is also important to help him understand that crying and whining for attention will make his life a little more difficult. The next time the whining starts, drop your car keys, Dr. Hunthausen suggests. Put a few coins in an empty soda can and give it a loud shake. Toss a book on the floor. Turn on a hair dryer or vacuum cleaner. When he discovers that crying and whining cause these horrible sounds, he will be more likely to pipe down.

For dogs that won't quit whining, vets sometimes recommend a special training halter, such as the Halti collar. Sold in pet supply stores, the halter is attached to a long lead. When your dog whines, give a slight tug on the lead. This gently presses the mouth closed, giving your dog the message that his vocalizations aren't welcome, says Michael Moore, D.V.M., associate professor of specialty medicine at Washington State University College of Veterinary Medicine in Pullman.

Some pets get extremely anxious when their owners leave, a condition that vets call separation anxiety. Making noises won't keep them quiet, Dr. Hunthausen says. In fact, the noises may make them even more anxious than they were before. What you can do, however, is help them understand that the world doesn't end when you walk out the door. Here is a technique you may want to try.

Act like you are leaving the house, even when you aren't. Pick up your car keys, for example, or put on your coat. But rather than leaving, sit down next to the door. Your frightened pet will discover that leaving isn't so bad after all. If you do this repeatedly—over a period of days or even weeks—your pet will gradually get less anxious when you approach the door.

As your pet becomes more at ease, take his training one step further by actually leaving the house. Go outside for a minute or two, and then come back in. Once again, your pet will discover that leaving isn't the same thing as leaving for good. If you keep practicing, leaving and coming back, and gradually increasing the length of time that you are gone, your pet will feel increasingly secure and less likely to cry and whine, says Dr. Hunthausen.

WHAT YOUR VET WILL DO

Anything that causes pain, from arthritis or tooth decay to cancer, can make dogs and cats cry. So if your pet's noise-making is persistent and getting worse, you will certainly want to see a vet, says Dr. Riordan.

If there isn't a physical problem and all your efforts at home haven't worked, your vet may decide to give your pet anti-anxiety medications like fluoxetine (Prozac). These medications have little effect on your pet's natural personality but will help take the edge off his anxiety so that he is less likely to be insecure and whiny.

Anti-anxiety medications are safe for long-term use, but often they are only needed for a few weeks—such as when your pet is crying because of a recent move or after the arrival of a new baby. Once he is feeling calm again, he probably won't need the medications, says Dr. Riordan.

See also Chapter 5: Barking, Fear of Being Alone, Fear of Loud Noises

CRYING WHILE USING THE LITTER BOX

Clues

- Your cat is a male.
- The litter is dry after he leaves the box.

Cats are quiet creatures, and the only way you can tell that they are using the litter box is by the soft scratching as they rearrange the sand.

Sometimes, however, they may cry or yowl when using the box, and it is a sound you shouldn't ignore. "Crying in the litter box always requires a veterinarian's attention," says Ellen Miller, D.V.M., a veterinarian in private practice in Fort Collins, Colorado. "It means that something is hurting them and something is wrong."

A variety of urinary tract problems, such as infections or stones in the bladder or urethra (the tube through which urine flows), can make urinating extremely painful. If your cat is crying and trying to urinate but is only able to produce a few drops, he could have a condition called feline lower urinary tract disease, in which debris in the urine forms a plug, making it difficult to urinate. "All cats can get this condition, but the plumbing of male cats makes them very prone to blockages," says Malcolm Riordan, D.V.M., a veterinarian in private practice in Santa Barbara, California.

Lower urinary tract disease is extremely serious, especially for males, adds Dr. Miller. If you even suspect that your cat is in pain because he can't urinate, get him to the vet right away.

How can you tell if your cat is straining to urinate (which is a serious problem) or is constipated (which probably isn't serious)? The trick is to watch his back, says Dr. Riordan. Cats keep their backs straight when they are trying to urinate. During a bowel movement, however, their backs will be hunched. If you are not sure, play it safe and call your vet, he advises.

WHAT YOU CAN DO

When your cat is constipated and uncomfortable, you may want to give him a high-fiber pet laxative, available in pet supply stores, which will help get things moving again. Or put a little petroleum jelly under his nose. He will lick it off, and it will help the stools move more smoothly, says Dr. Riordan.

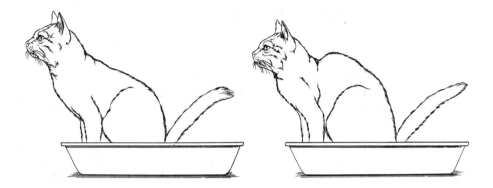

In cats, straining to have a bowel movement usually isn't serious, but straining to urinate can indicate a life-threatening problem. To tell the difference, look at your cat's back. Cats keep their backs straight when urinating and hunch their backs when having a bowel movement.

Another way to relieve constipation is to give your cat more dietary fiber. Fiber absorbs tremendous amounts of water in the intestine, which makes stools softer and easier to pass, Dr. Riordan explains. Veterinarians and pet supply stores sell a variety of fiber-rich foods. Or you can add vegetables such as broccoli or carrots to his plate. Many cats like the taste, although you will have to experiment to see if he prefers his vegetables raw or cooked. Adding small amounts of bran cereal or canned pumpkin will also give your pet a fiber boost.

Cats don't drink a lot of water, and sometimes this can lead to constipation. You can't make your cat drink more, but you can get more water into his system simply by giving him canned food now and then. Unlike dry food, which contains little water, canned food is 70 to 90 percent water, says Dr. Riordan.

Another reason to encourage your cat to drink is that water dilutes the urine. While concentrated urine may help prevent bacterial infections, it can lead to other, more serious urinary problems. "If your cat has a tendency to form crystals or stones, concentrated urine creates the right sort of environment for more to form," says Dr. Miller.

Encouraging your cat to urinate more often may also prevent pain in the litter box since the longer that urine stays in the bladder, the more likely it is to harden into pain-causing little stones. "Some cats don't want to go outside, especially in bad weather, and if they are not used to using the litter box, they just won't go," says Dr. Riordan. Even if your cat spends most of his time outdoors, you should still get him used to a litter box. Mixing a little dirt with the sand will make it more similar to what he is used to outside.

WHAT YOUR VET WILL DO

Since crying in the litter box can often be a sign of serious problems, you will want to take your cat to the vet right away. If your cat does have an obstruction in the urinary tract, your vet will probably use a catheter to remove the blockage and release pent-up urine. She will also take blood and urine samples to test for infections or other problems. Finally, she may recommend a test called a cystourethrogram, in which dye is injected into the bladder and urethra to reveal abnormalities.

If your pet seems to be stone-prone, your vet will check to see if he has high levels of magnesium, ammonium, phosphate, or calcium—all of which can turn into stones. If your pet is high in one of these minerals, your vet may recommend giving him a special food that corrects the mineral imbalance, says Dr. Miller.

When painful urination is caused by a urinary tract infection, your vet will give him antibiotics, which will relieve the pain within a day or two and eliminate the infection within two weeks. Your vet may also give him muscle relaxants, which will make using the litter box less painful while the underlying problems are being taken care of.

See also Chapter 6: Constipation; Chapter 9: Urinating Difficulty

FEAR OF BEING ALONE

Clues

- **Your pet is only destructive when you are gone.**
- **There has recently been a change in your lifestyle.**

It's no fun to leave for work in the morning and hear your dog barking and howling as you drive away. It's even less fun to come home and find that he has torn up papers, dug a hole in your couch, or chewed at the door.

Some dogs are so terrified of being left alone that they will essentially go off the deep end, howling with misery or, worse, destroying whatever comes within reach. This condition, called separation anxiety, sometimes occurs when dogs have recently moved to a new home or when there has been another upsetting change in their lifestyle, says Steven Diller, adjunct professor of applied animal behavior at Mercy College in Dobbs Ferry, New York, and director of the Center for Animal Behavior and Canine Training in Elmsford.

Cats, especially Siamese and Abyssinians, can also get nervous about staying alone, but generally they fare better on their own than dogs do.

"Dogs are naturally very social creatures," Diller explains. Even though most dogs eventually get used to being alone, for others, enforced isolation always remains a traumatic experience. It's as though they are convinced that you are never coming back. This is especially true in young dogs or those that have been abandoned or those that have changed owners frequently, Diller says.

WHAT YOU CAN DO

"Most pets lose their fear of being left alone with experience," says Diller. After you have walked out the door (and returned) a few times, they begin to understand that you are not abandoning them and that it is okay to curl up and go to sleep.

One way to help them understand that leaving doesn't mean leaving for good is to avoid fussing over them before you go. For dogs that are already nervous, the extra attention will make them suspect that something serious is going on. When you are ready to leave, Diller says, it is best to do it quickly and unobtrusively.

To help your dog get used to your absences, you may want to practice a few departures. Start out by leaving the house for a minute or two and then coming back in. He will be so relieved you are back that he will

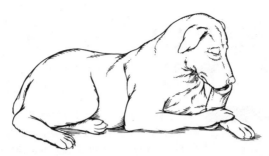

Dogs that have something to do are less likely to be lonely or destructive when they are left alone. Giving them a hollow sterilized bone filled with peanut butter is a great way to keep dogs quietly busy for hours. You can also buy hollow chew toys at pet supply stores.

hardly be able to contain himself. Then leave again, this time for a little longer. If you do this repeatedly over a period of weeks, leaving for longer and longer periods of time, your dog will come to understand that no matter how often you leave, you will always come back—and that can make all the difference.

For young dogs, crate training is an excellent way to help them stay calm when you leave. Dogs naturally feel safer when they are in secure, small spaces, which is why they climb under the bed or burrow into the closet when they are frightened. Keeping your puppy in a crate has the added advantage of preventing him from getting into mischief when you are gone. Your vet will help you plan a crate-training schedule that's right for your dog.

Another helpful strategy is to give your dog a vigorous workout before you leave. The more tired he is, the less likely he will be afraid. It is also a good idea to leave something for him to chew on—a hollow chew toy or a sterilized, hollow bone (both available at pet supply stores) stuffed with peanut butter, for example. This will keep him busy for a while, and if he can make it through the first few minutes alone, he will probably be fine after that, says Barbara Simpson, D.V.M., Ph.D., a veterinarian in private practice in Southern Pines, North Carolina, who specializes in animal behavior.

<u>What Your Vet Will Do</u>

Nearly all dogs can be taught to get over their fears, but it isn't always easy, Diller says. Your vet may recommend that you see a professional specializing in behavior problems, who will create a customized plan to decondition your dog so that he is no longer terrified of being left alone. At the same time, your vet may recommend giving your pet anti-anxiety medications to help him stay calm while the training is in progress.

"You have to stop the blasts of adrenaline that contribute to the fear, and these drugs help do that," Diller explains.

FEAR OF LOUD NOISES

Clues

- Your pet is afraid of some noises but not others.
- He gets panicky or destructive when he hears "bad" sounds.

Vets aren't sure why, but some dogs are so terrified of thunderstorms—or gunshots and other loud noises—that they will do anything, including jump through closed windows, in a desperate attempt to get away. Cats aren't fond of loud noises either, but they don't have the extreme reactions that some dogs do.

"Most of the time the fear appears to develop spontaneously," says Barbara Simpson, D.V.M., Ph.D., a veterinarian in private practice in Southern Pines, North Carolina, who specializes in animal behavior. Some dogs, such as terriers, may be genetically prone to being afraid of loud noises, she adds. In addition, dogs that have had bad experiences, such as getting hit by a bullet, may be terrified by similar noises when they hear them.

WHAT YOU CAN DO

There isn't a quick solution for helping a pet get over his fears. "The best thing to do is to create a safe space for him to go," says Dr. Simpson. For cats, putting an old sweater in a box and tucking it in the back of the closet will provide a soothing hiding place. For dogs, making a bed under your bed, in a closet, or in their own crate can be very comforting, says Steven Diller, adjunct professor of applied animal behavior at Mercy Col-

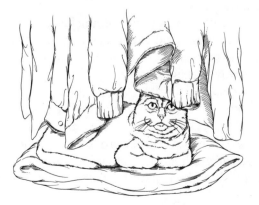

When your pets are frightened, having a secluded place for them to retire to, such as a closet, will make them feel safer and more secure.

lege in Dobbs Ferry, New York, and director of the Center for Animal Behavior and Canine Training in Elmsford.

One thing that you don't want to do—and this is hard for most people—is give them too much reassurance when they are afraid. "This does them a disservice because it is rewarding them for being fearful," Dr. Simpson says. In fact, making a fuss when your pet is frightened will probably make the problem worse instead of better.

"It's better simply to act as if everything is normal," says Kathalyn Johnson, D.V.M., clinical associate in companion animal behavior at Texas A&M University College of Veterinary Medicine in College Station. The next time your pet is quivering and shaking, speak calmly and give him a pat or two, she advises. Throw a ball or a stuffed mouse. The more you act as though everything is normal, the less likely he is to be afraid.

If your pet is truly terrified by loud noises, your vet may recommend that you plan a complete desensitization program, in which you gradually expose him to the noises that he is afraid of while helping him understand that there is nothing to be nervous about. The therapy works best in young animals but can also be used in older pets, says Craig N. Carter, D.V.M., Ph.D., head of epidemiology at the Texas Veterinary Medical Diagnostic Laboratory at Texas A&M University in College Station. Here's how it works.

1. Go to a music store and buy a tape or CD featuring the "bad" sounds, such as thunder.
2. As a test, play the recording for a second or two at a high volume to see if your pet gets nervous. If he doesn't, you may need to find a recording that more closely resembles the sound that he is afraid of.
3. When your dog is feeling comfortable and relaxed, turn on the recording at a very low volume.
4. If he stays calm, give him a treat and praise every couple of minutes. (If he is getting nervous, the volume is probably too loud. Cancel this session and try again the next day.)
5. As long as he stays calm, you can turn up the volume just a little bit. Continue giving him lots of praise and encouragement for staying calm. Don't give praise or treats when he gets frightened because this will reinforce the negative behavior.
6. Repeat this exercise every day. Each time, turn up the noise a little louder. When he starts getting nervous, distract him by practicing some commands—"Sit," for example, or "Lie down." When he is calm again, give him praise. The idea is to reward him only when he is not acting nervous. He will gradually learn that loud noises really aren't a problem, and you should see good results within a month or two.

You can use a similar strategy to cope with other noise-related fears. Many dogs are afraid of vacuum cleaner noise, for instance. To help him get over it, put the vacuum in the middle of the floor. Don't turn it on but put a few treats around it, Diller suggests. When he comes over to take a treat—and it may take him awhile to work up the courage—praise him lavishly. Continue doing this until he approaches the vacuum without fear. The next step, of course, is to turn the vacuum on. He will probably jump back, but that's okay. Continue giving him praises and treats. If you do this often enough, he will gradually be less nervous about the noise. He may even get excited when it is time to vacuum the rug.

WHAT YOUR VET WILL DO

While many pets dislike loud noises, for some the fears are extreme. To keep your pet safe, Dr. Simpson says, you are going to need some help.

Your vet may recommend that you see a trainer or a professional specializing in pet behavior problems, who will work with your pet to help him overcome his fears. In addition, she may recommend giving your pet anti-anxiety medications. He probably won't need these forever, but they can be very helpful when they are combined with training or other behavioral approaches, she says.

Of course, loud noises don't occur every day, so your vet may recommend using the medications only when they are absolutely necessary—when the Fourth of July is approaching, for example, or when you are in the season for rough weather. "Once thunderstorm season starts, you can have your dog treated. Then have him taken off drug therapy over the winter," says Dr. Simpson.

FEAR OF OBJECTS

Clues

- Your dog barks at or shies away from objects.
- He acts fearful in unfamiliar surroundings.

Your dog sees a tent in the backyard and barks as if it were an intruder with an ax. He sees a hose on the sidewalk and stops in his tracks. He sees a skateboard in the hallway and approaches with fear. What's going on?

"Dogs often become fearful of objects that they have never seen before," says Steven Diller, adjunct professor of applied animal behavior at Mercy College in Dobbs Ferry, New York, and director of the Center for Animal Behavior and Canine Training in Elmsford. All your dog knows is that this thing—whatever it is—looks strange and threatening. Maybe he will approach it, then turn and run away. He may let loose a few barks. Or he may crouch low to the ground and creep toward it, stretching his nose out as far as possible.

Dogs usually get over their fears—or phobias, as more serious fears are called—as the object becomes more familiar. In some cases, however, they are never truly at ease.

The fear of objects is rarely a problem in cats. They tend to be more curious than afraid of unfamiliar objects, although there are exceptions. "If you put a carpet deodorizer on the rug, some cats will lose it," Diller says. "Cats like sameness and get nervous when things change."

WHAT YOU CAN DO

Unless your dog is afraid of something that he is encountering every day, such as the stairs leading to the basement or a pile of books on a table, the fear of certain objects isn't necessarily a serious problem. Still, dogs should be filled with healthy curiosity rather than fear, so it is a good idea to tackle fears before they go too far, Diller says.

Since a dog is usually afraid of things that he hasn't seen before, sometimes all you need to do is make the introductions and then reward him for showing spunk. The next time he encounters something "terrible," such as a flight of stairs, stick around for a while, Diller says. Don't drag him to the stairs, but don't let him drag you away either. Just relax for a few moments and let him investigate the object in his own way, even if that means from 10 feet away.

When your dog starts calming down a bit, reward him with a treat, says Diller. This tells him that you respect his courage, so he will want to show you more of it.

It also helps if you demonstrate that the object isn't as frightening as he thinks it is. Sit on it, stand by it, or pick it up yourself. Act happy and unconcerned. If your dog comes over to investigate with a sniff, give him

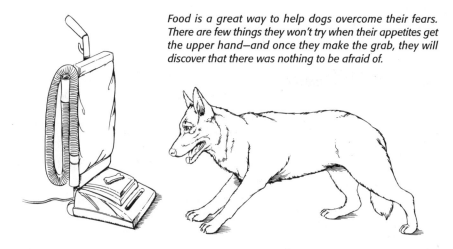

Food is a great way to help dogs overcome their fears. There are few things they won't try when their appetites get the upper hand—and once they make the grab, they will discover that there was nothing to be afraid of.

a treat, Diller says. If he isn't willing to make that final step, that's fine. Just try again another day.

Another way to help a dog overcome fears is to make a direct appeal to his stomach. Put some tasty treats on or near whatever it is that he's afraid of. He will be nervous at first, but he will find it very difficult to stay away. And once he gets his treat *and* lives to tell about it, he will be much less likely to be afraid in the future.

When your dog is still young, it is important to expose him to a wide variety of places and things, adds Wayne Hunthausen, D.V.M., a veterinarian in private practice in Westwood, Kansas, who specializes in behavior problems. Dogs form many of their impressions during their first three months. Taking your dog exploring on city streets, in the park, or on a busy playground will make him more confident later on.

WHAT YOUR VET WILL DO

Just as some humans never get over their fears, some dogs never really get comfortable around certain objects. And some dogs get truly panicky, hurting themselves or others as they try to escape whatever is frightening them. That's when you are going to need professional help.

Training and behavior modification are often essential steps for helping dogs overcome their fears, says Barbara Simpson, D.V.M., Ph.D., a veterinarian in private practice in Southern Pines, North Carolina, who specializes in animal behavior. Most dogs can be helped, she adds, but it takes time and patience—along with the help of a behavior specialist. Your vet will be able to recommend a behaviorist in your area.

To make things easier, your vet may prescribe anti-anxiety medications. But when your pet is just starting out, they can help keep him calm and more receptive to learning new things. As his fears diminish, he will gradually go off the medication, she says.

FIGHTING

Clues

- One pet approaches another's food.
- The tail looks tense.
- A pet is making strong eye contact.

It would be nice if pets settled their disagreements in a peaceful fashion. But since they can't sign treaties or talk things out, they often resolve their differences with a show of teeth or a slash of claws.

Fighting is almost always sparked by the pursuit of dominance, says Wayne Hunthausen, D.V.M., a veterinarian in private practice in Westwood, Kansas, who specializes in behavior problems. Whenever two or more pets meet, their first order of business is to establish a social hierarchy, with one pet being top dog (or top cat) and the others playing second fiddle.

"Usually the relationships are obvious as soon as they meet," says Dr. Hunthausen. "But if two pets are more or less matched in size, breed, and gender, fighting may be the only way they have to prove their superiority."

In addition, fighting may occur when a dog or cat invades another pet's territory by coming into the yard, for instance, or nosing too close to the food bowl.

Among males, fighting is virtually inevitable when a female is in heat, says Steven Diller, adjunct professor of applied animal behavior at Mercy College in Dobbs Ferry, New York, and director of the Center for Animal Behavior and Canine Training in Elmsford. Not surprisingly, fighting is much more common in unneutered pets than among their fixed friends, he adds.

Even among housemates who usually get along famously, fighting may occur when they are taken by surprise, such as when one of the pets comes home from the vet or groomer, bringing with him new smells that the other pets may find threatening, says Dr. Hunthausen.

WHAT YOU CAN DO

Most fights are mercifully brief, consisting more of bluster than actual physical contact. But dogs and cats can inflict serious injuries in a surprisingly short time. That's why you have to make every effort to prevent fighting before it starts.

To prevent fighting in household pets, it is essential to respect—and reinforce—their natural pecking order. In other words, don't treat your pets equally. The pet that is dominant—usually the older, bigger, or stronger one—should be given special treatment. Feed him first at mealtimes, suggests Dr. Hunthausen. When you come home, greet him before the other pets. It is even a good idea to let him in or out of the house first. This unequal treatment may strike you as unfair, but it is entirely natural for dogs and cats. The more secure they are in their respective roles, the less likely they are to struggle for social position.

Fights commonly occur when a new pet enters the family since his housemates will perceive him as a potential threat. To keep the peace, introduce your new pet slowly. Feed him separately at first and don't give him the run of the house. Instead, give him his own space away from the other pets and periodically bring them together for supervised get-acquainted sessions.

Don't be surprised if there are occasional flashes of temper, Dr. Hunthausen adds. Dogs and cats have to work things out in their own ways. By bringing them together slowly, however, they will have more time to peacefully establish their respective positions in the family.

Supervised visits are particularly helpful at mealtimes, Dr. Hunthausen says. Dogs and cats can be intensely protective of their food. To keep the hackles from rising, it is a good idea to place their bowls far apart or in separate rooms. As time goes by, you can gradually bring the bowls closer together. Once they realize that their food is safe, they will feel less threatened and should start getting along.

What works in the family, of course, won't be helpful when you are meeting other pets in the park or on the street. With dogs especially, be prepared to move quickly if tempers start to flare. "Look for growling, erect hair, a tail held high, and a stiff determined wag rather than a friendly, relaxed wag," says Dr. Hunthausen. "Also look for ears directed forward, strong eye-contact, and any sign of teeth."

When you sense trouble brewing, don't hesitate. Quickly lead your dog a safe distance away and command him to sit, says Dr. Hunthausen. This will break off the eye contact between the two dogs and, in most cases, will keep a fight from occurring.

If a fight does break out, it is essential to stop it fast. Pulling on the leash often doesn't help, and grabbing the collar will probably get you bitten. A better strategy is to grab one or both of your dog's hind legs or even the base of the tail, and lift him up and back, says Barbara Simpson, D.V.M., Ph.D., a veterinarian in private practice in Southern Pines, North Carolina, who specializes in animal behavior. This will pull him away from the fight while keeping your hands out of harm's way.

If both dogs are on leashes, the owners can work together to pull them apart by walking in opposite directions, adds Dr. Simpson.

Most cats don't go for formal walks, but given the chance, they will do plenty of wandering—and sometimes fighting—on their own, says Dr. Simpson. Cat fights can result in serious injuries, she adds. It is really best to keep cats, and particularly toms, inside and away from trouble.

WHAT YOUR VET WILL DO

If your pet hasn't already been neutered, this is the first thing your vet will recommend, Diller says. Intact males are not only more aggressive than their neutered kin, but the constant need to find a mate and fend off competitors leads them into dangerous situations.

Neutering doesn't significantly change male pets' personalities, Dr. Simpson adds. "If anything, they tend to be more people-oriented, and that's a plus."

If your pet is already neutered but still getting into fight after fight, your vet may recommend using drugs to curb his scrapping instincts. In many cases, vets use the same mood-altering medicines that are used for people, such as diazepam (Valium) and fluoxetine (Prozac). In addition, since fighting is potentially dangerous not only for pets but also for their human owners, your vet may recommend that you consult with a professional who specializes in pet behavior problems.

See also Chapter 5: Aggression

GROOMING EXCESSIVELY

Clues

- Your pet's coat is getting darker or thicker.
- There are bare patches in fur.
- Your pet is mainly grooming only in one spot.
- She is licking her whole body all the time.

They don't lounge in the tub on Saturday nights or spend their paychecks on expensive shampoos, but cats—and to a lesser degree, dogs—love being clean. Several times each day, they lick and rub their coats, removing dirt and loose hairs until their fur is clean and shiny.

Some pets, however, take cleanliness a little too far. They will lick, rub, or bite their coats for hours at a time. Sometimes they get so absorbed in grooming that they lose interest in all the other fun things in life, like eating or going for walks. The constant licking can result in bare spots in the fur, and the skin may even get raw and sore.

This condition, as well as such things as endless tail-chasing, is known as an obsessive-compulsive disorder, says Nicholas Dodman, B.V.M.S. (bachelor of veterinary medical surgery, the Scottish equivalent of D.V.M.), director of the animal behavior clinic at Tufts University School of Veterinary Medicine in North Grafton, Massachusetts, and author of *The Dog Who Loved Too Much.* "Sensitive, anxious, and nervous pets seem more likely to develop obsessive-compulsive disorders," he says. "And if you breed a dog with this condition, her offspring have a better-than-average chance of also having it."

Pets usually develop this problem after stressful events, such as following a move or the arrival of another pet. It can also be caused by boredom. Pets that are alone all day sometimes groom themselves simply as a way of passing the time. This is especially common in Doberman pinschers, says Bob Maida, a dog trainer and behavior counselor in Manassas, Virginia. "Some dogs can't handle inactivity. They get stressed because they are alone all day. This can be hard for them because of their history as pack animals."

Obsessive-compulsive disorder is fortunately quite rare. But it is not the only reason that pets will sometimes groom themselves raw. Another, more common cause of excessive grooming is allergies. Many pets are allergic to fleas, pollen, and even certain foods, says James C. Blakemore, D.V.M., professor in the department of clinical sciences at Purdue University School of Veterinary Medicine in West Lafayette, Indiana. In fact, as much as one-third of all dogs and quite a few cats develop food allergies, he says.

Anything that irritates the skin, such as a burr or a splinter, can cause pets to lick and worry the area until the discomfort goes away, says Wayne Hunthausen, D.V.M., a veterinarian in private practice in Westwood, Kansas, who specializes in behavior problems.

Finally, there are a number of medical problems that can cause pets to groom themselves too often. Pets with arthritis or cancer sometimes get itchy and will lick themselves to get relief. A condition called hypothyroidism, in which the thyroid gland produces too little hormone, is a very common cause of itchy skin. In fact, many pets that lick their skin excessively have this condition, says Richard Rossman, D.V.M., a veterinarian in private practice in Glenview, Illinois. Changes in the coat's color or thickness are also signs of thyroid disease, he adds.

WHAT YOU CAN DO

You can often figure out what the problem is simply by seeing where your pet is licking. If she is focusing on one place, something is probably irritating the skin, says Jacque Schultz, director of companion animal services for the American Society for the Prevention of Cruelty to Animals, headquartered in New York City. "Make sure that your cat doesn't have any hair knots that she is trying to get to," she says. In fact, anything that gets into the skin or coat, from a burr to masking tape from your child's art project, can cause pets to groom themselves silly.

When grooming appears to be happening at random—your pet is licking one part of her body then moving on to another—she is probably just bored. This isn't always easy to fix, especially if you work and leave your pet alone all day. Having a long walk in the morning and evening will help burn off some of her surplus energy, Schultz says. At the very least, try to have a vigorous play session in the house or yard before leaving in the morning.

Cats aren't always as easy to entertain as dogs, of course. But there are ways to take her mind off her coat. "They are drawn to anything that has an erratic movement," Schultz says. "Buy a mobile. Glue a piece of string to a table-tennis ball and hang it just out of reach. Or cut holes in the top of a shoe box and put a ball inside. Your cat will be fascinated trying to get the ball out of the box. Most important, you can rotate their toys to keep them from getting bored."

If your pet is licking and biting her feet or rubbing against furniture, she probably has allergies. If her tongue goes into overdrive mainly in the warm months, there is a good chance that she is allergic to pollen. Keeping her indoors in the early morning and evening hours, when pollen counts are highest, will help relieve the itching. It is also a good idea to

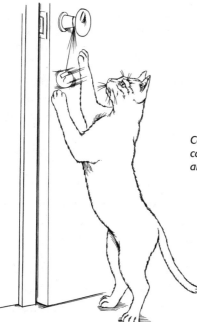

Cats get bored just like people do. Giving your cat something exciting to do, like batting a ball around, will help take her tongue out of gear.

keep her indoors after mowing the lawn, which stirs up enormous amounts of pollen and mold, explains Dr. Blakemore.

The only way to find out if your pet is allergic to food is to put her on a new diet, one with none of the ingredients in her usual chow, says Dr. Blakemore. Foods containing one protein (such as venison or lamb) and one carbohydrate (such as potato) may be worth trying. If her grooming habits return to normal, you may have identified the problem.

Fleas aren't that difficult to control, although it can be a time-consuming process. Pet supply stores sell a variety of flea sprays and powders. In addition, your vet may recommend giving your pet a medication such as Program or Advantage. Used monthly, both medications can help keep fleas from thriving.

If excessive grooming is accompanied by other symptoms, such as sore hips or lumps or swelling anywhere on the body, call your vet right away, says Dr. Hunthausen. Pets with cancer and other serious conditions sometimes get very itchy, and excessive grooming may be one of the warning signs.

What Your Vet Will Do

Since excessive grooming can be caused by so many things, be prepared to answer a lot of questions when you take your pet to the vet. He will want to know, for example, where your pet sleeps. Did you get a new carpet? If so, she could be allergic to chemicals in the backing. Do you leave the windows open? This could be allowing large amounts of mold or pollen to blow inside. The more information you can provide, the easier it will be to figure out the problem, Dr. Rossman says.

Your vet may recommend giving your pet a skin test to help pin down potential allergies. If she does have allergies, she may benefit from taking antihistamines, says Dr. Blakemore. These drugs aren't safe for pets with glaucoma or those taking antibiotics, however. To be safe, it is always a good idea to check with your vet before giving human medications to pets.

Since mites, fleas, and other parasites are common causes of excessive grooming, your vet may scrape off a bit of skin and examine it under a microscope, says Dr. Hunthausen. If parasites are present, they usually aren't that difficult to get rid of with the proper medications.

If the cause of the excessive grooming isn't quickly apparent, your vet may recommend x-rays to check for cancer or arthritis. He may also draw a little blood to check for thyroid problems. Untreated, thyroid problems can be serious, but with the proper medication, they are usually very easy to control—although your pet have may to take replacement hormone for the rest of her life.

When there doesn't appear to be a physical cause, your vet will probably suspect the grooming is caused by obsessive-compulsive disorder. Pets with this condition almost always need medications such as fluoxetine (Prozac) to keep the grooming under control.

See also Chapter 5: Chewing Skin, Coat, or Tail; Chapter 7: Scratching and Shaking; Chapter 13: Black Specks in Fur, Fur Loss

GROWLING

Clues

- **Your cat has been in a fight or another stressful situation.**
- **Your pet is salivating heavily, and his voice has changed.**

Pets that growl are often frightened, aggressive, or both. And they don't always stop with a growl. "Growling should be taken very seriously," says Sandy Driscoll, owner of the Academy of Dog Obedience in Los Angeles. "It may be a warning that precedes an actual bite."

Growling isn't always a sign of bad intentions. Pets that are in pain from arthritis, for example, may be short-tempered and quick to growl. Some older pets have trouble with their hearing or vision, which can make the world seem more threatening than it did before. And of course, it is natural for dogs to growl when they are merely playing, such as during tug-of-war or while wrestling on the living-room carpet.

A cat's growl doesn't seem as ominous as a dog's, but it can be equally dangerous. What's more, a growling cat isn't playing. He is either genuinely frightened or being aggressive, and if you don't watch out, a painful bite or scratch may not be far behind, says Ellen Miller, D.V.M., a veterinarian in private practice in Fort Collins, Colorado.

Cats have long memories, and sometimes they will get so upset by an earlier encounter, such as a fight with another cat, that they will growl at you later when you try to pet them or pick them up, says Victoria L. Voith, D.V.M., Ph.D., an animal behaviorist and veterinarian in private practice in Dayton, Ohio.

Some cats simply don't appreciate a lot of human contact and will growl when their well-meaning owners try to get more intimate. "Some cats are affection junkies, but some don't like being in a lap, ever," says Malcolm Riordan, D.V.M., a veterinarian in private practice in Santa Barbara, California.

WHAT YOU CAN DO

In dogs particularly, growling is really too serious a threat to handle without a veterinarian's help. "If you try to deal with it on your own, you may get hurt," Driscoll warns. In fact, your vet may recommend that you get professional assistance from a trainer or from someone who specializes in behavior problems.

In the meantime, you need to figure out what, exactly, is making your pet growl. Some pets growl mainly when they are startled, such as when you reach down to give them a quick pat or when you come around a corner and take them by surprise. This type of growling usually isn't a serious problem, and an expert will help put a stop to it fairly quickly, says William C. Beggs, D.V.M., a veterinarian in private practice in Colorado Springs, Colorado.

In some cases, however, pets simply have an angry personality and will growl or bite at a moment's notice. If your pet seems to be unusually short-tempered, it is essential to get professional help before you or someone else gets seriously hurt, says Dr. Beggs.

One thing you don't want to do is reward your pet for his temperamental personality. It is normal for people to respond to a growl with petting and reassurance. Rather than calming your pet, however, your good intentions could have the opposite effect by rewarding him for his misbehavior, says Dr. Beggs.

Cats can present a tougher training challenge than dogs not only for owners but also for professional trainers. If your cat is a growler, you may find that it is easier to change your routine than to change his personality, says Dr. Riordan. If you have children in the house, for example, you may decide that the best thing is to keep your cat in a different part of the house. At the very least you may want to put a baby gate between the temperamental cat and your cat-happy toddler, who doesn't understand that some cats don't love the extra attention.

WHAT YOUR VET WILL DO

While growling is usually a behavior problem, it can also be a sign that something is physically wrong. Your vet will begin with a thorough checkup. She will check your pet's joints to make sure that they are working smoothly. She will look at his paws to see if there is a cut or infection. She will also check for internal conditions such as thyroid disease, which can makes pets overactive and aggressive. Finally, she will probably check your pet's vision and hearing since pets with weakened senses are much more likely to be taken by surprise—and to react by growling.

Thanks to vaccinations, rabies is rare in dogs and cats. But if your pet's bad temper came on very suddenly or if he has other symptoms, like changes in his tone of voice or a lot of saliva, your vet will want to investigate this as well.

If your pet seems unusually aggressive or anxious, your vet may recommend giving him anti-anxiety medications. Most of the time, however, she will suggest that you see an animal behaviorist, who can help you and your pet interact more peacefully. "Often the problem comes down to the failure of the owner and the pet to understand one another," says Michael Moore, D.V.M., associate professor of specialty medicine at the Washington State University College of Veterinary Medicine in Pullman.

See also Chapter 5: Aggression

HEAD PRESSING

Clues

- Head pressing is accompanied by other types of odd behavior.
- Your pet seems ill or confused.

Pets use their heads the way people use their hands—for exploring, rubbing, or just saying "Hi." But sometimes they will act more like billy goats than dogs or cats. They will drop their heads and walk straight into walls, sometimes getting "stuck" for hours until their owners rescue them or until they come to their senses and walk away.

This condition, called head pressing, would be humorous if it weren't so serious. It is often caused by liver problems, explains Grant Nisson, D.V.M., a veterinarian in private practice in West River, Maryland. The liver is responsible for removing toxins from the bloodstream. When it isn't working properly, toxins stay in the blood and enter the brain. This can make dogs and cats act very strangely, with head pressing being one of the most common signs.

In young pets, head pressing is often caused by a liver shunt. This is an inherited condition in which they are born with an extra blood vessel that ships blood around, instead of through, the liver, says Karen Munana, D.V.M., associate professor of neurology at North Carolina State University College of Veterinary Medicine in Raleigh. Other symptoms of a liver shunt include drooling, loss of vision, and slow growth during the early months.

In older pets, head pressing may be a sign of cirrhosis, a serious breakdown of the liver that can be caused by dozens of different problems, from internal infections to the long-term use of certain medicines. Ear infections may cause it as well.

Brain diseases can also cause head pressing. Pets with encephalitis, for example, develop inflammation in the brain, which can make them do odd things, says Deena Tiches, D.V.M., a veterinary neurologist in private practice in Gaithersburg, Maryland. Viral infections such as distemper or rabies also affect the brain, as do some bacterial infections.

Brain tumors are always a possibility, adds Dr. Tiches. As they get larger, they may begin pressing on tissues within the brain, changing the way it works. Pets with brain tumors may act strangely in many ways, including walking in circles as well as engaging in head pressing.

WHAT YOU CAN DO

Head pressing is always a serious symptom, and you need to see your vet immediately. Don't be fooled if your pet starts acting normal again, Dr. Tiches adds. In pets with liver disease, strange behavior will often come and go. But the underlying problem won't go away; it will only get worse over time, she explains.

If you are unable to see your vet right away, switch your pet immediately to a high-carbohydrate, low-protein diet. Proteins are broken down into strong, sometimes toxic substances during digestion. When the liver isn't working right, this can lead to head pressing and other odd behavior. Instead of giving your pet her usual food, switch her to meals like cooked rice, pasta, or potatoes, maybe flavored with a little cottage cheese or meat broth. And try to get her to a vet as soon as you can, says Dr. Nisson.

WHAT YOUR VET WILL DO

Since head pressing is often caused by liver disease, your vet will begin his exam by feeling your pet's belly. This is a quick way to see if the liver is the normal size. He will also run blood and urine tests. If there is a liver problem, it will usually show up in one of these tests.

Since there are many conditions that affect the liver, the treatment options will vary widely. Pets with liver shunts will always need surgery to close off the extra blood vessel and reroute the blood in the proper direction. Other liver diseases, such as cirrhosis, are much more difficult to diagnose and treat. The only way to find out what's causing cirrhosis is to take a biopsy of the liver, which is usually done under general anesthesia.

There's isn't a cure for cirrhosis. But with a low-protein diet and medications that reduce the production of harmful substances in the intestine, many pets with cirrhosis will do just fine for a long time.

Brain diseases are even harder to diagnose, says Dr. Munana. You will probably need to take your pet to see a specialist, who will do a variety of tests, including an MRI (magnetic resonance imaging), to look for tumors inside the brain. In addition, your pet will probably be given a spinal tap to check for infections.

Many brain diseases can be treated and cured, says Dr. Tiches. Infections, for example, are usually treated with several weeks of antibiotics. Tumors that are growing fast enough to damage brain tissue might be removed surgically, although your vet may give medications such as prednisone, which can shrink tumors from the inside out.

Head Shaking or Head Tilting

Clues

- Your dog has large, floppy ears, which are red inside.
- There is a discharge or strong odor.
- The head shaking is accompanied by frequent scratching.

Just as former President Ronald Reagan often cupped his hand to his ear when listening to questions, dogs and cats give their heads a little tilt in order to hear better. But when they are cocking their heads even when everything is quiet or they are shaking their heads all the time, you can bet they have an ear problem that is making them uncomfortable.

Head shaking and head tilting are usually caused by an outer-ear infection called otitis externa. Caused by bacteria, yeast, or other organisms, this condition is particularly common in dogs with large, floppy ears because the insides of the ears get hot and humid, creating a perfect environment for infection, says Stephen Simpson, D.V.M., associate professor of neurology at Auburn University College of Veterinary Medicine in Auburn, Alabama.

Pets with ear mites will also shake or tilt their heads. Dogs aren't immune to ear mites, but they get them much less often than cats do.

Food allergies are a common cause of ear problems. Unlike people, who often get upset stomachs from eating foods that they are allergic to, dogs and cats can get downright itchy. When they aren't scratching, they may give their heads a quick shake for temporary relief.

While the occasional shake or tilt isn't anything to worry about, pets that are constantly tilting their heads may have problems with their sense of balance. This can be caused by an inner-ear infection or even by a brain infection called encephalitis, says Dr. Simpson. Brain injuries or tumors can also cause head tilting.

In dogs, head tilting will occasionally have a simpler explanation: They may be doing it for no other reason than that people think it is cute—especially if their little "show" gets rewarded with a tasty treat, says Wayne Hunthausen, D.V.M., a veterinarian in private practice in Westwood, Kansas, who specializes in behavior problems.

What You Can Do

Since head shaking and tilting are often caused by ear problems, take a look inside the ear. If you see something that doesn't belong, like a burr or grass seed, you may have solved the problem. It is generally easy to re-move small objects from the ears with your fingers, says Katherine Houpt, V.M.D., Ph.D., professor of physiology and director of the Animal Be-havior Clinic at the College of Veterinary Medicine at Cornell University in Ithaca, New York.

In cats and dogs, ear mites, which create a dark, brown discharge that looks like coffee grounds, are very likely the cause of the problem. Pet supply stores sell a variety of products that will ease the itching and kill the mites. Follow the directions on the label, and your pet should start feeling better in a few days.

It's important to clean the ears before using the medication, says Craig N. Carter, D.V.M., Ph.D., head of epidemiology at the Texas Veterinary Medical Diagnostic Laboratory at Texas A&M University in College Sta-tion. If the ears are unusually hairy, you may want to pluck out some of the hair from the canal with your fingers or tweezers, which will help the ear canal dry. Then flush the canal with an ear cleanser, available from vets and pet supply stores, and massage the base of the ears to distribute the fluid. Cleaning the ear will help the medication go where it is supposed to, says Dr. Carter. In addition, ear-cleaning solutions can help prevent germs from multiplying. Don't use cotton swabs to clean your pet's ears since they can damage the eardrum, he adds.

If the ear looks red, raw, or swollen or if there is a sticky or smelly dis-charge, there is probably an ear infection, and you will want to call your vet.

WHAT YOUR VET WILL DO

Vets, like pediatricians, see lots of ear problems, which usually aren't hard to treat. Your vet will begin by taking a look inside your pet's ears with an otoscope, an instrument that makes it easy to see inside. If she can't see anything in the outer portions of the ear, she may recommend taking an x-ray to see if anything is wrong deep inside.

If your pet does have an ear infection, she is going to need antibiotics. In addition, your vet will probably give you an ear-washing solution and perhaps a bottle of anti-inflammatory drops to use at home. Once you begin treatment, ear infections usually feel better within a day or two and are entirely gone in a week to 10 days.

If your pet doesn't get better and she continues tilting or shaking her head, call your vet right away, Dr. Simpson says. She could have a more se-rious, neurological problem that needs immediate attention. If food aller-gies are the problem, you are going to need your vet's help figuring out what ingredient is causing the symptoms and what you need to do to avoid it.

See also Chapter 7: Dirty Ears, Discharge, Odors

HISSING

Clues

- Your cat hisses when other animals are around.
- He is hissing much more often than usual.
- The hissing started after an illness or injury.

Nature provides a lot of warning signs to keep us safe. A red burner on the stove means "don't touch." A dark sky means "storms ahead." And a hissing cat means "keep your distance—or you may get scratched."

Cats almost always hiss because they are nervous or angry—when another animal enters their territory, for example, or when someone reaches out too suddenly and gives them a scare. Some cats, of course, are extremely mellow and rarely hiss. Others hiss all the time. In either case, cats are much more likely to hiss at other cats than people. Through a survey of almost 900 cat owners, researchers found that about 80 percent of cats will occasionally hiss at other cats, and about 25 percent occasionally hiss at people.

If your cat has always hissed a lot, he is probably just temperamental. But if he is gradually hissing or growling more often and you can't figure out why, there may be something physically wrong. Cats with infections may be in pain, making them short-tempered and likely to hiss. In rare cases, cats can have neurological problems that affect their personalities. Even more rare, thankfully, is rabies, which can make cats aggressive, says Victoria L. Voith, D.V.M., Ph.D., an animal behaviorist and veterinarian in private practice in Dayton, Ohio.

WHAT YOU CAN DO

Since hissing is a normal part of a cat's vocabulary, you usually don't have to worry about it—although you will want to keep your distance until he calms down.

The one thing you don't want to do is try to comfort a hissing cat, cautions Dr. Voith. When cats are worked up, they may scratch or bite with little provocation. The best thing to do is leave him alone, she says. When cats get upset, it can take hours before they settle down.

Cats often hiss when a new pet enters the family. Sometimes, unfortunately, cats simply take a dislike to each other. In most cases, however, they hiss because they are unsure of each other. Once they get used to each other's presence, the aggression will fade.

One way you can help them adjust is to slowly acquaint them during feeding time. Set their bowls very far apart, but within eyesight of each other. Then, before the next feeding, move the bowls slightly closer. If you do this slowly over time, cats will usually start getting used to each other. If the bad feelings are intense, however, you may have keep them in separate parts of the house or even find another home for one of them, says Dr. Voith.

Cats will sometimes hiss at threats they see outside, such as a visiting cat on the lawn. To keep your cat calm, you may want to make his world a little less scary by restricting his view, says Wayne Hunthausen, D.V.M., a veterinarian in private practice in Westwood, Kansas, who specializes in behavior problems. He recommends taping paper over the windows that your cat usually looks out of. Or, if you don't want to restrict your view along with your cat's, you may want to try moving furniture away from the windows.

Hissing at other cats is unsettling enough, but when your cat is hissing at visitors or members of the family, it can be downright scary. In some cases, you can train cats to be less nervous and more accepting. Dr. Voith recommends sitting nearby while your cat is eating. Don't get too close—give him plenty of space. After a while, move a little bit closer and sit still again. If you do this gradually—over a period of days or even weeks—your cat will get used to your presence and realize that you are not a threat, she explains.

Don't get discouraged if he periodically gets threatened and starts hissing, she adds. Just back up and give him more space. When he is feeling calm, begin the process again.

Even though hissing can be frightening, it is not something that you should punish your cat for, says Dr. Hunthausen. Cats can't be taught not to hiss. In fact, punishing a hissing cat will only make him feel more threatened and more likely to hiss, he says.

WHAT YOUR VET WILL DO

A veterinarian faced with the problem of a hissing cat will first have to decide whether a physical or behavioral problem is to blame. Since cats may get extremely agitated after a run-in with another cat (or dog), your vet will check him for injuries or infections, says Malcolm Riordan, D.V.M., a veterinarian in private practice in Santa Barbara, California.

Male cats that haven't been neutered tend to be much more aggressive and territorial than fixed cats. Neutering is a relatively simple, safe procedure that lower levels of testosterone. This can help your cat be less assertive toward pets as well as people, making him less likely to hiss, explains Barbara Simpson, D.V.M., Ph.D., a veterinarian in private practice in Southern Pines, North Carolina, who specializes in animal behavior.

When the hissing and accompanying aggression seem to be serious, your vet may give your cat anti-anxiety medications such as fluoxetine (Prozac), which will help him calm down. In addition, he may recommend that you see an experienced animal behaviorist. Behaviorists are trained to look at the cat's total environment to see what may be causing the problem and to suggest ways to resolve it.

HOUSE SOILING

Clues

- You have a spayed female who leaks a little urine after sitting or lying down.
- Your pet is having trouble getting around.
- The accidents occur only when your pet is excited.
- You have recently moved the litter box.

Just about every dog (and most cats) will occasionally have accidents in the house, especially when they are young. But when your formerly fastidious friend suddenly forgets his manners, and then the problem persists, there is clearly something wrong, says Wayne Hunthausen, D.V.M., a veterinarian in private practice in Westwood, Kansas, who specializes in behavior problems.

Pets with diarrhea, for example, often have a viral infection, which can make it impossible for them to get outside or to the litter box on time. Some pets lose muscular control as they get older, making them accident-prone. For pets with hip problems or other forms of arthritis, getting up and walking can be very painful, so they are unable to go where they should.

Female dogs that have been spayed will occasionally dribble small amounts of urine or even leave puddles after sitting or lying down. This is because the hormone estrogen helps strengthen the holding power of a muscle in the urethra, the tube through which urine flows. And after spaying, estrogen levels decline dramatically, making accidents more likely to occur.

House soiling isn't caused only by physical problems, of course. Some dogs simply get very excited, such as when people visit, and temporarily lose control. In addition, dogs, like people, have different levels of control. Some can go all day without needing to go outside, while others get uncomfortable after just a few hours. Cats also have different levels of control, but they tend to have accidents much less often than dogs, says Dr. Hunthausen.

House soiling isn't always an accident. Dogs and cats that haven't been neutered, for example, will sometimes mark their territory with sprays of urine, especially when they are feeling threatened, says Dr. Hunthausen. If your dog has recently begun lifting his leg on the furniture, or your cat is spraying the walls, you need to figure out what is bothering him.

Visits from other pets will sometimes cause pets to mark their territory. Even an unauthorized visit, such as from a stray dog that crosses the lawn, can cause house soiling.

In cats, house soiling may be related to their litter boxes, Dr. Hunthausen says. Even small changes in their routine—such as letting the litter box get dirty or moving it to a different room—can cause them to seek out forbidden spots like behind the couch or in a potted plant. Even changing brands of litter will send some cats in search of new places.

WHAT YOU CAN DO

House soiling is an unpleasant problem, but there are ways of dealing with it. With dogs, usually what they need is a refresher course in basic training.

"It's very simple. You act as though your dog hasn't been housebroken before, and you start again," says Sandy Driscoll, owner of the Academy of Dog Obedience in Los Angeles. Keep an eye on your dog whenever he is in the house. Your goal is to catch him *before* he lifts his leg or squats on the carpet since it is more effective to praise good behavior when he goes in the right place than to punish him for making a mistake, she says.

You don't have to wait until he is almost in the act before heading for the door, Driscoll adds. Letting him out more often will give him more opportunities to take care of business, and the praise you give will help him understand what he is supposed to do in the future.

Unless you work at home (and stay awake all night), you can't supervise your dog all the time. That is why vets often recommend keeping accident-prone dogs in a large, comfortable crate during the training period. The crate should be large enough so that your dog can stand and turn around comfortably. Dogs are very reluctant to soil the area where they sleep, and they will do their best to wait until you let them out. If your pet isn't already crate-trained, ask your vet for advice.

For crate training to be effective, however, it is essential to let your dog out often, always praising him when he goes in the right place, Driscoll says. To prevent accidents, be sure to let him out first thing in the morning and again after eating, when the urge to have a bowel movement is strongest. Don't forget to let him out before you go to bed, which will allow him to get ready for the long night ahead.

Unlike dogs, when cats are making messes in the house, there is usually a reason for it—but it is not always easy to figure out what the reason is. "There are probably a thousand reasons that cats decide to go someplace other than their litter box," says Dr. Hunthausen.

Since cats are creatures of habit, it is a good idea to get into a routine and stick with it. When you are using a brand of litter he likes, think twice before making changes, Dr. Hunthausen says. Don't move the litter box unless you have to since some cats will refuse to visit the new place. If you do move the box, don't put it too near his food since most cats prefer to keep the two separate.

Some cats won't use their boxes unless this area is scrupulously kept clean. Vets recommend removing the solid wastes every day and changing the litter at least once a week. And since cats are sensitive to odors, avoid covered boxes or scented litter, both of which may offend your cat's fastidious sense of smell, says Dr. Hunthausen.

Some outdoor cats have trouble getting used to the sandy feel of litter boxes. "You can appeal to their little cat minds by putting some dirt in with the sand," says Malcolm Riordan, D.V.M., a veterinarian in private practice in Santa Barbara, California.

As a last resort, you may need to temporarily confine your cat and his litter box to a small area, like the bathroom or the utility room. "When there is nowhere else to go but the bare floor, most cats will usually use the litter box," explains Dr. Hunthausen. This isn't meant to be punishment, he adds. Let him out often for fun and games, but always return him to the enclosed area. Within a few weeks, he will be used to the litter box and more likely to use it in the future.

It is essential to clean messes thoroughly to prevent your pets from returning to the "scent of the crime," Dr. Hunthausen adds. You can begin the job with ammonia, vinegar, or other household cleaners, but these should be followed by an odor-neutralizing product such as KOE. You can get odor-neutralizers from vets and pet supply stores.

WHAT YOUR VET WILL DO

House soiling usually has more to do with behavior and lifestyle issues than with physical problems, so don't be surprised if your vet wants to know exactly what has been going on at home since just before the problem began. If she is still stumped, she may refer you to a specialist in animal behavior, who is trained to deal with house soiling and other common problems.

Before you spend a lot of money on specialists, however, your vet may recommend giving your pet a thorough going-over. She will probably begin by taking a urine sample to test for a bladder infection. In addition, she may look at the possibility of bladder cancer, neurological or spinal problems, and in cats, feline leukemia. In older pets, arthritis, dementia, or other mental problems may cause pets to lose control.

If your dog is leaking urine due to low estrogen levels, hormone replacement pills may be necessary, says Dr. Riordan. And of course, when pets are spraying or urinating to mark their territory, neutering is often the best solution.

See also Chapter 5: Spraying

HUMPING

Clues

- Humping is accompanied by growling or biting.
- Your pet is having difficulty urinating, or there is blood in the urine.

Dogs aren't at all shy about getting intimate with other pets or even with people's legs. Even cats will sometimes engage in embarrassing displays of affection, usually with inanimate objects such as blankets, small towels, or teddy bears.

"A few cats may mount your arm or leg, but people are usually too big for them," says Katherine Houpt, V.M.D., Ph.D., professor of physiology and director of the Animal Behavior Clinic at the College of Veterinary Medicine at Cornell University in Ithaca, New York.

Even though humping—vets call it mounting behavior—appears to be sexual, it is usually a pet's way of showing that he is top dog. It is more common in males, but females do it, too.

Aggressive breeds of dogs, such as Rottweilers, German shepherds, and Doberman pinschers, do the most humping. "It is sexual harassment by dogs," says Dr. Houpt. "If a dog mounts you, he is saying, 'I'm dominant over you.' This often happens when a dog has nothing else to do," she adds. "It's an attention-getter."

Even though humping is natural for dogs and, to a lesser extent, for cats, it sometimes occurs when there is an underlying physical problem. Dogs with anal sac infections will sometimes emit an odor that, to other dogs, will smell like a female in heat, says Dr. Houpt. Cats can develop bladder or kidney stones, and humping may ease the discomfort.

But most often, they just do it because they do it. As long as they are not humping people or inanimate objects, it is probably not a big deal. "It's between them, as far as I'm concerned," says Jacque Schultz, director of companion animal services for the American Society for the Prevention of Cruelty to Animals. "If neither of them cares, fine."

WHAT YOU CAN DO

Pets don't always limit their attentions to other pets. When your dog is showing interest in the limbs of people or if he is growling and threatening other pets, you will want to put a stop to it, says Bob Maida, a dog trainer and animal behavior counselor in Manassas, Virginia.

"The best way to discourage humping is to not encourage other dominant behaviors such as roughhousing or tugging games," Maida says. Letting your dog indulge his aggressive tendencies in one way invariably encourages him to try other, less-acceptable methods, he explains.

The next time your dog gets ready to hump, interrupt him with a firm "No!" says Wayne Hunthausen, D.V.M., a veterinarian in private practice in Westwood, Kansas, who specializes in behavior problems. If he doesn't respond to your commands, try putting a few coins in an empty soda can and giving it a vigorous shake. Dogs hate the noise, and it will usually distract them from their misbehavior, he says.

Just be sure to reward your dog when he obeys your command, Dr. Hunthausen adds. Giving him a treat or extra attention will help him understand that it is in his best interest to obey you. Eventually, he will get the idea that *not* humping brings better rewards than his usual carrying-on.

With cats, you'll want to try a different approach. Scolding your cat isn't a good idea—not only because it is unlikely to change his behavior but also because cats take discipline very personally and may become fearful of their owners.

What you should do is anticipate when your cat is getting ready to make his move and then distract him. Roll a ball across the floor or dangle a piece of string, suggests Dr. Houpt.

For cats, it's also a good idea to check for blood spots in the litter or to see if there have been any changes in his urinating habits. These are signs of urinary tract infections, which need to be treated by a vet right away. One thing you may want to try, however, is to occasionally give your cat canned food. It contains substantially more water than dry food, and the extra fluids can help prevent the onset of some urinary problems. Or you can try adding a little broth to your pet's water, which may encourage him to drink more.

WHAT YOUR VET WILL DO

Since humping occurs most often in unneutered pets, vets have a simple solution. "If your dog hasn't been neutered, I'd recommend doing it," says Dr. Hunthausen. "That will take care of the humping problem in 60 percent of the cases."

If your dog isn't in heat but has still been on the receiving end of another dog's attentions, your vet will probably check her anal sacs for infection. This isn't a serious problem and will usually clear up when an antibiotic ointment is applied. If the infection has spread, your dog may need oral antibiotics as well, says Dr. Houpt.

Since humping is fairly rare in cats, your vet will begin by checking for physical problems, especially problems in the urinary tract. She will probably recommend a urinalysis as well as x-rays to check for kidney or bladder stones or tumors.

SYMPTOM # RESTLESSNESS

Clues

- Your pet is restless mainly at night.
- The restlessness is a recent problem.

She lies down. Gets up. Licks her paw. Licks the other paw. Paces. Barks or meows. Jumps up. Lies down. This could go on all day. With the way your pet is squirming around, you are beginning to suspect that she has been hitting the Mr. Coffee.

Restless dogs and fidgety cats usually don't have anything physically wrong. Like some people, they simply have more energy than they know what to do with, and they are burning it off as best they can.

Certain breeds of cats, such as Siamese and Abyssinians, tend to be very restless. The same is true of working dogs like Border collies and Labrador retrievers, says Kathalyn Johnson, D.V.M., clinical associate in companion and animal behavior at Texas A&M University College of Veterinary Medicine in College Station. "If these dogs are left alone a lot and don't have big yards to play in, they will end up doing what dogs do—bark, chew, or dig—because the energy has to come out some way," she says.

Occasionally, an imbalance of hormones or of chemicals in the brain (a condition that vets call hyperkinetic activity) can cause extreme restlessness. And in rare cases, pets with food allergies will get very restless. "Pets may be allergic to beef or chicken or even something as small a flavored heartworm pill," says Dr. Johnson. When they eat the wrong thing, they will suddenly act as though constant motion is the only way to be comfortable.

WHAT YOU CAN DO

Unless your pet has a physical problem, regular exercise is about the only way to keep her from feeling restless. How much exercise depends on your pet. If you have a German shepherd, for example, walking a mile or two a day is probably enough. "But that's not enough for working dogs," says Dr. Johnson. They typically need three to five miles of running or walking a day.

You can give dogs and cats a great workout without leaving the yard. For cats, rolling a ball, tossing a catnip-filled mouse, or swinging a piece of string will keep them moving for as long as you care to play. And most dogs will chase balls until your arm gives out. After 20 to 30 minutes, however, they will usually be plenty pooped and more likely to rest than be restless.

For dogs, regular training sessions are a great way to burn off energy. "It's a good social activity, and the training will help calm the dog," says Dr. Johnson. Plus, training makes it easier to control your dog when she is constantly asking for your attention. Having her obey a command before you reward her will make her more attentive to you and less wrapped up in her own nervous energy.

When giving your dog commands, it is important to use an even, neutral tone of voice and reward her without too much excitement, says Dr. Johnson. If you get excited, she will get excited. But if you are calm, that will rub off on her, too.

For dogs with unusually high energy levels, you may want to consider competitive sports, such as Frisbee or agility courses. You can get information on these activities from vets and some supply stores. "These games are high energy, and dogs love them," says Dr. Johnson.

Apart from exercise, you can train your dog to stay calm, says Barbara Simpson, D.V.M., Ph.D., a veterinarian in private practice in Southern Pines, North Carolina, who specializes in animal behavior. Don't allow vigorous play in the house. When you are in the mood for some energetic activity—such as wrestling or throwing a ball—do it only outside, she advises. When you are spending time inside, keep the fun and games sedate. Eventually, your dog will learn to be calm indoors, knowing that she will have a lot of fun when you go outside.

Of course, dogs that get worked up outside often have trouble calming down once they come back in. A few minutes spent in crate will often make the transition a little easier. If your dog isn't already crate-trained, your vet will advise you on the best ways for getting started.

While such training is a great way to control a restless dog, it doesn't work for cats. If you have an active young cat, you may want to consider getting another young cat. There is a good chance that they will entertain each other for hours—and when they are done, they will usually curl up in a nice, warm place and fall asleep.

It's also helpful to give your cat her main meal late at night, especially if she does most of her racing around after hours, says Craig N. Carter, D.V.M., Ph.D., head of epidemiology at the Texas Veterinary Medical Diagnostic Laboratory at Texas A&M University in College Station. In cats as in people, a big dinner at night makes them sleepy, and when they are sleeping well, so will you.

What Your Vet Will Do

Since restlessness can be caused by a hormonal imbalance, poisoning, or other physical problems, your vet will want to do a checkup to make sure nothing is seriously wrong. If your pet gets a clean bill of health (as she probably will), your vet will help you come up with some fun ways to tire her out a bit.

As a last resort, your vet may advise giving a dog or cat small doses of tranquilizers to take the edge off her nervous energy, says Dr. Johnson.

If tranquilizers don't work, your vet may try the opposite approach and give her a stimulant. "Some pets respond to stimulants and calm down," says Dr. Simpson.

Since food allergies occasionally cause restlessness, your vet may recommend putting your pet on a special diet—one that contains none of the ingredients in her usual chow. Called an elimination diet, this will help you figure out if a food allergy is really the problem. These diets usually take 8 to 10 weeks to show results. If your pet starts calming down, you may have found a solution. "We'll try to find a commercially prepared food that contains the appropriate ingredients and is convenient to use," says Dr. Johnson.

SCRATCHING FURNITURE

Clues

- Your cat keeps scratching the same place.
- Your dog scratches while listening intently.

You paid good money for your living-room furniture, but your cat has no respect for credit card bills. She thinks the recliner and the couch with matching ottoman are her personal scratching posts, and with gleeful abandon she is ripping them to shreds. Even your dog is getting into the act, jumping on the couch and scratching away at the cushions. What's attracting your pets to the decor?

Dogs are chewers rather than scratchers, so when your dog's feet go to work, she is probably just trying to retrieve a toy that slipped under a cushion or to "bury" a toy where no one will find it. Or she may be scratching to make a spot more comfortable for a good nap. Less often, dogs scratch when something piques their curiosity, like the scampering of little mouse feet behind a wall. If she listens intently before she starts scratching, maybe that's why. "Sometimes there are funny things going on that we don't realize," says Kris Kates, owner of Animal Manners, a pet-training and consulting company in Davis, California.

Cats, on the other hand, often do the real damage with scratching furniture. When the urge to scratch strikes—as it does many times a day—they don't really care if they sink their claws into a tree trunk or the sides of your new couch.

A cat's nails are layered, and scratching removes the top layer, uncovering the sharper nail beneath. "Scratching is very natural to cats," Kates says. "When we look around the house, we see a sofa, a chair leg, or a shoe. When your cat looks around, she sees scratching post, scratching post, and scratching post."

More is involved than just nail care. Cats have scent glands inside their paws, and scratching is one way they leave their marks, says Wayne Hunthausen, D.V.M., a veterinarian in private practice in Westwood, Kansas, who specializes in behavior problems. In your cat's mind, the house is her domain, and she wants everyone to know it. Scratching furniture guarantees that the word gets out.

WHAT YOU CAN DO

Just as birds gotta fly and fish gotta swim, cats gotta scratch. The best way to stop the damage is to give them something they like better than the furniture, namely, a sturdy scratching post.

Forget the short, rickety posts you will sometimes find in bargain stores. Cats need a post that's tall enough to reach up to and stout enough that it doesn't tip over when they use it. Some cats enjoy carpet-covered posts, but most prefer a rougher texture—made from burlap, for example, or even coiled rope, says Dr. Hunthausen. You can make your own post by anchoring a bark-covered fireplace log with three long wood screws and some wood glue to a plywood base. "Cats really like it, and it's inexpensive," he says.

Since cats scratch as a way of marking their territory, be sure to put the post in a place that's important to them, preferably near the furniture that has their attention. To make the post doubly attractive to them, start out by spreading a little anchovy paste on top, Kates suggests.

"Cats respond to rewards just like dogs do, so give them praise and a treat when they use the scratching post," Kates says. You don't have to keep using the treats. Once the cats are in the habit of using a post, they will return to it again and again.

Some cats, of course, will continue their furniture attacks no matter how many scratching posts you have around. One strategy to get them to back off is to make the scratching less satisfying than it was before. Try applying a strip of double-sided tape to areas where your cat is scratching. Cats don't like sticky sensations on their paws, and eventually they will turn to other, more satisfying locations, Dr. Hunthausen says.

Another form of ambush is to drape a towel or a pillowcase over a

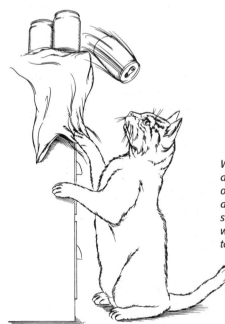

When your cat won't leave the furniture alone, try setting a booby trap. Drape a piece of cloth over the area that she is scratching and put a few empty soda cans on top. When she reaches up for a good scratch, the cans will clatter down, and she will soon learn to take her claws somewhere else.

corner of furniture and put empty soda cans on top. When your cat reaches up for a good scratch, she will pull down the material and get an unexpected surprise, says Dr. Hunthausen.

For stubborn cats, you might try a motion detection alarm like the Critter Gitter, which sound a shrill bleep when your cat starts scratching. You can also swab scratched areas with an odor neutralizer, available in pet supply stores. (Test the product on an inconspicuous area first to make sure that it doesn't stain the material.) When cats can't smell where they have been, they are less likely to return to that spot in the future.

WHAT YOUR VET WILL DO

You may be able to redirect a cat's aim, but there is simply no way to stop them from their natural activity of scratching. Some owners, after reupholstering a few chairs and couches, finally give up and ask their vets if declawing is a sensible solution.

Declawing is a serious operation in which the bone holding the claws is cut off beneath the skin. The procedure is done under general anesthesia, and pets may spend a day or two in the hospital afterward and take several weeks to fully recover.

Declawing *is* major surgery, Dr. Hunthausen adds, and some vets are reluctant to perform the procedure. "Try other things first," he advises.

SCRATCHING PEOPLE

Clues

- Your cat just started getting aggressive.
- Scratching is accompanied by an arched back or twitching tail.
- She seems sick, sore, or cranky.

When your cat is purring in your lap and rubbing her head against your hand, it is easy to forget that her ancestors were aggressive hunters. The tamest house cat still has the instincts of a predator and the speed and reflexes to match. That is why cat scratches can occur so quickly that you never see them coming.

Cats use their paws and claws all the time for hunting, fighting, and playing with other cats. And since you are part of their family, they will sometimes use their claws on you, says Wayne Hunthausen, D.V.M., a veterinarian in private practice in Westwood, Kansas, who specializes in behavior problems.

Cats usually don't mean any harm when they scratch people, says Dr. Hunthausen. In fact, most scratches occur when cats are play-hunting, and your ankles or fingers are the prey. Young cats are particularly fond of stalking their human owners, leaping out from behind doors or from under the bed to deliver a quick scratch or bite.

Cats aren't always playing when they use their claws, however. They often scratch when they are feeling irritated, such as when you are rubbing their belly and they suddenly decide that they have had enough. A quick scratch is their way of saying "Get back!" says Kris Kates, owner of Animal Manners, a pet-training and consulting company in Davis, California. Some cats are naturally crankier than others and will extend their claws at the slightest annoyance. All cats may scratch when they are feeling trapped or frightened, she adds. Look out for an arched back or twitching tail, which may mean an attack is on the way.

Cats will also scratch when they are feeling sick, a problem that vets refer to as pain aggression. "Any cat that suddenly starts scratching people should be examined for painful medical problems, such as sore ears or abscesses," says Dr. Hunthausen.

Even though most cat scratches aren't particularly deep, they often get infected, Dr. Hunthausen warns. So it is not the kind of behavior that you want to encourage, even when it is done in play.

WHAT YOU CAN DO

Young cats are much more likely to indulge in rough play than their older (and calmer) kin. Even when they start out as enthusiastic ankle-

and finger-scratchers, they generally learn to keep their claws in as they get a little older.

It's very difficult to stop the scratching entirely. What you can do is give them something else to focus on, Kates say. Rather than letting them play with your fingers or toes, try giving them "active" toys, like table-tennis balls or a stuffed toy attached to a springy pole. Cats enjoy batting moving toys, and when they can work out their aggression in safe ways, they are less likely to take a swipe at you. If you do get scratched, wash the area well with soap and water and apply an antibiotic cream. Cats scratches often get infected, so you may need to call your doctor as well.

You can't train cats the way you do dogs, but there are ways to help them understand that their rough behavior isn't appreciated. The next time your cat takes a claws-extended swipe, firmly say "No!" says Dr. Hunthausen. To make the message even more emphatic, put a dozen coins in a soda can and give it a vigorous shake. Cats hate the sound and will eventually learn that scratching can have unpleasant (and noisy) consequences. After awhile they will take the hint and keep their claws in.

A more direct reproach is to give her a quick spritz from a water bottle, Dr. Hunthausen says. Cats love to play rough, but they dislike getting wet even more and will eventually learn to behave.

While play-scratching is fairly easy to control or at least avoid, scratching caused by aggression is a more serious problem. If your cat seems to be angry or threatening and is biting and hissing as well as scratching, you will need to talk to your vet.

WHAT YOUR VET WILL DO

If your cat has only recently started scratching, your vet will probably recommend bringing her in for a checkup so that he can see if something is physically wrong. Conditions like arthritis, ear infections, or abscesses can be extremely painful, making cats short-tempered and cranky. In most cases, however, scratching people is a behavioral problem, and your vet may recommend that you see a professional who specializes in deconditioning negative behavior.

If your cat simply won't quit scratching, your vet may recommend having her declawed, a procedure that requires surgery and sometimes several days in the hospital. Although declawing will protect you from scratches, it will leave your cat vulnerable to attacks from other animals, Dr. Hunthausen says. In order to be safe, cats that have been declawed will usually spend the rest of their lives indoors.

See also Chapter 5: Aggression, Biting, Hissing

SPRAYING

Clues

- Other cats have been in the yard.
- There has been a change in your routine.
- The litter box is dirty.

Cats can't write (they never get the hang of holding a pencil), but that doesn't mean they don't leave messages. All too often, they do—on the drapes, furniture, or living-room walls.

Spraying urine is a cat's way of marking his territory, says Wayne Hunthausen, D.V.M., a veterinarian in private practice in Westwood, Kansas, who specializes in behavior problems. When there are other cats living in the house or neighborhood cats are visiting the yard, your cat may start feeling jealous and protective of his turf. So he will leave his scent in the house and yard so that the "intruders" will know who is boss.

All cats may occasionally spray in the house or outside, but it is most common in unneutered males. Dogs also mark their territory, but they don't spray, and they rarely do it indoors, says Dr. Hunthausen.

It is not only jealousy or competition that causes spraying. Anxiety can cause it, too, Dr. Hunthausen says. Scolding your cat, for instance, can hurt his feelings and result in damp walls later on. In fact, anything that upsets his routine, from moving to a new house to giving him less attention, can cause him to spray.

Adding another cat to the family is a common cause of spraying. "The chance of your cat spraying goes up with each new cat you bring into the house," says Kris Kates, owner of Animal Manners, a pet-training and consulting company in Davis, California.

In addition, indoor cats will occasionally spray as a way of expressing their dislike of the current litter-box situation—if it hasn't been cleaned, for example, or if it has been moved to a location they don't like. Cats may also spray simply because they are worked up or excited. In males, this often occurs when a female is in heat, Kates says.

While spraying is usually a behavioral problem, a number of physical conditions, like diabetes or urinary tract infections, can cause it, too.

WHAT YOU CAN DO

Since spraying is a natural part of a cat's behavior, punishing him won't make him stop. In fact, the extra anxiety caused by punishment can make him do it even more, says Dr. Hunthausen. What you can do, though, is figure out what is making him spray and then try to remove the cause.

Since cats are very territorial and nervous about other cats, it is worth taking a few minutes to make your yard less attractive to wandering felines by keeping garbage cans closed, for example. You can rearrange the furniture so that your cat isn't able to see interlopers in the yard, says Dr. Hunthausen. At the very least, you may want to hose down trees, the walkway, and other areas outside where visiting cats have been. By removing their smell, your protective puss may never even know they were there.

If you suspect the problem is due to sibling rivalry, you may want to keep your cats in separate rooms until the bad feelings have had time to fade. "Some cats will only tolerate living with a certain number of cats," adds Dr. Hunthausen. In fact, some cantankerous cats will never accept living with another cat and will show their displeasure—sometimes for years—by spraying.

One trick you may want to try is to move your cat's food bowl near the area that he is spraying. Cats are very particular about their food, and this can cause them to hold their fire. Pet repellents are also helpful, although your pet may simply find another place to spray, Dr. Hunthausen adds.

Incidentally, it is not always easy to tell where your cat has been spraying, although the bad smell makes it obvious what he has been up to. One way to find the spot is to turn out the lights in the house and turn on a black light. "Urine shows up lighter than the surrounding surface," explains Jill O. Kulig, V.M.D., a veterinarian in private practice in Harleysville, Pennsylvania. "Once you have found a place where he has sprayed, clean the area thoroughly so that his scent won't tempt him to spray there again," she says.

WHAT YOUR VET WILL DO

Spraying can be very difficult to stop on your own. Vets, however, have an effective solution. Neutering cats, both males and females, will dramatically reduce the urge to spray. In fact, many cats that are neutered will never spray again.

If your cat is already neutered and is still causing trouble, your vet will probably recommend that you bring him in for testing. The vet usually performs urine tests to see if there is an infection or another problem in the urinary tract, says Dr. Hunthausen.

As a last resort, vets sometimes will use medications, especially anti-anxiety drugs like diazepam (Valium) or fluoxetine (Prozac), to stop the spraying. "They are often very effective and very safe," says Dr. Hunthausen.

COMMON BEHAVIOR-RELATED CONDITIONS

Allergies. You wouldn't think that what your pet breathes, steps in, rubs against, or eats for breakfast would affect her behavior, but allergies can cause problems that go way beyond a little itchy skin or a runny nose, says Barbara Simpson, D.V.M., Ph.D., a veterinarian in private practice in Southern Pines, North Carolina, who specializes in animal behavior.

Pets with allergies will often scratch themselves for hours at a time, pawing and rubbing their skin, ears, or eyes. They may have trouble sleeping and can get irritable or aggressive, Dr. Simpson says. You may notice your pet cocking his head, as though he were listening to something you can't hear—all because there is an itch in his ear that won't go away.

It can be difficult to figure out what pets are allergic to, Dr. Simpson says. Like people, many dogs and cats are allergic to airborne irritants, like pollen or house dust. Some pets are allergic to beef, eggs, wheat, or other ingredients in their food. They can even be allergic to the bowl itself, particularly plastic bowls, which sometimes harbor potential allergens around the edge. Dogs and cats also experience contact allergies, in which they react to things they step in or rub against—a carpet shampoo, for example, or the dyes in certain towels. Allergies to fleas are very common, she adds.

The best treatment for allergies is to avoid whatever it is that's causing them. When that's not possible, your vet may give antihistamines to relieve the symptoms. In more serious cases, your vet may advise giving your pet a series of allergy shots, which can build up the body's tolerance so that the allergy-causing substances are no longer a problem.

Boredom. People who are bored may daydream, watch the shopping network for hours, or browse the real estate section of last Sunday's paper. Dogs and cats, however, look for more entertaining pursuits, like chewing your shoes, tipping over the trash, or having a scratch-a-thon on the new leather couch. Boredom can cause more serious problems as well. Pets without enough to do may spend hours licking their feet, biting their flanks, or chewing their tails, which can result in rashes or infections.

All pets get bored sometimes, but it is more likely to be a problem for pets that spend their days alone. Being alone is particularly hard on dogs since they are social creatures who prefer being close to humans or other dogs. Cats are better than dogs at amusing themselves, but they need stimulation as well, says Jacqui Neilson, D.V.M., a veterinarian in private practice in Portland, Oregon.

Bored pets are frequently destructive pets, adds Kris Kates, owner of Animal Manners, a pet-training and consulting company in Davis, California. "Dogs will chew, and if you don't supply chew toys, they will find something on their own." Some cats are chewers, too, although they often have other ways of working off energy, like shredding the drapes. Or they will simply get irritated and make sure that you are aware of their displeasure, possibly by avoiding the litter box in favor of other, less appropriate places.

Unless you spend your days at home, it is not always easy to keep dogs and cats entertained. If you suspect that boredom is causing behavior problems, however, you may want to consider making an arrangement with a neighbor to drop in once or twice a day to play with them or take them for a quick walk. Or you can hire a professional pet sitter, who will drop by on a regular basis.

At the very least, you will want to leave out a few toys when you are gone, says Dr. Neilson. For dogs, durable chew toys will help keep them entertained, while cats will enjoy catnip-filled mice.

More important than giving your pets toys, says Dr. Neilson, is making sure they get plenty of exercise when you are home. The more energy you help them burn off, the more relaxed they will be when you are gone all day. A tired pet, vets agree, is a happy pet.

Dominance. A growl. A show of teeth. A look that says, "I'm in charge, and don't you forget it."

Whether you are living with a toy poodle or a Great Dane, a dog that tries to be dominant over his human owners can cause serious problems. (While cats may strive for dominance over other cats, it is less likely to affect the people in the family.) Even if your dog isn't growling or biting, the quest for dominance can contribute to many forms of misbehavior, from lifting his leg in the house to humping people's legs.

Your dog's ancestors lived in packs, and in every pack there is a hierarchy, with some dogs having more prestige and status than other dogs. This works fine in the wild but can lead to problems in the living room. "People sometimes develop problems with their pets because they consider us just another dog in their social pack," says Dr. Neilson.

Unless you establish yourself as the leader of the pack—and many pet owners don't—your dog may assume that role himself. This can lead to a very common problem called dominance aggression. "If the pet owner hasn't established himself as the leader, then when he tries to remove a food item or a pet's favorite toy or when he wakes the dog to move him off the bed, the dog may growl, snarl, or bite," Dr. Neilson explains.

There are many forms of aggression that are related to dominance, she adds. Dogs can get very protective of their food (food aggression), hostile to other dogs (inter-dog aggression), or simply too rough when they play (play aggression). But dominance aggression is the most common form, she says, and the one that often causes the most difficulties.

The only way to stop your dog from pushing you around is to make it clear from the start that you are the one in charge. He should come when you call, sit when you tell him to, and get out of your way rather than expecting *you* to move.

Regular training is the best way to control the quest for dominance, Dr. Neilson says. "When you get a dog, young or old, make the dog work for everything in life. Make him sit before he gets a pat on the head or you give him his food dish. Always reinforce your position as being dominant," she says.

Pain. Your wonderfully patient dog suddenly shows his teeth when your nephew touches his tail. Your old, sleepy cat has started hissing when people come too close. What's causing these sweet-tempered Dr. Jekylls to turn into surly Mr. Hydes?

When dogs and cats start getting cranky, crotchety, or aggressive, one of the first things your veterinarian will suspect is pain. Pets are more stoic than people, and it is not always easy to tell when they are hurting—from arthritis, for example, or a cut on the paw. In some cases, however, they will have changes in their personality that will tip you off that something is wrong, says Dr. Simpson.

Pets in pain may pace a lot and seem restless because they are unable to find a position that's comfortable, says Patti Schaefer, D.V.M., a veterinarian in private practice in Olympia, Washington. They may quit eating, whine or meow constantly, or be short-tempered and aggressive. And because pain weakens the immune system, they may be more susceptible to infections as well.

Veterinarians can often control or eliminate pain by using some of the same medications that work for people, says Dr. Simpson. In addition, there are many home remedies, from acupressure and massage to hot-water bottles, that can help dogs and cats feel better. Pain is serious business, she adds, so it is worth calling your vet as soon as you suspect that something is wrong.

Phobias. Vets aren't sure why, but dogs will occasionally develop an intense fear, or phobia, of perfectly harmless things, like thunder, vacuum cleaners, or even stairs. Dogs have been known to jump off balconies or chew through doors in their desperate attempts to escape. Cats also may develop phobias, but they do so much less often than dogs do.

One of the most common phobias for dogs is the fear of thunderstorms, says Dr. Neilson. It is not just the noise, she adds. There is the lightning, the sound of rain pouring down, and the dramatic changes in air pressure. Many dogs will dive under the bed or go into a barking frenzy at the first rumble of thunder.

Other common phobias include the fear of fireworks, gunshots, or other loud noises; the fear of being left alone; and the fear of unfamiliar objects—anything from a stairwell to an umbrella stand.

Some pets naturally get over their phobias as they get older. In many cases, however, the phobias never go away, or they even get worse over time. To reduce the fears, vets often recommend a procedure called desensitization, in which pets are gradually exposed to whatever it is that they are afraid of—by using a tape recording of thunder, for example—until the fears begin to diminish. Desensitization can be very effective, but it is time-consuming, usually requiring daily practice sessions that may continue for weeks or even months, says Dr. Neilson. You can do it at home if you are truly committed. Or you can ask your vet to refer you to a pet behaviorist, who is trained to handle this sort of problem.

When phobias are severe, your vet may recommend giving your pet an anti-anxiety medication such as fluoxetine (Prozac). These drugs alter the balance of chemicals in the brain, making pets calmer and easier to work with. The medications are often used temporarily, Dr. Neilson adds—during the desensitization period or at times when the fears greatest, such as during fireworks season.

Stress. Pets don't seem to have a lot of worries. They sleep a lot, get fed regularly, and never have to worry if the bills are late or the car needs new tires. But dogs and cats are very sensitive to their owners' moods and the changes around them. When you are upset, your pets get upset, too. When you have moved the furniture or had out-of-town visitors, they notice the change in routine, and they don't like it.

"Our pets can be so close to us and so in tune to us that if we are stressed, they feel it, too," says Dr. Schaefer. Stress can affect your pets' behavior in a variety of ways. They often get irritable or depressed, and this, in turn, can cause them to do things that they wouldn't normally do, such as chewing, pacing, barking, or avoiding the litter box in favor of the potted plants.

Dogs and cats can't talk about what is bothering them, so it is important to be attuned to changes in their behavior, especially during times of turmoil, Dr. Simpson says. Giving them extra attention is very important in times of stress. Regular exercise is also helpful because it helps dissipate energy that might otherwise go in more destructive directions.

"Some pets thrive on new situations and seem stimulated," Dr. Simpson explains. "But others are shy and appear to develop anxiety with change. You must give these pets space and time to adjust to stressful events."

Digestive System

The digestive system is your pet's power plant. It converts food into the energy that keeps your dog or cat active. It's a big job, which is why the digestive system is so complicated and takes up so much room. The small intestine alone is about 3½ times the length of your pet's entire body.

The digestive tract has four main parts. Food slides down your pet's esophagus into the stomach, where it is mixed with powerful compounds that break it down into smaller parts. Then it moves into the small intestine, where the nutrients are absorbed into the bloodstream. What's left travels into the large intestine, where the last drops of fluid and nutrients are removed. The rest is stored as stool until it passes out of the body.

Unlike many parts of the body, the digestive system is always working. It doesn't matter whether your pet is digesting dinner or running around in the yard. The intestines are always contracting and expanding, churning food and mixing it with enzymes. At the same time, organs such as the pancreas and liver are creating hormones and digestive enzymes, making sure that harmful substances are filtered out and helpful substances are being used the way they should be. At the same time, the digestive system is constantly regulating blood sugars to keep metabolism and energy at a steady pitch.

Because the digestive system performs so many different jobs in so many locations, it is not always easy to tell when something is wrong. Pets with digestive problems may lose their appetites, vomit, or have changes in their stools. Sometimes the symptoms are more subtle—a little bit of cramping, an extra bit of gas, or temporary (and hard-to-detect) dips in energy. Or your pet may have a sudden increase in appetite that you can't understand, or she will start turning away from her food even though she always ate eagerly before.

The digestive system is so complex and is responsible for so many symptoms that the only way to be sure that something is wrong—and to find out exactly what it is—is to call your vet. You can do your part by taking note of any changes in your pet's usual routine, appetite, and so on. Is your pet hungrier than she used to be? Does she vomit only after meals or when she hasn't eaten for a while? Has her stool changed color or consistency? Is your pet more (or less) energetic than she used to be? Your vet can only do so much with lab tests and an exam. He will depend on you to provide many of the necessary clues.

Most digestive problems aren't serious. Nearly every pet will have diarrhea now and then or a bad case of gas or a sudden eruption of hair balls. Some dogs and cats aren't very careful about what they eat. They dig into the trash with the same enthusiasm that they show for a bowlful of premium canned food, and they lap up water from the most unsavory locations. It is not surprising that their digestive systems act up now and then.

Even though you would have to be an expert to understand all the potential digestive problems pets may encounter at some time in their lives, there are only a few that you have to understand and know how to recognize. Once you know what is normal for your pet and what things are likely to go wrong, you will have a pretty good idea of what you can do to help her feel better right away. Just as important, you will know what symptoms you can treat yourself and when you need to call your vet.

See Your Vet If:

- Pushing on your pet's belly causes her pain.
- Your dog or cat hasn't eaten for 24 hours or more.
- Her abdomen appears bloated.
- She has eaten rodent poison, antifreeze, houseplants, or other harmful substances.
- Your pet has been vomiting for more than a day or is vomiting blood.
- There are worms or other parasites in the stool.
- She has had diarrhea for 24 hours or more.
- There is blood in the stool or it looks dark and tarry.
- She is scooting across the floor, or the anal area looks swollen.
- Your pet has gained or lost substantial amounts of weight.
- She is having side effects from medication, like appetite loss or vomiting.
- There are growths in the anal area.
- There is a bulge in her throat.
- She is drooling much more than usual.
- Your pet vomits shortly after eating.

BLOAT

Clues

- Your dog's stomach suddenly expands.
- She tries but is unable to vomit.
- She is restless and may be drooling.

Vets aren't sure why it happens, but occasionally a dog's stomach may suddenly fill with air, doubling or even tripling in size within an hour. This condition, called bloat, is extremely serious because as the stomach expands, it can put pressure on the heart, kidneys, and other organs. If it is not stopped quickly, your pet could go into a shock, which is a life-threatening condition.

Fortunately, bloat is easy to recognize, says Howard Rothstein, D.V.M., a veterinarian in private practice in Saugerties, New York. "Her abdomen will be very hard, and it will look like it has a balloon in it," he says. In addition, dogs that are bloating will often be restless and trying (but not being able to) vomit. They will also be drooling, he says.

Even though vets have been studying bloat for more than 20 years, it is still something of a mystery. While any dog can bloat, it is most common in large, deep-chested dogs like Labrador retrievers, Doberman pinschers, and Great Danes. (Cats, however, don't get this condition.) Bloat may occur if your pet has vigorous exercise soon after eating or, conversely, if she eats soon after exercising. It can also occur when a dog eats or drinks a lot more than usual.

"I've usually seen bloating in dogs that gorged themselves—for instance, after getting into the bin where their food was stored," says Michael

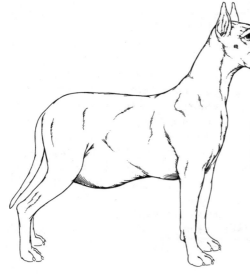

If your dog's abdomen suddenly swells and feels hard and drumlike, there is a good chance she is bloating, and you need to call your vet immediately.

Brothers, D.V.M., a veterinarian in private practice in Middletown, Connecticut.

Some dogs may be sensitive to certain brands of dry dog food. "If the kernels of food are filled with air, it may make some dogs more prone to bloat," says Dr. Brothers. In addition, there is some evidence that dogs with slow motility (the rate at which food moves through the intestine) are more likely to suffer from bloat than those that digest their food more quickly.

WHAT YOU CAN DO

If you even suspect that your dog is bloating, it is essential to get her to the vet right away since every minute counts. But you can also take some action to make sure that it doesn't happen in the first place.

One way to help prevent bloat is to feed your dog two or even three times a day instead of giving her the daily ration all at once, says Karen Mateyak, D.V.M., a veterinarian in private practice in Brooklyn, New York. Having less food in her stomach at one time will help prevent large amounts of air from accumulating. Since a puppy's stomach is so much smaller than a grown dog's, you have to be even more careful with them. As a rule, puppies under a year old should be fed *at least* three times a day, she says.

"I recommend not giving a dog a lot of food or water an hour before or after vigorous exercise," adds Dr. Mateyak. You have to be particularly careful during the warm months since a hot, thirsty dog can drink a lot of water at one time. Even though it is important to always have water available, you should only let your dog drink small amounts—say, one or two cups—soon after long walks or energetic romps. After a half-hour or so, you can let her have more water if she wants it.

Another way to help prevent bloat is to store dog food in a place where your voracious pet can't get to it, such as under the kitchen counter or in the basement. Otherwise, her eagerness to eat may inspire a search for the stockpile when you are not around.

If you usually feed your dog dry food, it is a good idea to moisten it with a little water and let it sit on the counter for 10 minutes before letting her eat, Dr. Mateyak says. "I like the food to swell up on the outside, not inside the dog."

WHAT YOUR VET WILL DO

Bloat is one condition that won't get you and your dog a backseat in the waiting room. When you get to the veterinarian's office, you will be rushed into an examination room almost immediately.

The first thing that your vet will do is flick a finger against the side of your dog's stomach. "If the animal is bloated, the stomach will be filled with air, and you will hear a hollow sound that resonates," says Dr. Brothers. The vet will also feel your dog's abdomen to see if the spleen or kidneys are where they are supposed to be. If they are not, there is a good chance that a swelling stomach has pushed them out of place.

Your vet will probably recommend x-rays to see how serious the problem really is. In some cases, for example, bloat simply causes the stomach to get distended with air. A more serious problem occurs when the stomach actually twists and kinks from all the pressure. Not only does this make it more difficult to get the trapped air out, it can also put pressure on nearby organs like the kidneys or spleen.

Once these tests are completed, your vet will have to work quickly to remove the air. This is usually done by inserting a tube through the dog's mouth and into the stomach. "I'll put a roll of tape in the dog's mouth so that I don't get bitten," says Dr. Brothers. "Then I'll put a tube through the opening in the roll of tape down to the stomach. This lets the air and water come out, takes the pressure off the internal organs, and decreases the potential for shock."

If your dog won't hold still for this procedure, your vet may take a shortcut and insert several large needles through the abdomen and into the stomach, which can help the air escape.

In some cases, removing the air is all that is required. More often, however, surgery is also necessary—either to unkink the stomach or to anchor it more firmly to the walls of the abdominal cavity, which will help prevent it from getting twisted if bloat occurs in the future. This is important because dogs that have an episode of bloat are likely to have another one later on, says Dr. Mateyak.

BLOOD IN STOOL

- The surface of your pet's stool has spots or smears of blood.
- His stool is dark and tarry-looking.

Few things are more frightening than seeing blood in the stool because this is sometimes a warning sign of cancer, at least in people. But in dogs and cats, it generally isn't quite that serious, says Michael Brothers, D.V.M., a veterinarian in private practice in Middletown, Connecticut. Still, blood in the stool is not normal; it always means that something is wrong.

When the blood is bright red and on the surface of the stool, there is a good chance that something sharp, like a bit of bone, scraped the lining of the large intestine and made it bleed. The bleeding may continue for a day or two, but it probably won't last much longer. Even small scrapes can cause a lot of bleeding, so don't be surprised when the stools appear quite red.

Blood in the stool may also be a sign of parasites, like whipworms, which are irritating the intestine wall. "They are like mosquitoes that make many tiny bites until your pet bleeds," says Dr. Brothers.

When the blood looks dark, dry, or tarry and is mixed with the stool, there may be a problem in the small intestine. Some viral infections can temporarily irritate the walls of the small intestine and make it bleed. Blood in the stool can also be a sign of colitis, an inflammation of the large intestine.

Finally, bleeding may be caused by an infection of the anal sacs—two sacs on either side of the anus that contain a strong liquid that pets use to mark their territory. These sacs normally empty whenever your pet has a bowel movement. When the sacs are infected, however, they don't empty the way they should, causing them to swell. Having a bowel movement can irritate the area, causing blood to flow.

WHAT YOU CAN DO

There is no reason to panic at the first sign of blood. Even though it looks scary, it usually isn't serious, anymore than a bloody nose is. "If you see just a few specks of red blood, I wouldn't worry about it," says Dr. Brothers. In most cases, the problem will be minor, and the bleeding will stop in a day or two.

In fact, you can often prevent bleeding by taking simple precautions. For starters, skip the bones, says David Tayman, D.V.M., a veterinarian in private practice in Columbia, Maryland. No matter how much your pet loves them, bones generally do more harm than good. As pets crunch them into small bits, the bones often get sharp edges that can damage the intestine. As an alternative, he suggests rawhide bones for dogs. Make sure your pet is supervised while chewing on rawhide bones to see that he is not ingesting large pieces. Or you can buy nylon bones at pet supply stores.

If you enjoy sewing, be sure to keep the sewing box closed since cats love playing with yarns and threads—and the attached needles. It is not uncommon for cats to actually swallow sewing supplies, which can cause serious bleeding, says Dr. Brothers. It's not only the needles that create problems. Thread and string can wrap around the intestines, causing serious problems.

Reducing your pets' exposure to parasites can be very helpful for preventing bleeding. One way to do this is simply to stop your pets from sniffing (or, worse, eating) other pets' stools. "Most parasites are contracted by sniffing the stool of other pets," says Howard Rothstein, D.V.M., a veterinarian in private practice in Saugerties, New York.

It is a good idea to clean the yard after every bowel movement and to scoop out the litter box every time it has been used. "That way they can't reinfect themselves," says Dr. Rothstein.

If you live in the country or go for hikes in the woods with your pet, pack enough water for the day—for you and him—since streams and ponds are common sources of parasites. Even stagnant water in your yard, under a rainspout, for example, may harbor parasites.

Even though blood in the stool usually indicates a minor problem, sometimes it is a serious warning sign. Don't take chances if there is a lot of blood or if the stool looks dark and tarry. Take a stool sample when you notice the problem, and make an appointment to see your vet as soon as possible, says Karen Mateyak, D.V.M., a veterinarian in private practice in Brooklyn New York. It's best if the sample is less than 24 hours old at the time of your appointment, she adds.

WHAT YOUR VET WILL DO

The appearance of the blood tells a lot about what the problem is, so your vet will ask a lot of questions: Was it bright red or a darker color? Were there just a few drops or a dramatic splash? Did it appear on the surface of the stool or was it mixed up inside?

Your vet will examine the stool sample under a microscope to see if there are parasites. This isn't as easy as it sounds since the only sign of some parasites will be their eggs, which only appear in stools periodically—the parasites themselves may be anchored inside the intestine. So even if the test is negative, your vet may ask you to bring additional stool samples on different days.

If parasites are the problem, there are a number of medications that will eliminate them, usually within 24 to 48 hours. You may be asked to repeat the treatment in three weeks and again in three months to make sure that the parasites don't come back.

When parasites don't appear to be the problem, your vet may take a look at the inside of your pet's intestines, using an instrument called an endoscope. This procedure can detect infections and other problems that may be causing the bleeding.

Anal sac infections are quite common, and, in most cases, easy to diagnose and treat. Most pets with infected anal sacs will need antibiotics to clear up the infection. Your vet will probably drain the sacs as well, which usually just takes a few seconds and can be done manually without special instruments or anesthetic.

In some cases, unfortunately, blood in the stool really is a sign of cancer. Your vet may use the endoscope to examine the pet's intestines for unusual lumps or growths. She may also check the outside of your pet to see if lumps have formed under the skin. If there are signs of cancer, your pet could need surgery, chemotherapy, or other treatments to bring it under control.

See also Chapter 9: Licking Hind End

SYMPTOM) BLOOD IN VOMIT

Clues

- Bloody vomit is accompanied by bleeding from her mouth, nose, or anus.
- Your pet is being treated for arthritis.
- The vomit resembles used coffee grounds.

It is not their most pleasant characteristic, but dogs and cats vomit much more often than people do. It is nature's way of coping with their free-wheeling appetites. They often eat things that don't agree with them, and as soon as they empty their stomachs, they feel better.

But when blood is coming up along with the vomit, you need to call your vet. Bloody vomit doesn't always indicate a serious problem, but sometimes it does—and moving quickly can make all the difference, says A. David Scheele, D.V.M., a veterinarian in private practice in Midland, Texas.

Stomach ulcers are often to blame, says Dan M. Jordan, D.V.M., a veterinarian in private practice in Houston. Pets with ulcers are typically being treated for arthritis or other long-term problems, and the medications they are taking, such as aspirin, are irritating their stomachs and causing bleeding. "We see more ulcers in older pets because they are the ones most likely to be taking the medications," he says. Blood that is vomited from the stomach usually resembles used coffee grounds, although in some cases it will be bright red, he adds.

Bleeding can also be caused by eating the wrong foods. Pets that raid the trash or root around in the compost pile may suffer from food poisoning and get miserably nauseated. Their retching can break blood vessels in the esophagus, the tube that carries food from the mouth to the stomach. This isn't a serious problem, but it will cause the vomit to look a little bloody.

One of the most serious—and all-too-common—causes of bloody vomit is getting into rodent poison. "These poisons can interfere with the blood-clotting process, which can cause bleeding," says Dr. Jordan. Pets that have eaten poison will often bleed from the mouth, nose, or anus as well.

Sometimes what appears to be bloody vomit is really bloody saliva caused by periodontal disease, for example, or a cut from a sharp bone or stick. "Pets are incredibly stoic and will often continue to eat with very sore teeth and gums," says Dr. Scheele. "You may not realize they have trouble until you see blood."

WHAT YOU CAN DO

You can't treat bleeding caused by periodontal disease at home, but you may be able to prevent it. Brushing your pet's teeth several times a week, or better yet, every day, is one of the greatest favors you can do for her. "Not only will you prevent the bleeding that may eventually occur with periodontal disease but you will also save her teeth," says Dr. Scheele.

There is no easy way to tame your pet's adventuresome appetite. What you can do is to provide safer things for her to raid. Most dogs enjoy gnawing on artificial bones from pet supply stores, which are much safer than meat bones or sticks, says Dr. Scheele. "If your dog has oral bleeding from chewing on rough or sharp objects, it is a good idea to soften her dry dog food for a few days by adding warm water and allowing the food to sit for 10 to 15 minutes," he adds. "This will give the gums a chance to heal. Or you can feed her a good quality canned food for a few days."

It is essential to put potentially dangerous items, from the kitchen trash to rodent bait, well out of reach. But dogs and cats are intrepid explorers, Dr. Jordan remarks. "No matter how carefully you place this poison, pets seem to find it." It is best to forget the poison and try some other means of pest control instead.

Even though blood in vomit isn't uncommon, you always need to call your vet, says Dr. Jordan. "Although it usually isn't caused by anything serious, sometimes it is, and then it can threaten your pet's life."

WHAT YOUR VET WILL DO

Depending how much blood your pet has lost (your vet can tell exactly by checking her blood pressure), she may need an emergency blood transfusion as soon as you bring her in. Once she is out of danger, your vet will run a variety of tests to see what is causing the bleeding. He will probably do blood tests to see if the blood is clotting properly and will take a stomach x-ray. In addition, he may need to do a procedure called endoscopy, in which a tube is inserted into your pet's stomach to see what's causing the bleeding. Endoscopy is uncomfortable, and your pet will need to be sedated first.

If your pet has gotten into the type of rodent poison that causes bleeding, she will probably be given an injection of vitamin K_1, says Dr. Jordan. This should eventually reverse the effects.

Pets with ulcers are usually treated with the same types of medications that people take. These drugs work in different ways. Some reduce the amount of acid that is present in the stomach, while others lay down a protective layer to coat the stomach lining. Of course, your vet will also want to know why your pet is getting ulcers in the first place. When they are caused by harsh medications, he will try to find another drug that will provide the same benefits without the side effects.

BOWEL-CONTROL PROBLEMS

Clues

- Your pet is having trouble walking.
- There have been changes in her diet.
- There has been a recent change in your routine.
- The litter box is in a new location.

You expect puppies and kittens to make mistakes, but when an older, well-trained pet leaves a surprise on the living-room floor or behind the drapes, you know that something is wrong.

Anything that upsets their digestion can cause a loss of bowel control. Dogs and cats are very sensitive to changes in their diets. If you have recently begun giving them a different food or feeding them leftovers, they could have diarrhea that is impossible to hold in. Unauthorized trips to the garbage may also upset their stomachs.

It probably doesn't happen often, but some pets may "lose" control as a way of telling you that they are unhappy, says Michael Brothers, D.V.M., a veterinarian in private practice in Middletown, Connecticut. Dogs—and cats, too (despite their feline independence)—crave your attention and are unhappy when they don't get enough of it. They aren't able to talk things out and tell you what they want. So if something has interrupted your usual loving routine, such as when you are working longer hours or are spending more time with people than with them, they may decide to leave you a sign of their displeasure. "They realize that it is a way to get back at their owners," he says.

For cats, bowel-control problems may be caused by problems with the litter box. Leaving dirty litter in the box, for instance, is like putting out a Do Not Enter sign. If you have more than one cat, box sharing can cause problems since cats often refuse to use a litter box that has had another visitor. Even moving the litter box to a new location, such as near the food bowl, can cause cats to take their business elsewhere. The same is true if the litter box is too far away. A cat that spends her days in the living room may not want to walk down a flight of stairs to use a litter box in the basement.

There are a number of physical problems that can also cause pets to have poor bowel control. Dogs and cats with arthritis, for example, simply may find it too painful walk to the door or the litter box. And it is not uncommon for older pets to have less bowel control than they had when they were younger. In fact, they may be just as surprised as you are when they discover what they have done.

WHAT YOU CAN DO

Since pets that are unhappy or lonely may start having accidents, the solution may be as simple as giving them a little extra attention, says Dr. Brothers. "When you are at home, try to take your dog out every couple of hours," he says. (It is especially helpful to take them out 20 to 30 minutes after eating since that is when the urge to have a bowel movement is strongest.) Plan some extra play sessions. Even taking a few minutes to groom them once or twice a day will reassure them that they are still important in your life.

Even slight changes in your pet's diet can cause bowel-control problems. It is a good idea to give your pets the same food all the time. If you do change brands or try another food, make the change gradually by mixing a little bit of the new food in with their old. By phasing in the new diet over a period of weeks, they are much less likely to have digestive complaints that can lead to messes.

For older pets, it is a good idea to give them "senior" foods containing high-quality protein made from fish, meat, or poultry. Some vets also recommend giving older pets premium foods such as Hill's Science Diet Canine Senior, which are easier to digest than the standard supermarket brands, says Karen Mateyak, D.V.M., a veterinarian in private practice in Brooklyn.

Whatever you do, don't give in to those sad eyes and pass along a delectable bit of meat or other treats from the family's table, says Howard Rothstein, D.V.M., a veterinarian in private practice in Saugerties, New York. Human foods are really too rich for pets, and tonight's treat can easily become tomorrow's headache for you.

For cats, keeping the litter box clean is the best way to encourage them to use it more often. Vets advise removing solid wastes every day and replacing the litter every three to four days, washing the box well with soap and water before pouring the fresh litter in. Another strategy is to put an extra litter box in the house so that your cat always has a place nearby. And don't change brands of litter too often. Cats like things to be predictable, and changing litter can cause them to express their displeasure in an unmistakable way.

When your pet does make a mess, clean the area thoroughly with an odor-removing spray or liquid, such as Lambert Kay Pet Odor Destroyer. "Dogs and cats are sniffing constantly, and if they smell a place where they have soiled before, they may think that they can do it again," says Dr. Brothers.

Finally, if your pet seems to be in pain and is having trouble getting around, get her to a vet right away. Her messes could be a warning sign that something more serious is going on.

WHAT YOUR VET WILL DO

Since bowel-control problems are sometimes caused by emotional turmoil, your vet will want to know if there have been big changes in either of your lives. Did you recently get a new pet? Are you spending more time away from home? Is there a new baby in the house? If your pet's loss of control occurred at about the same time as your lifestyle changes, you will have a pretty good idea of what the problem is.

The most important thing, of course, is to discover if there is a physical problem that is making your pet lose control. Your vet will probably ask that you bring in a stool sample (it should be no more than 24 hours old) so that he can test for parasites. If this turns out to be the problem, consider yourself lucky, says Dr. Rothstein. Parasites are easy to get rid of with the appropriate medications.

There are a number of serious problems, including cancer, that can cause a loss of bowel control. Your vet will probably perform a rectal examination to see if there are any lumps or growths inside the rectal area. If any are found, your pet will probably need surgery to remove them.

Don't be surprised if during the visit your vet walks to the far end of the hallway and watches as you and your pet walk toward him. He will be watching to see if your pet is stiff or has trouble moving, which can be signs of joint or spinal problems. If your pet does have trouble walking, your vet may recommend anti-inflammatory medicines, which can help her stay more limber. "Sometimes we also give a shot of cortisone to help relieve the pain," says Dr. Brothers.

See also Chapter 6: Diarrhea

CONSTIPATION

Clues

- The litter box is dirty.
- Your pet is trying to have bowel movements with increasing frequency.
- He has been chewing on splintery bones.
- He is drinking or exercising less than usual.

If anything, most dogs and cats are a little bit *too* regular, which is why you have to change a cat's litter box every day or let the dog out at 2:30 A.M. But sometimes they wait . . . and wait. Then, when they finally do have a bowel movement, they have to strain to get things done.

In pets (as in people), constipation that lasts a day or two isn't a serious problem. They will return to normal soon enough, says Karen Mateyak, D.V.M., a veterinarian in private practice in Brooklyn, New York.

In cats, constipation sometimes occurs if they have swallowed too much hair during their normal grooming. When hair gets into the digestive tract, it binds to the stool, making it harder and more difficult to pass.

Cats can be extremely fussy about their litter boxes, Dr. Mateyak adds. "If the cat box is dirty, they may not want to use it," she says. While they are waiting for fresh litter, stool in the intestine is getting dry and hard, which will make it difficult to pass later on.

Take note of when your cat is making frequent trips to the litter box but without any results. "A cat that is constantly straining may be suffering from obstipation"—a severe form of constipation in which the stool won't move without a veterinarian's help, says Alan Green, D.V.M., a veterinarian in private practice in Katonah, New York.

In dogs, constipation may be caused by their snacking habits. When your dog munches bones, for example, he may swallow small particles that irritate the large intestine, causing stools to move more slowly, says Dr. Green. In addition, bone chips may bond together into rock-hard lumps, making stools especially difficult to pass. This tends to be a problem with smaller dogs since their digestive tracts can be upset even by small particles.

Both dogs and cats may get constipated when they don't get enough to drink. The intestines need large amounts of water to keep things moving smoothly. When water levels fall, stools get harder and drier and are more likely to stay in place.

One of the most common causes of constipation for both dogs and cats is not getting enough exercise, says Dr. Mateyak. If your pet has been lounging on a windowsill or sleeping under the kitchen table all week, his entire body, including the digestive tract, will slow down. "And the longer they hold the stool in, the harder it gets," she says.

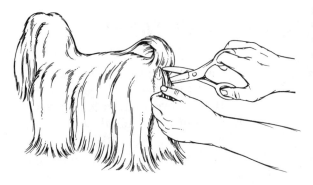

Keeping your pet's backside neatly trimmed will make it easier for stools to get out. Just be sure to use a pair of blunt-tipped scissors so that you don't accidentally cut this delicate area.

You wouldn't think that your pet's hairstyle could cause constipation, but in cats and small dogs it may be a problem. When hair around the back end gets long and unruly, it can literally block the passage of stool, making bowel movements painful. Simply keeping the hairs trimmed will help prevent this from happening, says Dr. Mateyak.

Finally, constipation may be a warning sign of other, more serious problems, such as kidney disease, infected anal sacs (two sacs on either side of the anus that contain a strong-smelling liquid that pets use to mark their territory), or muscle weakness caused by old age or other conditions. In addition, what looks like constipation may in fact be something else, like a hernia.

WHAT YOU CAN DO

One of the easiest ways to treat and prevent constipation is simply to give your pets more water, says Dr. Mateyak. No matter what is causing the constipation, drinking more water will help lubricate the intestine so that stools pass more easily.

Of course, you can't make your pets drink when they don't feel like it. But if you make sure that water is always available, they will naturally get enough, says Michael Brothers, D.V.M., a veterinarian in private practice in Middletown, Connecticut.

Another way to relieve constipation is to get more fiber in their diets. Since fiber isn't absorbed by the body, it passes more or less intact into the large intestine, where it absorbs large amounts of water. As the stools get larger and softer, the body gets the message that it is time to move them along.

To add fiber, mix two to three teaspoons of bran flakes in their food. Or give them a few tablespoons of canned pumpkin (preferably the kind with no added ingredients) once a day until the constipation ends. "Canned pumpkin is high in fiber, and they like the taste," says David Tayman, D.V.M., a veterinarian in private practice in Columbia, Maryland.

Another strategy is to give them a little bit of Metamucil. This over-the-counter product contains psyllium, which is very high in fiber. For cats and small dogs, give about a half-teaspoon of Metamucil twice a day. For larger pets, give one to two teaspoons twice a day until they pass a normal stool, advises Dr. Mateyak. To be safe, ask your vet what dose is right for your pet.

While giving your pet more fiber will help relieve constipation, keep in mind that bones are not on the list of fibrous foods. If your dog enjoys munching on bones, try giving him nylon bones that you can buy at a pet supply store.

Getting more exercise will often prevent constipation. And it doesn't take a lot to get the benefits. Going for a walk or having a vigorous play session once or twice a day for 15 minutes will help speed up your pet's metabolism and keep the digestive system working smoothly.

For cats, it is essential to keep the litter box clean. "You should scoop it out once a day and clean the whole thing once or twice a week," says Dr. Mateyak. In addition, be sure to brush your cat every day since the less loose hair he has in his coat, the less he will swallow during grooming. You may also want to buy an over-the-counter hair-ball remedy available at pet supply stores or from your vet, which will help prevent hairs from accumulating in the digestive tract.

WHAT YOUR VET WILL DO

Constipation usually isn't a serious problem. But when it doesn't go away within a few days, your vet may decide to clear things out.

She may begin with an x-ray to see what's going on inside and then follow that with an enema. Enemas often require an overnight stay at the veterinarian's office. "Animals often have to be anesthetized to sit still for an enema," says Dr. Mateyak.

If the enema doesn't help, your vet may prescribe a laxative such as Propulsid, which lubricates the digestive tract and stimulates the large intestine so that it works more vigorously. And since constipation may be caused by dehydration, your vet may give your pet intravenous liquids as well. Even if your pet isn't dehydrated, the extra fluids can help the intestine work more efficiently.

See also Chapter 5: Crying While Using the Litter Box

DIARRHEA

Clues

- Your dog has been raiding the trash.
- Your pet has been eating table scraps or unfamiliar foods.
- He has been exposed to parasites.

Perhaps the worst thing about diarrhea is the element of surprise: It often comes on so quickly that even conscientious pets aren't always able to make it outside or to the litter box in time.

Dogs and cats have sensitive digestive tracts. When they eat something that they shouldn't—from leftovers in the trash to a shoelace they found on the floor of the closet—the body tries to get rid of it, and diarrhea can be the messy result. Cats occasionally get diarrhea, but it is much more common in dogs, mainly because of their adventuresome appetites, says Alan Green, D.V.M., a veterinarian in private practice in Katonah, New York.

"We see a lot of diarrhea in dogs around Thanksgiving and Christmas because people give them high-fat foods that they don't usually eat," adds Dr. Green.

Diarrhea isn't caused only by your pet's culinary indiscretions. It can also be a sign of tapeworms, hookworms, or other parasites, which interfere with the body's absorption of nutrients, says Dr. Green. Diarrhea caused by parasites is more common in puppies and kittens than in older pets because their immune systems aren't yet strong enough to keep the pests under control.

Less often, diarrhea is a symptom of other, more serious illnesses, like parvovirus (an intestinal infection in dogs), kidney disease, diabetes, or an inflammation of the large intestine. When diarrhea lasts longer than a day or two, it could mean that something is seriously wrong, and you should call your vet right away, says Dr. Green.

WHAT YOU CAN DO

Since diarrhea is the body's way of saying no thanks to food or water in the digestive tract, you can often stop it simply by putting your pet on a one-day fast, says Karen Mateyak, D.V.M., a veterinarian in private practice in Brooklyn, New York. Fasting lets the digestive system rest, reducing the irritation that is causing the diarrhea.

Assuming your pet is healthy in every other respect, don't feed him food for 24 hours. But be sure to keep plenty of water available for him throughout the day. Water eliminates the risk of dehydration.

Fasting isn't recommended for puppies, kittens, or small dogs since they may not have enough sugar reserves to tide them over until they eat again, Dr. Green adds.

After your pet has fasted for a day, you can begin giving him small amounts of baby food. "It's bland, very digestible, and extremely nutritious," says Dr. Green. "Most dogs and cats will devour it." They like it so much, in fact, they will probably beg for more, but don't give in or the problems may start all over again.

The best baby foods are those containing lamb or poultry. (Avoid baby foods made with vegetables since they can make the diarrhea worse.) Dr. Mateyak recommends giving cats and small dogs a jar of baby food a day, spread over two or three feedings. Medium-size dogs can eat two jars a day, and larger dogs can have three jars.

An alternative to baby food is to boil some chicken or hamburger and mix it with cooked white rice. Like baby food, it is very easy to digest. Each serving should contain about one-third meat and two-thirds rice, says Dr. Mateyak.

After your pet's stool has returned to normal, you can start giving him small amounts of his usual food, mixing it with the baby food. Gradually start giving him more and more of his usual food until he is back on his regular diet.

For severe diarrhea, vets sometimes advise limiting for about 12 hours the amount of water that your pet is allowed to drink. You want him to have *some* water, however, to replace the body's essential fluids that diarrhea takes out and to soothe his dry mouth. Dr. Mateyak recommends giving him one ice cube every hour. Many dogs and cats enjoy munching ice, and it is a great way to get additional water into their systems without giving them too much.

You can often control diarrhea with diet alone, but sometimes you need to stop it fast. "I'd use Pepto-Bismol or Imodium A-D right away," says Harold Rothstein, D.V.M, a veterinarian in private practice in Saugerties, New York. When using Pepto-Bismol, give one-half tablespoon of the liquid for every 15 pounds of dog, two or three times a day, he says. For Imodium A-D, give one teaspoon of the liquid for every 15 pounds of dog, two or three times a day.

Neither of these medications should be given to cats, he adds, since they contain ingredients that can be toxic to them.

Diarrhea isn't difficult to treat, and preventing it is even easier. If your pet is having any kind of bowel-control problem, including diarrhea, don't give him snacks from the dinner table since human foods are really too rich for him to digest. And if your pet is an incorrigible scrounger, keep the garbage can away from nose level or at least make sure that it has a tight-fitting lid.

It's not always easy to do, but you should try to protect your pet from harmful parasites like tapeworms and hookworms. If your cat is a hunter, for example, you may want to keep him inside or fit him with a bell collar to scare off birds and mice since they often harbor parasites. You will also want to keep the yard clean since dogs often get parasites from nosing (or eating) other pets' wastes, says Dr. Rothstein. Finally, keep your pets away from pond water or stagnant streams, which are breeding grounds for many parasites. Even stagnant water in your yard may be contaminated, he adds.

What Your Vet Will Do

Before you take your pet to the vet, collect a recent stool specimen, which can be used to check for parasites, says David Tayman, D.V.M., a veterinarian in private practice in Columbia, Maryland. Parasites are killed relatively easily with prescription medications, he says. Don't spend money on over-the-counter worming medications, however, because they are usually not as effective as drugs that you will get from the vet, and they only work for certain kinds of worms, he says.

If your vet suspects that something is wrong in the intestine, she may use an instrument called an endoscope to take a peek inside. In addition, she may run blood tests to see if something serious—like internal bleeding or problems with the kidneys or other organs—is causing the diarrhea.

When diarrhea has been severe, your vet may keep your pet overnight, giving him extra fluids through an intravenous tube. In most cases, however, your pet will go home right away and will probably be better within a few days.

See also Chapter 6: Bowel-Control Problems

FLATULENCE

Clues

- There are white specks or round strands in your pet's stool.
- You have been feeding your pet milk.
- He has been losing weight or having diarrhea.

Your pet's digestive tract is full of enzymes and bacteria, which the body uses to transform kibble into energy. A little gas is a natural part of this process. When your pet is unusually flatulent, however, or the smell is unusually foul, you can be pretty sure that something is putting his bowel out of balance.

"A gassy pet is often a worm-infested pet," says John Brooks, D.V.M., a veterinarian in private practice in Fork, Maryland. Tapeworms and roundworms are often to blame because they irritate the lining of the intestine and interfere with proper digestion. White specks or spaghetti-like strands in the stool are common signs of worms, he explains.

When worms aren't to blame, your pet's diet often is. Many pet foods contain beans, bran, whole wheat, and fat, which are difficult for the body's digestive enzymes to break down. As a result, these and other ingredients collect in the colon and ferment, causing large amounts of gas.

Also, dogs and cats love milk, but it doesn't love them back. Many pets, like humans, lack the enzyme (lactase) that the body uses to digest the sugar (lactose) in milk, says Jane Brunt, D.V.M., a veterinarian in private practice in Towson, Maryland. A bowl of milk will often make dogs and cats very gassy, she explains. They may have diarrhea as well.

Food allergies cause problems, too, says Dr. Brooks. If your pet is allergic to ingredients in his chow, the intestines won't work as well as they should. Eating too fast can also cause gas because pets will swallow a lot of air, which has to go somewhere—so out it goes, many times a day.

Dogs don't always discriminate between an open garbage can and their food dish, and spoiled, smelly food doesn't get sweeter when it wafts into the air hours after a garbage raid. Cats don't go after trash as much as dogs do, although canned cat food can also cause some fairly noxious emissions.

It takes a healthy intestinal tract to absorb nutrients properly. Pets that are sick with intestinal viruses, intestinal cancer, or other digestive problems will often have a lot of flatulence. Pancreatic problems may also be to blame. The pancreas is the organ responsible for producing digestive enzymes. When it isn't working well, your pet won't properly digest his food, causing gas, loose stools, and possibly weight loss, explains Dr. Brunt.

What You Can Do

When your pet is especially odoriferous, write down everything that he has had to eat in the last 24 hours, suggests Jim Hendrickson, V.M.D., a veterinarian in emergency private practice in Rockville, Maryland. If you discover a connection, perhaps he is only gassy after eating his favorite treats, you will know what to avoid in the future.

Your vet may recommend changing his entire diet. Try giving him easy-to-digest foods like cottage cheese and rice for a few days, suggests Dr. Hendrickson. If the air clears, you will know that food was causing the fumes, and you may want to put him on a new diet permanently. One commercial food that is very digestible is Hill's Prescription Diet I/D. Or check with your vet about other foods, either homemade or store-bought, that may help.

If you have more than one pet, it is smart to feed them separately. Otherwise, they often gobble their food to make sure the other one doesn't get it. Feeding them one at a time or in different rooms allows them to eat more slowly, and they will then swallow less air. Feeding them several small meals a day instead of one big meal can also reduce greedy gobbling, says Joanne Hibbs, D.V.M., a veterinarian in private practice in Powell, Tennessee. Some vets advise putting a large object, such as a baseball, in the bowl. This forces the pet to eat more slowly as he nibbles around the ball.

As a last resort, you might want to ask your vet about a product called CurTail. Available from vets, it contains digestive enzymes that help the intestines work more efficiently. Adolph's Tenderizer has a similar effect. "That's usually what I try first," says Dr. Brooks. He recommends using one-half teaspoon per cup of food, mixing it in, and letting it sit for 10 minutes to give it time to work.

What Your Vet Will Do

Flatulence that occurs frequently should always be checked by a vet. But before you go to her office, collect a fresh stool sample. This will allow your vet to test for worms or other parasites, says Dr. Brooks. She will also check the stool for undigested fats, which are a sign of pancreatic problems.

Worms are easy to treat. Your vet will probably prescribe an oral medication containing fenbendazole (Panacur), which eliminates worms in three days, says Dr. Brooks. Pancreatic problems are potentially serious, but they also may be easy to treat, in some cases, just by giving your pet digestive enzymes to replace the ones that he is not making on his own.

Finally, when flatulence is accompanied by serious diarrhea or weight loss, your vet may recommend taking a biopsy of the bowel to check for cancer or inflammatory bowel disease.

SPECKS IN STOOL

Clues

- Your pet has been eating stools, either in the yard or from the litter box.
- She often eats bones or sticks.

Dogs and cats aren't always careful about what they eat, which is why almost anything—from bone chips to buttons to strips of aluminum foil—can appear in their stools. "What comes out is exactly what's taken in," says Michael Brothers, D.V.M., a veterinarian in private practice in Middletown, Connecticut.

Most of the time, specks in the stool are simply food particles that weren't digested, like the whole corn in some dog foods or bits of fat from the leftovers that you slipped in her breakfast bowl.

If your pets spend a lot of time outdoors or manage to catch mice or birds, specks in the stool are frequently a sign of roundworms or tapeworms. Although tapeworms live inside the intestine, they periodically shed small portions of their bodies, which appear in the stool. Roundworms, however, come out whole. They look like strands of thin spaghetti, while tapeworms look like flattened bits of rice.

WHAT YOU CAN DO

Since specks that appear in the stool are most likely food particles, you probably don't have to worry about them, says Craig N. Carter, D.V.M., Ph.D., head of epidemiology at the Texas Veterinary Medical Diagnostic Laboratory at Texas A&M University in College Station. On the other hand, the specks mean that your pet's food isn't being thoroughly digested, and you may want to ask your vet if a premium food might be a better choice.

It is still a good idea, however, to take a close look now and then because specks in the stool can tell you what your pet has been getting into—and whether you need to be concerned. "If your dog is passing little bits of twigs, I wouldn't worry about it," says Dr. Brothers.

If you see bits of bone, however, you will know that your pet has been swallowing sharp, abrasive particles that could damage the digestive tract—and you would be wise to limit her munching to safer things, like the nylon bones that you can get in pet supply stores. says David Tayman, D.V.M., a veterinarian in private practice in Columbia, Maryland.

Parasites, of course, can also be a problem. While there is little that you can do to treat parasites at home,because over-the-counter remedies don't work as well as medicines that you get from your vet, there are ways to prevent them from getting into your pet's system. One of the easiest things is simply to keep the yard clean since many pets get worms from nosing (or eating) stools, says Howard Rothstein, D.V.M., a veterinarian in private practice in Saugerties, New York.

WHAT YOUR VET WILL DO

If you can't identify the specks in your pet's stools, you may want to collect a sample and take it, along with your pet, to the veterinarian's office. (Stool samples should be no more than a day old.)

If your pet does have intestinal parasites, your vet will give you a prescription for a deworming medication. This is given orally and will clear things up within a few days. Or he may recommend switching to a heartworm medication that also contains ingredients that kill common intestinal parasites.

A more worrisome situation is when specks in the stool appear to be coming from a larger object still inside. Your vet may recommend an x-ray to see what, if anything, is inside her digestive tract. Even if your pet has swallowed something that she shouldn't have, like a large stone or a piece of wood, it isn't necessarily a problem. In fact, it will probably pass on its own without causing further difficulties.

If the object is unusually large, however, or it looks like it might damage her insides, your vet may recommend surgery to remove it, rather than letting it pass on its own. "Once we did surgery on a dog and found a pair of chopsticks inside," says Dr. Brothers.

See also Chapter 4: Eating Objects

VOMITING

Clues

- Vomiting occurs first thing in the morning.
- Your cat does a lot of grooming.

Pet food isn't very appealing (to humans, that is) even when it is fresh from the store. It is a lot less appealing when it reappears on the carpet.

For dogs in particular, who often love nothing better than a snack from the garbage can, vomiting may be nothing more than a bad restaurant review. The combination of rancid food and overindulgence can empty their stomachs in a hurry, says Joanne Hibbs, D.V.M., a veterinarian in private practice in Powell, Tennessee.

Dogs have another unappetizing trait. They will occasionally greet the day by bringing up a little yellow liquid. This "bilious vomiting" is caused by going all night without food and getting an upset stomach. It isn't serious; once your dog throws up, he will feel just fine again, says Dr. Hibbs.

Cats aren't prone to this kind of vomiting, and they are a lot less likely than dogs to raid the trash. They do, however, spend hours grooming themselves, swallowing a lot of hair in the process. When the hair doesn't pass through the digestive tract, it irritates the stomach and comes back up.

Ulcers and bacterial infections can also cause dogs and cats to vomit. You should suspect that your pet has an ulcer when the vomit looks black and grainy, like used coffee grounds. This is a sign that your pet is throwing up digested blood, and he needs to see a vet, says Dr. Hibbs.

Vomiting can also be caused by more-serious conditions like cancer, infections, or problems with the liver or pancreas, says Dr. Hibbs. Vomiting is a common symptom of poisoning as well. If your pet vomits time after time or if he seems dizzy or disoriented, call your vet right away.

WHAT YOU CAN DO

Except for keeping the lid to the garbage closed, there isn't a lot you can do to stop your dog from adventuresome dining. Dogs prone to "morning sickness," however, will often feel better if you give them a few dry dog biscuits or another bedtime snack, says Dr. Hibbs. If he needs a little more help, you can give a little Maalox to neutralize stomach acid.

You can give a 60-pound dog one tablet (no more than eight tablets a day), a 30-pound dog one-half tablet (no more than four tablets a day), and a 15-pound dog one-quarter tablet (no more than two tablets per day), says Dr. Carter. Be sure to consult your vet before giving antacids on a regular basis, however. Antacids will reduce the effectiveness of tetracycline, which is often prescribed for Lyme disease.

For cats with the habit of heaving hair balls, there are several remedies

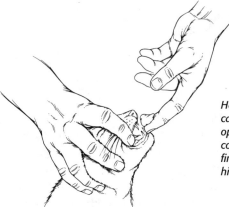

Hair-ball remedies are effective, but many cats won't swallow them. To get the gel down, open your cat's mouth by gently pressing the corners of his jaw with your thumb and fore-finger. Use your other hand to coat the roof of his mouth with the gel.

you may want to try. "I like Vetasyl, which comes as a gelatin capsule filled with powdered fiber," says Jane Brunt, D.V.M., a veterinarian in private practice in Towson, Maryland. Available from vets, Vetasyl helps keep the stomach full and calm and helps hair balls move through the system more quickly.

Another option is to use hair-ball remedies that come in the form of a gooey gel, which lubricates the hair so that it passes through the digestive tract with less irritation. Put a dab on your finger and wipe it on the roof of his mouth. Don't bother putting it on his paws, Dr. Brunt adds. "That just annoys your cat and makes a mess."

One of the best ways to stop hair balls for good is to brush your cat at least once a day. Hair that is brushed away can't get swallowed—or vomited up later on, says J. M. Tibbs, D.V.M., a veterinarian in private practice in District Heights, Maryland.

What Your Vet Will Do

Some vomiting is normal, but when it occurs frequently, there is probably a problem. Veterinarians have identified more than 70 different causes of vomiting, many of them quite serious. Your vet is likely to take blood samples to check for kidney disease, infection, or other whole-body illnesses. She may recommend x-rays to see if your pet's digestive system is blocked or if there are lumps that may be intestinal cancer.

Since there are many possible causes of vomiting, there are also many cures. For ulcers, your vet may prescribe an acid-lowering drug such as ranitidine (Zantac) or a medication that protects the stomach lining such as sucralfate (Carafate). For poisoning or other serious problems, your pet will need further tests and may need to be hospitalized.

See also Chapter 6: Blood in Vomit

COMMON DIGESTIVE SYSTEM CONDITIONS

Exocrine pancreatic insufficiency. The pancreas is a small, complex organ that produces powerful chemicals that dogs and cats (and humans) need to survive. One part of the pancreas secretes insulin, the hormone that helps the body absorb the sugars found in foods. The rest of the pancreas secretes enzymes that are shipped to the intestines to aid in digestion.

When the pancreas doesn't produce enough of these digestive enzymes (a condition called exocrine pancreatic insufficiency), food will pass through the intestines without being broken down and absorbed. Pets with this condition will be hungry all the time. They will also lose weight and pass large amounts of soft, poorly formed stools. The stools may look greasy because of the large amounts of undigested fats they contain.

Without treatment, this is an extremely serious condition. Once it has been diagnosed, however, it is very easy to manage. Generally, all you will need to do is add a pancreatic replacement enzyme, such as Viokase or Prozyme, to your pet's food each time she eats, says Grant Nisson, D.V.M., a veterinarian in private practice in West River, Maryland.

Hair balls. Cats get a lot of pleasure from grooming and will spend hours luxuriating in self-engrossed cat-baths. Not surprisingly, they swallow a lot of hair. Fur doesn't digest well, so it often stays in the stomach until, with a lot of noisy retching, it is propelled back up again.

Hair balls aren't pleasant for cats or for people, but these fur-and-fluid concoctions aren't usually a problem. "It's the hair that doesn't get thrown up that is the biggest worry," says Joanne Hibbs, D.V.M., a veterinarian in private practice in Powell, Tennessee. Hair in the stomach often passes into the intestine, where it can create a blockage that requires surgery to remove.

Most cats don't have any trouble coughing up hair balls. If the wad of fur is too large, however, it can get stuck on the way up, possibly blocking the flow of air. It is normal for cats to make loud, dramatic noises when vomiting up hair balls. But if your cat is also pawing frantically at her face, her gums are turning blue, or she passes out, get her to the vet emergency room immediately, says Dr. Hibbs.

Intestinal obstructions. Dogs and cats don't always think before they eat. "I've seen pets eat gloves, panty hose, corncobs, string, and lots of other indigestible stuff," says Dr. Hibbs. Unfortunately, the inside of your pet's digestive tract is smaller than her mouth, which means that things that slide down the hatch don't always pass through the other end.

You should suspect that your pet has something blocking the digestive tract if she is trying to vomit but isn't bringing much up or if she is straining without success to pass a stool. Her abdomen may be tender, and she may be contorting herself into unusual positions to reduce painful pressure on her insides.

It is not uncommon for foreign objects in the digestive tract to move around, causing the blockages to come and go. Dogs have big stomachs, for example, and a ball or some other object can drift around for a long time without causing symptoms until it blocks the outlet to the intestines. These occasional obstructions are not as serious as complete ones, but in the long run they can still make your pet very sick.

Cats often swallow thread or string, adds Dr. Hibbs. When strings get into the digestive tract, they can wrap around the intestines, sometimes cutting them open.

In most cases, surgery is the only way to remove foreign objects from the digestive tract. "Once the obstruction is out, pets usually get well very quickly," says Dr. Nisson.

Pancreatitis. Another illness that can affect the pancreas is pancreatitis, in which its powerful digestive enzymes, rather than being sent to the intestines, spill inside the pancreas itself. When this happens, they begin digesting tissue in the same way they would pet food.

A number of infections, including feline infectious peritonitis (FIP) and toxoplasmosis, can cause pancreatitis, but most of the time vets don't know what is behind it, says Dr. Hibbs. It is most common in middle-aged, overweight pets, and it often begins right after a fatty meal or snack. Pets with a sudden onset of pancreatitis will vomit violently and have diarrhea, and their bellies may be very tender. Pets with a milder, long-term form of this condition won't appear quite as sick, but they will have similar symptoms for months or even years.

The treatment for pancreatitis depends on how sick your pet already is. If she has a mild case, your vet may recommend putting her on a 24-hour fast, followed by a week of small, bland meals. After that, she should be okay, says Dr. Hibbs. In more serious cases, your pet will need to be hospitalized, put on a fast, and given intravenous fluids and injections of antibiotics.

Parasites. The digestive tracts of dogs and cats are warm, dark, and full of nutrients—perfect havens for hookworms, tapeworms, giardia, and other parasites.

Pet can often have parasites for years without having any symptoms whatsoever. But when the parasites thrive and multiply, they can cause weight loss, bloody stools, weakness, and fatigue. "They irritate the bowel, so your pet can't absorb the nutrients from her food," says Dr. Nisson. Parasites such as hookworms also suck blood, which can make pets anemic and weak.

Most parasites are highly contagious. The eggs are shed in the stool, which contaminates the ground and water. When your pet drinks contaminated water or runs across grass and then licks her feet, she will ingest the eggs and get infected herself. Tapeworms, which are among the most common parasites, are transmitted differently. They live inside fleas as well as in rabbits, mice, and other rodents. When dogs and cats lick themselves and swallow an infected flea or if they regularly hunt outdoors, they will eventually come down with tapeworms.

Pet supply stores sell a number of medications for controlling parasites, but they are mainly designed to kill roundworms and hookworms and won't touch other parasites, says Dr. Nisson. The only way to be sure that you are using the right medication is to take a fresh stool sample to your vet. Knowing what parasites your pet has will make them much easier to treat.

Parasitic worms can be killed with a drug called fenbendazole (Panacur), which is available by prescription from vets. Non-worm parasites such as coccidia and giardia are treated with antibiotics. Your vet has other medications to choose from as well.

When fighting worms, don't forget about the next generation. It is important to clean up stools in the yard, says Dr. Nisson. It is also a good idea to wash your pet's food and water dishes often and to keep your house and yard as flea-free as possible.

Parvovirus. If you have ever seen a puppy with full-fledged parvo, you won't soon forget it. This viral infection can make pets miserably ill, causing yellow or white foamy vomit and bloody diarrhea.

For all its fearsome power, parvovirus hasn't been around very long. Vets believe that a virus that originally caused diarrhea in cats mutated in the late 1970s. It quit bothering cats and began infecting dogs. Any dog can get parvovirus, but it is most common in puppies 16 weeks and younger, probably because their immune systems aren't fully developed. Vets aren't sure why, but certain breeds such as Rottweilers, Doberman pinschers, and English springer spaniels tend to get exceptionally ill when they get parvo.

As with many viral infections, parvo is highly contagious. Particles of the virus are shed from the body in the stool and are readily passed from dog to dog. It is an extremely serious illness that requires prompt treatment. "Parvo kills a lot of dogs each year, so if you suspect that your dog might have it, see a vet right away," says Dr. Hibbs.

Dogs with mild cases of parvovirus are usually treated with antibiotics at home. In more serious cases, dogs may need to be hospitalized in order to receive intravenous fluids and injections of antibiotics.

Even though the virus that causes parvo is very common in the environment, the illness is easy to prevent by getting your dog vaccinated once a year. "This is a bad disease, so avoid it if you can," says Dr. Hibbs.

Ears

Cats and dogs are known for their exquisite sense of hearing. No matter where they are in the house, they perk up when they hear the rustle of a bag or the whir of a can opener. Even when pets are snoozing, their ears will move around to pick up the slightest sounds.

Those ears are sensitive to more than just sounds, however. They are also sensitive to health problems. "This is especially true in dogs, whose internal ear structure is very complex," says Jay W. Geasling, D.V.M., a veterinarian in private practice in Buffalo, New York.

Cats (and occasionally dogs) will sometimes get ear mites, tiny little creatures that can make the ears sore and itchy. And because the insides of the ears are warm and moist, they are also a good environment for bacteria, fungi, and other organisms that may set up shop and cause infections. Even allergies can cause your pet's ears to itch, triggering a whirlwind of head shaking and ear scratching.

Ear problems usually aren't that difficult to treat with home remedies and with veterinary care. The hardest thing is recognizing what, exactly, is causing the problem. Here are some things to look for.

See Your Vet If:

- There is bleeding inside or on one of the earflaps, or the ears are swollen.
- Your pet is frequently tilting her head or having trouble with balance.
- There is a bad smell or discharge in one or both ears.
- There is fur loss around the ears, or the ears are scabby.
- Your pet seems to be having trouble hearing.
- Her ears are unusually tender or itchy.
- The tips of her ears are cold, white, and dry, which are signs of frostbite.
- Your pet is frequently scratching one or both ears.

DIRTY EARS

Clues

- Your pet's ears have a strong smell.
- There is grit in her ears that looks like coffee grounds.

Cats and dogs are renowned for their sharp sense of hearing. Not only are their ears large, they are also mobile: Depending on the breed, they can be raised, rotated, and adjusted to pick up the faintest signal.

The problem with ears is that they are constantly exposed to grit and grime. To keep them clean, the body produces earwax, a sticky substance that traps particles before they get into the ear canal. While earwax usually isn't a problem, some pets produce too much of it, making the ears dirtier instead of cleaner. This can make it difficult for them to hear and can increase the risk of infection.

Cats rarely get dirty ears—and not just because they are fastidious creatures. The design of their ears essentially makes them self-cleaning. Dogs, however, have "two-directional" ears, meaning that there is a bend in the ear canal that traps dirt and debris. "Heavy hair in the ear canal also promotes dirtier ears," says Merry Crimi, D.V.M., a veterinarian in private practice in Milwaukie, Oregon. This can cause problems in hairy-eared breeds like poodles, schnauzers, and Old English sheepdogs.

Dirty ears are often a sign of infection, particularly if there is a strong smell or a discharge that doesn't resemble earwax, says Dr. Crimi. Even if your pet doesn't have a full-blown (and potentially serious) infection, organisms in the outer ears may be multiplying, gradually creating a buildup of waxy dirt.

When the ears are filled with a black, dry material that looks like coffee grounds, there is a good chance that your pet has ear mites, although allergies can also cause an accumulation of debris.

WHAT YOU CAN DO

It is important to keep your pet's ears clean, if only to reduce the risk of infection. And if your pet has ear mites, cleaning the ears will help the medicine work much more efficiently. "While cats are much better than dogs at keeping their ears clean, even they need help at times," says Ernest K. Smith, D.V.M., a veterinary allergist and dermatologist in private practive in Tequesta, Florida.

Keeping ears clean doesn't have to be a messy business. Dogs such as cocker spaniels, for example, sometimes have a problem because their long, floppy ears trap wax and oils. One way to keep their ears clean is to air them out. If your dog will put up with it, once a week or so pull her ears over her

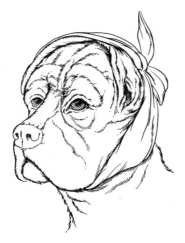

Some dogs are prone to infections because their long, floppy ears trap moisture inside, creating a perfect environment for bacteria and other germs. Airing out the ears periodically by wrapping them on top of her head will help keep them infection-free.

head and bind them with a strip of soft cloth around the head and under her chin. Letting the ears ventilate for a few hours will lower the humidity inside.

Keeping ears clean reduces the risk of infection, says Dr. Smith. It is also a good idea to periodically trim or pluck the hair inside the ears, in the area where the earflap meets the canal. This will help air get in and let ear secretions out, he says.

To trim the ears, hold your pet's ear with the flap turned up. Using a pair of blunt-tipped scissors, trim the hair, being careful not to slip the end of the scissors into the ear canal. You can also pluck the hair with your fingers or tweezers, although this may be a little painful, he says.

Most pets will benefit from having their ears cleaned periodically, says Dr. Crimi. (Cleaning them too often, however, will strip away the protective wax, making the ears raw and sore.) Don't bother with cotton-tipped swabs, which can be dangerous if they go in deeper than you can see, she adds. Instead, swab out the outer portions of the ears with a dry cotton ball, she says.

If your pet has gotten yeast or bacterial ear infections in the past, you may want to clean the ears using a solution made from equal amounts of vinegar and water. This will kill germs before they have a chance to multiply, Dr. Smith explains.

As a final precaution, you may want to apply an ear-drying product after washing your pet's ears. Sold in pet supply stores, ear-drying powders, according to Dr. Smith, will help lower moisture in the ear canal and check the growth of bacteria and fungi. Some people use drying solutions every time their dogs swim or have a bath.

Even though people sometimes clean their own ears with hydrogen peroxide, it is generally not a good idea for pets, says Dr. Smith. Once the bubbles disappear, there is a lot of water left behind, making a perfect breeding ground for organisms to flourish.

If you suspect that your pet has ear mites, remove a bit of debris from inside the ear and look at it with a magnifying glass or, if you have one, through a microscope. If you see little crablike creatures, your pet has mites, and you will have to get rid of them. The first thing to do is clean the ears thoroughly with an ear-cleaning formula. Then apply a few drops of a medicated solution designed to kill ear mites, available at pet supply stores, following the directions on the label.

What Your Vet Will Do

If your pet's ears continue getting dirty even after regular cleanings or if you see that there is a lot of discharge, she probably has an ear infection, and you need to call the vet, says Jay W. Geasling, D.V.M., a veterinarian in private practice in Buffalo, New York.

Ear infections can be very painful, so it is not always easy for veterinarians to take a look inside. If your pet won't hold still, your vet may have to give her a sedative or even a general anesthetic so that he can complete the examination.

He will begin by swabbing some of the gunk from the ear and examining it under a microscope. "This will quickly tell if the ears are infested with mites, or if there is a bacterial or yeast infection," says Dr. Crimi. If your vet suspects that there is a bacterial infection, he may culture some of the material from inside the ear to identify the organism. This makes it possible to select the most effective antibiotic. Since it takes a few days or even longer for an ear culture to be completed, your vet may apply an antibiotic ointment, which will kill some of the bacteria immediately. The rest will die once your pet starts taking antibiotics, she says.

See also Chapter 7: Discharge, Odors

SYMPTOM DISCHARGE

Like humans, dogs and cats have a bit of wax inside their ears to trap grit before it gets into the ear canal. But when you see a runny or crusty discharge, which may be white, brown, green, or tinged with red, it is time to be concerned.

In cats, a discharge that is dark and dry-looking is often caused by mites, tiny organisms that burrow into the delicate tissue inside the ear to lay their eggs. (Dogs, however, rarely get ear mites.) Mites can cause extreme itchiness, so frequent scratching is another common sign.

Discharges can also be caused by allergies, says Merry Crimi, D.V.M., a veterinarian in private practice in Milwaukie, Oregon. "Dogs and cats can have an allergy to plant pollens, especially those that are abundant in the spring and fall. And just as a person gets a runny nose from pollen allergies, a pet can develop waxy and itchy ears." Food allergies can also cause problems, she adds.

Infections are a common cause of ear discharges, Dr. Crimi says. In cats, the discharge will probably be light brown or yellow; in dogs, it will probably be brown, green, or white, possibly with a little blood mixed in. Labradors and other dogs that love the water are prone to bacterial or yeast infections because wet ears are a perfect breeding ground for bacteria, fungi, or other organisms. Sometimes, just giving your dog a bath can start an infection brewing.

In some cases, an ear discharge can actually be caused by medications used to treat an ear infection, says Jay W. Geasling, D.V.M., a veterinarian in private practice in Buffalo, New York. "If your pet's ears ooze after you start treatment, she could be allergic to the antibiotic." This type of problem is especially common with ointments containing neomycin, he adds.

An ear discharge can also be caused by a foreign object like a burr or grass seed that gets inside the ear and starts festering, says Dr. Crimi.

WHAT YOU CAN DO

If you suspect that your pet has mites, look for their telltale sign—dark specks in the ear that look like coffee grounds. (It is not always easy to distinguish mites from other ear problems, so don't hesitate to ask your vet for advice.) The only way to get rid of them is with a mite-killing medication, which is available from vets and pet supply stores.

Before treating your pet for mites, it is essential to thoroughly clean the ears. Otherwise, the mites will hide under the debris, out of reach of the medication. Following the directions on the label, use an ear-cleaning solution to remove the debris. Then apply the medication.

"Always treat both ears, even if you detect ear mites in just one," Dr. Geasling adds. In fact, it is a good idea to give your pet a bath and use a mite-killing shampoo. Otherwise, mites that wandered into the fur may migrate back into the ear, causing another infection. Be sure to treat other pets in the family, too, since mites can easily travel from pet to pet. If you don't get them all, you will have to start all over again.

If your pet likes spending time in the water—or you are simply planning to give her a bath—it is a good idea to pack her ears with cotton balls, which will help prevent harmful organisms from getting in. Dogs and cats have narrow ear canals, so the cotton balls won't get stuck "as long as you don't cram them in," says Rene van Ee, D.V.M., a veterinarian in private practice in Buffalo, New York.

"To form a good seal, put a little petroleum jelly or water-based lubricant such as K-Y jelly on the cotton balls first," says Dr. Geasling.

Allergies aren't easy to diagnose yourself. But if your pet only has ear problems during the warm months, it is possible that she has hay fever, and you may want to keep her indoors during peak pollen times, usually the early morning and evening hours.

Food allergies can also cause a discharge. The only way to tell if this is the problem is to work with your vet to create a special diet that contains none of the ingredients in her usual chow. If the problem disappears within 8 to 10 weeks—about the time it takes the old food to leave her system—you will know what your pet needs to avoid in the future, says Dr. Geasling.

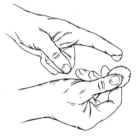
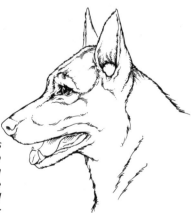

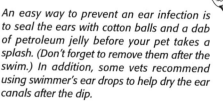
An easy way to prevent an ear infection is to seal the ears with cotton balls and a dab of petroleum jelly before your pet takes a splash. (Don't forget to remove them after the swim.) In addition, some vets recommend using swimmer's ear drops to help dry the ear canals after the dip.

If it turns out that the discharge is caused by a thistle or some other object in your pet's ear, you can try to ease it out gently with your fingers. "If the object doesn't come out easily, don't attempt to extract it yourself," says Ernest K. Smith, D.V.M., a veterinary allergist and dermatologist in private practice in Tequesta, Florida. Get some help from your vet.

What Your Vet Will Do

Unless an ear discharge is caused by mites or certain allergies, there is not a lot that you can do to treat this condition at home. Your vet will need to examine your pet and look at the discharge to learn what the problem is, says Dr. Geasling.

"We will look at it under a microscope, and this will tell us if the discharge is caused by mites, bacteria, yeast, or something else," says Dr. Crimi.

When the discharge has been heavy, your vet may flush the ear canal, using a cleaning solution and a bulb syringe. "Definitely don't do this on your own because you can puncture your pet's eardrum," Dr. Geasling warns.

Sometimes, your vet can't tell what is causing the problem just by looking, and he may recommend skull x-rays to see if deeper portions of the ear canal are infected.

If your pet does have an infection, your vet will prescribe a medication—probably antibiotics—that will clear it up within a week or two, says Dr. Crimi. In addition, she will probably give you an antibiotic (or in some cases, an antiyeast) ointment to apply at home.

It doesn't happen often, but if your pet actually gets worse instead of better after you leave the vet, she may be having a reaction to the antibiotic ointment, says Dr. Geasling. This usually isn't a serious problem, and you don't need to worry. Your vet simply will recommend using another medication instead.

Allergies can be tough to diagnose, so your vet may recommend that you see an allergy specialist. In some cases, antihistamines may be needed to relieve the problem. For pets with more serious allergies, your vet may recommend desensitization shots, which can essentially cure the allergy. "This can save the pet repeated aggravation," says Dr. Crimi. Allergy shots don't work for all pets, however, so be sure to ask your vet for advice.

See also Chapter 7: Dirty Ears, Odors

Hearing Loss

Clues

- Your pet seems less responsive than usual.
- There is a foul smell coming from one or both of his ears.

Dogs and cats have very sharp hearing, and some sounds, like the jingle of the leash or the front door opening will bring them running no matter how far away they are. That is why you should pay attention if your pet suddenly isn't responding to his favorite sounds. There is a good chance that he is losing his hearing.

"At first, many owners think that their pet is ignoring them or misbehaving," says J. Pat Mims, D.V.M., a veterinarian in private practice in San Antonio. Dogs and cats that are losing their hearing won't only be unresponsive, Dr. Mims adds. They also may seem unusually needy, always following you around sticking nearby so that they can see your expressions and hand movements.

Hearing loss is occasionally caused by a buildup of wax in the ears, which can block the opening to the eardrum. It can also be caused by an ear infection. If there is a discharge coming from one or both ears or if you notice a bad smell, there is almost certainly an infection, and you should get your pet to the vet. "These are the most difficult types of deafness for a pet to deal with because they don't have time to adjust," says Peter S. Sakas, D.V.M., a veterinarian in private practice in Niles, Illinois. "They will often get frustrated, anxious, and flighty."

What You Can Do

Once your pet loses his hearing, there is usually not a lot you can do at home to get it back. But there are many ways to help him adjust to the change. For example, you should never approach a deaf pet from behind. He won't hear you coming, and your sudden presence is sure to startle him, says Dr. Sakas.

Outdoor pets should be moved inside or at least kept in a securely fenced yard. This is especially true for cats, which depend on their hearing to detect danger such as an approaching car or the quiet steps of dogs or some other predators.

You can protect your pet's ears by keeping them clean. Regular cleaning will remove excess earwax that can block the ear canal. It is also a good way to prevent infections, especially in dogs. "Dogs' ears are hairy and closed off to air and light, which makes them perfect moist breeding grounds for bacteria and fungi that cause ear infections," Dr. Sakas explains. Cleaning them regularly will help prevent infections from getting started.

He recommends cleaning your pet's ears once or twice a month with an ear-cleaning solution, which you can get from your vet or in pet supply stores. Fill the ear canal with solution, cover the opening with the earflap, and massage it for a minute or two. Or simply rub your finger at the base of the ear opening. This will circulate the fluid in the ear canal and help loosen dirt, grit, and wax. Then use a cotton ball to blot up the liquid. Don't use cotton swabs, Dr. Sakas adds, because they can damage the ear.

WHAT YOUR VET WILL DO

Pets can lose their hearing and still function quite well. But some of the underlying problems that cause deafness, such as infections, can be quite serious. If your pet is suddenly less responsive than he used to be, you will want to call your vet right away.

When an infection or damaged eardrum is causing hearing loss, a simple ear exam will usually show what the problem is. If it's an infection, your vet will begin by giving the ears a thorough cleaning. She will probably send you home with a bottle of anti-inflammatory ear drops and, perhaps, oral antibiotics.

Ear infections that aren't caught early can cause extensive damage, sometimes causing the ear canal to close. Your vet may recommend surgery to open it up again. "If done properly, this surgery may restore your pet's hearing," says Dr. Mims.

See also Chapter 7: Dirty Ears, Discharge, Odors

ODORS

Clues

- Your pet's ears are very itchy.
- She has been swimming or has had a bath recently.

Every day you hug your pet, rub her belly, and enjoy little canine (or feline) kisses. But lately—ugh!—her ears smell like old gym socks. You don't even want to be in the same room.

Ear odors aren't so good for intimacy, but they are a valuable warning sign. They usually mean that your pet has ear mites, an ear infection, or both, says Merry Crimi, D.V.M., a veterinarian in private practice in Milwaukie, Oregon.

Though dogs can get an infection caused by mites, they are more likely to get a bacterial or yeast infection. "Generally, such an infection develops after they have an allergic episode," says Dr. Crimi. In the warm months especially, when pollen in the air makes them itchy, dogs and cats may scratch their ears raw, allowing bacteria or other infection-causing organisms to move in.

Smelly ears can also occur after baths or when pets take a plunge in a nearby pond because wet ears provide a fertile environment for germs. This type of infection is most common in breeds with long, hanging ears, like cocker spaniels, since the earflaps trap moisture inside. Poodles are also prone to ear infections because they have narrow ear canals that trap bacteria-breeding wax and grime.

In some cases, dogs and cats develop polyps or tumors in the ears when they get older. If the growths prevent normal drainage, ear secretions can gradually accumulate, getting smellier over time. In fact, anything that gets inside the ear, like burrs or grass seed, can begin to fester, causing smelly sores or infections.

WHAT YOU CAN DO

If your cat has smelly ears, ear mites are the most likely suspects. To get rid of mites, in cats as well as dogs, use this two-step process: Clean the ear thoroughly with an ear-cleaning solution. Then apply a mite-killing medication, following the directions on the label. You can buy cleaning solutions and mite medications at pet supply stores.

When you are treating your pet for mites, it is important to give her a bath and wash her well with a medicated shampoo. (Shampoos that kill fleas and ticks will also kill mites.) Otherwise, mites in the fur may migrate back inside the ears, causing another infection later on. Wash the head and the fur around the ears thoroughly since that is where mites are

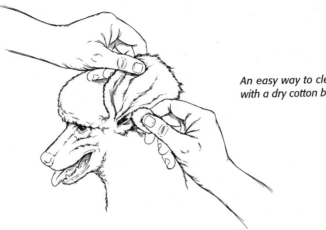

An easy way to clean your pet's ears is with a dry cotton ball.

likely to gather. And don't forget to wash the tail since cats sleep with their tails near their heads.

Even if your pet doesn't have mites, keeping her ears clean is one of the best ways to prevent infections and the resulting odors, says Jay W. Geasling, D.V.M., a veterinarian in private practice in Buffalo, New York. This is more important for dogs than cats since a dog's ears are more likely to harbor infection-causing grit and grime.

You don't have to clean the ears often, Dr. Geasling adds. Most pets will benefit from having the outer portion of their ears cleaned periodically with a dry cotton ball, Dr. Crimi says. (Cleaning them too often, however, will make the ears raw and sore.) Ask your vet to recommend a good cleaning regime based on your pet's particular needs. If your pet gets frequent ear infections, your veterinarian may recommend that you use a medicated cleaning solution to kill harmful organisms before they have a chance to multiply.

Many dogs love splashing in ponds and rivers. After your dog has taken a swim, it is a good idea to put swimmer's drops in her ears, which will help them dry more quickly, says Craig N. Carter, D.V.M., Ph.D., head of epidemiology at the Texas Veterinary Medical Diagnostic Laboratory at Texas A&M University in College Station. Swimmer's drops are designed to dry out the ear and to help prevent infections. They are available in pet supply stores.

Since allergies can set the stage for ear infections, you may want to keep your pet indoors during peak pollen times—typically the early morning and evening hours, says Dr. Crimi. Dogs and cats aren't allergic only to pollen, of course. If your pet is always itchy and you are not sure why, your vet may recommend an allergy test to identify the problem.

Finally, it is important to take a look inside your pet's ears to see if something is stuck inside. If you see a burr, grass seed, or any other foreign object, you can try to ease it out gently with your fingers, says Ernest K. Smith, D.V.M., a veterinary allergist and dermatologist in private practice in Tequesta, Florida. Lubricating the object with a few drops of mineral oil will help it slip out. The ears are very sensitive, however, so if the object doesn't come out easily, call your vet for advice.

WHAT YOUR VET WILL DO

Since smelly ears are often a sign of infection, it is always a good idea to see your vet. Don't clean the ears before you go, however, because what is inside will provide valuable clues to the problem, says Dr. Geasling.

After examining the insides of your pet's ears, your vet will examine some of the grit under a microscope. "This is the only way we can distinguish an allergy from an infection—and one type of infection from another," says Dr. Geasling. If there is an infection, your pet will probably need antibiotics, he adds.

Ear infections can be excruciatingly painful, and not many dogs or cats will hold still for the examination. Your vet may recommend giving her a sedative or even anesthetic. "This is the kind thing to do," says Dr. Geasling, "since it prevents the pet from making sudden movements while a medical instrument is within the ear canal."

See also Chapter 7: Dirty Ears, Discharge

SCRATCHING AND SHAKING

Clues

- Skin around your pet's ears is dry.
- There is dark debris in one or both of his ears.
- Your pet is scratching mainly during the warm months.

It warms your heart when your dog presses his head against your hand or your cat rubs his ear against your leg. But then you notice that he is also rubbing against the couch and the living-room carpet. Apparently, it wasn't affection he wanted, but simply a good scratch.

When your pets are using you—along with the furniture—as a rubbing post or they are pawing and shaking their heads, it is probably because something is tickling their ears and making them itch. And the more they scratch, the itchier they are going to get, says Dennis W. Thomas, D.V.M., a veterinarian in private practice in Libby, Montana. This cycle will continue until you figure out what's going on.

Anything that gets inside the ears—from fleas to water to tickly burrs—can set off a frenzy of head shaking and ear scratching. In cats particularly, itchy ears are often caused by ear mites, which are tiny, crab-like parasites that occasionally take up residence. When the mites scurry around, the ears can get intensely itchy. Dogs also get ear mites but much less often than cats do.

Allergies are the main reason that dogs and cats paw their ears and shake their heads. You can guess what's causing the itching by where they scratch. Ear and facial itchiness is usually caused by allergies to foods or airborne particles such as pollen, adds Ernest K. Smith, D.V.M., a veterinary allergist and dermatologist in private practice in Tequesta, Florida.

Some pets are prone to seborrhea, a skin condition that can make the ears extremely dry and itchy. Basset hounds, cocker spaniels, and Irish setters are particularly prone to seborrhea, as are springer spaniels, golden retrievers, and shar-peis.

Finally, there are a number of potentially serious conditions, including thyroid disease and polyps (small growths inside the middle ear), that can cause the ears to get extremely itchy.

WHAT YOU CAN DO

The problem with itchy ears is that the constant paw- and head-action can make the ears more itchy and possibly cause infection. To stop the

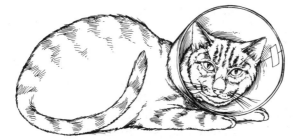

To give itchy ears time to recover, you may need to fit your pet with an Elizabethan collar to stop him from scratching. You can buy the collars in pet supply stores, or you can make your own collar by getting a bucket or a large tub and cutting a hole just big enough for your pet's head. Cover the sharp edges that will touch the neck with bandage tape. It should fit snugly but comfortably around his neck, keeping his ears out of paw's range. Just be sure that he is able to eat and drink normally while wearing the collar.

itch/scratch cycle, vets sometimes recommend putting a pair of socks on your pet's hind feet. He will still be able to scratch, but the socks will prevent the nails from irritating the ear. Your vet may also recommend fitting your pet with an Elizabethan collar, a paper or plastic cone that will prevent him from scratching the ears altogether until they have a chance to heal. Elizabethan collars look a little unusual, but they are very effective. The collars are available from vets and pet supply stores.

When ears are itchy and inflamed, your vet may recommend applying several drops of over-the-counter hydrocortisone liquid, which can help ease the discomfort. Every pet will need a different amount, however, and this medication is not recommended for all conditions. Be sure to check with your vet before using it.

Since allergies are so common, it is worth taking a few minutes to try to figure out what's causing the head-shaking, ear-pawing, furniture-rubbing frenzy. Dogs and cats can be allergic to all kinds of things, and it is sometimes difficult to discover the culprit.

If itching occurs mainly during the warm months, there is a good chance that pollen or grasses may be to blame. When it occurs at various times of the year, however, you should suspect that something in your pet's food may be to blame.

If you think that your pet might be allergic to mold, dust, or dust mites, you should clean the house thoroughly and then watch for signs of possible improvement in your pet. "Vacuum the heck out of the drapes and clean the air-conditioner filters," Dr. Smith suggests.

Food allergies can be a little more complicated to recognize and to treat. The only way to figure out what your pet is allergic to is to work with your vet to create a special diet that contains none of the ingredients in his usual chow. Keep him on the diet for 8 to 10 weeks. During that time, "you can't let him finish the cornflakes and milk after breakfast or give him any treats," Dr. Smith adds. If the scratching gradually subsides, a food allergy may have been the problem, and you will want to keep him on this new diet.

There isn't a cure for seborrhea, which causes oily, dandrufflike scales to accumulate on the skin, but it is usually easy to treat by using a medicated shampoo. Available from veterinarians and pet supply stores, medicated shampoos are designed to relieve itchy, dry skin. Selenium-based shampoos can be particularly helpful. In severe cases, your vet may recommend a brief course of steroids such as cortisone to control the itching and inflammation.

If you suspect that your pet has ear mites—a telltale sign is an accumulation of dark-colored debris in the ears—you will need to clean the ears thoroughly and apply a mite-killing medication, available at pet supply stores, following the directions on the label. Fleas and other pests, of course, can also be controlled with over-the-counter medications as well as with stronger, prescription medications.

Hairy-eared dogs like poodles and terriers sometimes have itchy ears because there isn't enough air circulation in the ear canals to keep them dry. Removing some of the hair will allow more air to get inside, says Dr. Thomas. He recommends plucking excess hairs with your fingers or tweezers. Only remove hair that is protruding from the canal itself, not inside the earflap, he adds. If your dog has floppy ears, trimming the hair at the base of the flaps will also help the air to circulate. Some vets even recommend tying long, floppy ears over the head with a bandanna to let air inside and help keep them dry.

For pets that are prone to ear problems, vets recommend cleaning the ears once a week, especially during allergy season or if you live in a humid climate. Cleaning the ears is also helpful after your pet has had a bath or has taken a swim because moisture from the water can result in swimmer's ear, an infection caused by bacteria or other germs. Drying the ears makes it harder for germs to thrive.

To give the ears a thorough cleaning, cup your hand around the base of the ear and then fill the ear with an ear-cleaning solution, available from pet supply stores, following the directions on the label. (You can make your own cleaner by mixing equal parts white vinegar and water.) "Massage the base of the ear and be sure that you can hear the liquid swooshing around," Dr. Thomas says. Then stand back: When he shakes his head, the liquid and dirt will come splashing out.

The one thing that you don't want to do when the ear is inflamed is to use alcohol to clean your pet's ears, adds Dr. Thomas. "Alcohol sets the ear on fire," he says. "Cats especially can get tremendous inflammation." There are other manageable ways to get the job done, he adds.

WHAT YOUR VET WILL DO

Itchy ears by themselves usually aren't a serious problem. The constant scratching, however, can set the stage for inflammation and infection. When your pet has been pawing his ears and shaking his head for more than a day or two, you will need to see your vet.

It probably won't be difficult for your vet to identify the problem. First, she will look inside your pet's ears with a viewing instrument called an otoscope. She may take an ear swab to check for mites or infection. She also will check for polyp growths in the ear that can lead to infections.

If your pet does have an infection, he is going to need antibiotics, which are usually taken for a week to 10 days. To relieve the itch, he may be given steroids, either in injection, pill, or drop form. Or if the itching is caused by allergies, he may receive antihistamines instead. Your vet will let you know what drug and dose is right for your pet.

It is always better to prevent allergies than to try to treat them. Your vet may recommend that you see a veterinarian specializing in allergies, who will run a series of skin tests to determine what, exactly, your pet is allergic to. These tests are extremely efficient and can test your pet's sensitivity to as many as 50 substances at one time.

If your pet has other problems, of course, such as thyroid disease, he is going to need medications to help control the problem.

See also Chapter 7: Dirty Ears, Discharge, Odors, Swelling and Redness

SWELLING AND REDNESS

Clues

- Your pet has been scratching more than usual.
- He is shaking his head frequently.

Unlike the furry outer parts, the insides of your pet's ears are very sensitive to such things as burrs and insect stings. Pets respond to ear problems by scratching, and the more they scratch, the greater the risk of infection. Such subsequent infections are the main cause of swelling and redness, says Cheryl Hedlund, D.V.M., chief of surgery at the Louisiana State University School of Veterinary Medicine in Baton Rouge.

Pets with allergies are particularly prone to ear infections because they will often scratch their ears raw. Over time, repeated infections can cause scar tissue to form inside the ears, making them permanently thick and swollen, says David Holt, B.V.Sc. (bachelor of veterinary science, the Australian equivalent of D.V.M.), assistant professor of surgery at the Veterinary Hospital of the University of Pennsylvania in Philadelphia. "The skin thickens due to chronic inflammation, and then in really bad cases, the cartilage hardens," he explains.

Swelling and redness can also be a sign of sunburn. This tends to be a problem for pets with fair skin and sparse fur, which make them especially vulnerable to the sun's burning rays, says Dr. Hedlund. When pets spend too much time outdoors, their ears can get red, blistered, and swollen.

In dogs, ear swelling sometimes occurs when they have been giving

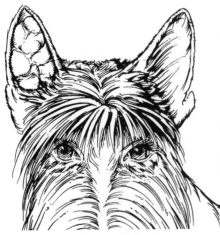

Dogs that shake their heads too hard can develop bulges or blisters on the ears. The bulges usually aren't serious, but they won't go away without help from your vet.

their heads frequent and vigorous shakes—so vigorous, in fact, that blood blisters or bulges form on the earflaps, a condition that vets call aural hematomas. Without treatment by a veterinarian, these bulges can cause the ear to be permanently deformed.

In cats, swelling and redness are sometimes (and indirectly) caused by polyps, small growths inside the middle ear. Even though you can't see the polyps, "they clog up the ear canal, and infection almost always follows," says Dr. Hedlund.

Swelling can also be caused by small growths underneath the skin in the earflaps. These growths are usually harmless, but cancer is also a possibility. This is why it is important to see your vet whenever you discover suspicious bumps, says Dr. Holt.

WHAT YOU CAN DO

Since swelling and redness are often caused by infections, this really isn't a problem that you can treat at home, says Dr. Holt. What you can do, however, is be especially alert whenever your pet's hind leg swings into high gear. Whatever is causing the itching may not be serious, but the scratching itself can lead to serious infections. The sooner that you can stop the scratching, the less likely it is that your pet will develop problems later on.

In cats, ear scratching is often caused by mites—tiny creatures that can make the ears unbearably itchy. (Dogs also get mites but much less often than cats do.) Take a look in your pet's ears. If you see a dark-colored discharge that looks like coffee grounds, he probably has mites, says Jay W. Geasling, D.V.M., a veterinarian in private practice in Buffalo, New York. You will want to pick up a mite-killing medication from your vet or at the pet supply store and carefully follow the instructions on the label. Before using the medication, be sure to clean the ears well with an ear-cleaning solution. This will help the medication work more effectively.

For pale-skinned pets that are vulnerable to sunburn, it is a good idea to apply a little waterproof sunscreen to the tips of their ears before letting them outside, says Dr. Hedlund. The sunscreen you use on your skin will work for your pets as well. Vets recommend using a sunscreen with a sun protection factor (SPF) of 15 or higher. Don't use sunscreens containing PABA as it can be dangerous for pets.

Since allergies are a common cause of itchy ears, it is worth trying to figure out what, exactly, your pet may be reacting to. Dogs and cats may be allergic to many things, from pollen to perfume to ingredients in their chow. Your vet may recommend specialized tests to figure out what the problem is.

WHAT YOUR VET WILL DO

When swelling and redness are caused by infection, a vet will often begin by cleaning the ears. She will usually apply an anti-inflammatory medication to reduce the swelling and follow that with putting your pet on antibiotics. "Once an infection is being treated, your pet will usually feel a whole lot better by the next day," says Dennis W. Thomas, D.V.M., a veterinarian in private practice in Libby, Montana.

If your pet has polyps or other growths or if his ear is constantly swollen and infected, he is probably going to need surgery to clear up the problem. Swellings called hematomas, for example, will sometimes respond to steroids, but they usually need to be surgically drained, Dr. Holt says. In fact, any growth that threatens to block the ear canal or is potentially malignant will have to be removed, he says.

See also Chapter 7: Discharge, Odors, Scratching and Shaking

Common Ear Conditions

Infection. Ear infections are among the most common and potentially serious problems that dogs and cats get. Although infections in the outer ear are easy to see and treat, inner-ear infections are entirely out of sight, so both detection and treatment are more challenging. The inner-ear infection can get extremely "hot" before you realize that something is wrong.

"You generally won't be able to detect these infections just by looking in your pet's ear because the infection is so deep inside," says Jay W. Geasling, D.V.M., a veterinarian in private practice in Buffalo, New York. Signs that your pet may have an ear infection include head tilting, fever, tenderness, and, less often, a loss of balance. In addition, there may be a strong odor coming from inside the ear, and possibly a discolored discharge.

Almost anything can cause ear infections, says Merry Crimi, D.V.M., a veterinarian in private practice in Milwaukie, Oregon. In cats, one of the most common causes is ear mites—tiny parasites that can cause ferocious itching when they wiggle around. Dogs also get ear mites but not as often as cats do. But because dogs like the water, they often get bacterial and yeast infections. Their wet ears are perfect breeding grounds for bacteria, fungi, or other organisms.

Infections in the outer ear can often be cured simply by cleaning the ear with a commercial ear-cleaning solution, available from vets and pet supply stores, says Craig N. Carter, D.V.M., Ph.D., head of epidemiology at the Texas Veterinary Medical Diagnostic Laboratory at Texas A&M University in College Station.

Inner-ear infections, however, are more serious and frequently require oral antibiotics. These medications usually clear up the infection in a week or two. When the infection is well-advanced, your vet may need to drain pus and other fluids from inside the ear, says Dr. Geasling.

Ears are always open to the elements, so it is not always easy to prevent infections. Periodically trimming excess hair from your pet's ears will help keep the ear canals dry and prevent moisture from accumulating inside. It is also important to treat outer-ear infections promptly. If you don't, the harmful organisms may move inside, causing a more serious problem, says Dr. Crimi.

Mites. They are so small that you can barely see them, but when mites get inside your pet's ears, they can cause some very obvious scratching.

Ear mites are little parasites that thrive in the dark, moist recesses of the ears. The problem with mites is that they tickle as they scurry around inside the ears. As a result, cats will scratch and scratch to ease the itch. They will scratch so much, in fact, that they will sometimes rub off the fur around their ears, making the skin raw and sore. Over time, this can lead to serious infections.

Even though it is very hard to see mites, you can see the dirt they leave behind. "Ear mites produce a distinctive, brown-black waxy substance," says Dr. Crimi.

Pet supply stores and veterinarians sell different kinds of liquid drops that will help kill ear mites. Be sure to follow directions on the label and to use the medication as long as recommended—usually one to two weeks. If you have more than one pet in the house, the best way to get rid of mites is to examine all your pets and treat each animal if necessary, Dr. Crimi says. If even a few mites get away, the problem will start all over again.

Other bugs or objects in the ear. Dogs and cats spend their lives a lot closer to the ground than people do. They run through tall grass, scurry under shrubs, and investigate burrows in the dirt. Along the way, their hairy ears are natural basins for all sorts of things, including burrs, twigs, or even stones. Insects such as ticks and fleas find the ears a very comfortable place to set up shop. And if the object or insect slips down into the ear, it can cause problems. "If it is not removed right away, the object can travel down the ear canal and set up inflammation or infection or puncture the eardrum," says Dr. Crimi.

If your pet is pawing her ear or shaking her head and you can't see anything inside, there is a good chance something has slipped into the ear canal, and you will need to call your vet, says Ernest K. Smith, D.V.M., a veterinary allergist and dermatologist in private practice in Tequesta, Florida. You should also make the phone call if there is a bad odor in the ear, which is a common sign of infection.

Eyes

Dogs and cats use their eyes to great effect—to con you out of another treat, for example, or to coax you out the door for an evening walk. But the eyes do more than tell you what your pet is feeling. They are also a valuable window into your pet's inner health. "Many eye symptoms are a reflection of something more serious going on inside your pet," says David A. Wilkie, D.V.M., associate professor and head of ophthalmology at the Ohio State College of Veterinary Medicine in Columbus.

Even something as simple as bloodshot eyes could be a sign of glaucoma, cancer, or other serious conditions. "While there are quick, easy, and safe home remedies to try for some problems, symptoms that don't go away should be seen by your vet," says Nick A. Faber, D.V.M., a veterinary ophthalmology resident at the University of California School of Veterinary Medicine, Davis.

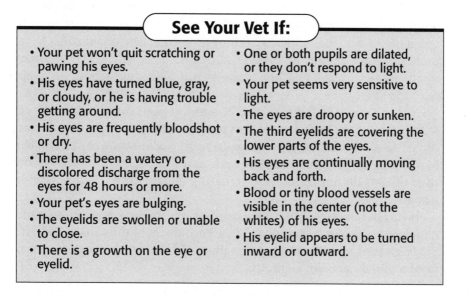

See Your Vet If:

- Your pet won't quit scratching or pawing his eyes.
- His eyes have turned blue, gray, or cloudy, or he is having trouble getting around.
- His eyes are frequently bloodshot or dry.
- There has been a watery or discolored discharge from the eyes for 48 hours or more.
- Your pet's eyes are bulging.
- The eyelids are swollen or unable to close.
- There is a growth on the eye or eyelid.
- One or both pupils are dilated, or they don't respond to light.
- Your pet seems very sensitive to light.
- The eyes are droopy or sunken.
- The third eyelids are covering the lower parts of the eyes.
- His eyes are continually moving back and forth.
- Blood or tiny blood vessels are visible in the center (not the whites) of his eyes.
- His eyelid appears to be turned inward or outward.

BLOODSHOT EYES

Clues

- Your pet's eye seems sore and irritated.
- She has been riding in the car.
- Your pet has been sprayed by a skunk.

If you hadn't been watching when your pet curled up and went to sleep, you would swear that she spent the night at the corner bar. Her eyes are so red and bloodshot that they look like road maps.

Don't put a lock on the liquor cabinet just yet. Bloodshot eyes are a common occurrence for the simple reason that dogs and cats are energetic, curious creatures that approach the world headfirst. They don't always have time to duck or blink when running face-first through high grass, under branches, or under the bed. Even a little scratch or irritation in the eye can cause major redness in their eyes, not just for an hour or two, but sometimes for a few days.

There is another reason that they are prone to bloodshot eyes. Unlike people, dogs and cats have third eyelids, which are designed to protect the eyes from foreign objects, says Paul M. Gigliotti, D.V.M., a veterinarian in private practice in Mayfield Village, Ohio. Sometimes, however, bits of wood or other debris get trapped under the lid, making the eye sore and irritated. "A foreign body in the eye is the most common cause of bloodshot eyes," he says. In fact, when only one eye is bloodshot, you should suspect that's the cause.

When both eyes are bloodshot, however, you can be pretty sure that something is happening elsewhere in the body. Pets with allergies, for example, will sometimes get red eyes. In dogs, high blood pressure may be to blame. And in dogs and cats, serious problems such as glaucoma or tumors can cause bloodshot eyes, says Nick A. Faber, D.V.M., a veterinary ophthalmology resident at the University of California School of Veterinary Medicine, Davis.

Minor causes of red eyes also abound. If your dog rides in the car with her head out the window, ears plastered back, and a look of ecstasy on her face, her superdog pose can cause bloodshot eyes, says Dr. Faber. Many dogs are permitted to place their heads out open car windows, but their owners do not realize how irritating this can be to their pets' eyes, he adds.

If you live in the country or suburbs, there is a very good chance that bloodshot eyes may be caused by close encounters of the stinky kind. "If a pet is sprayed by a skunk at close range, her eyes will become very irritated and red," says Dr. Gigliotti.

WHAT YOU CAN DO

Since bloodshot eyes are usually sore, irritated eyes, it is a good idea to flush them thoroughly with saline solution, says Dr. Faber. Hold the eye open with one hand and use the other to pour in a generous amount of the solution. "This might be easier with two people—one to hold the pet's eyes open and the other to rinse," he says.

If your dog has been joy-riding and now has windburned eyes, flushing them with saline solution will be very soothing. Or you may want to soak a washcloth in warm water, wring it out, and hold it over her sore eyes for a few minutes several times a day. "Most pets will settle into the soothing comfort that this affords," says Dr. Faber. In the future, of course, you may decide to keep the windows closed when driving with canine company. Or you can combine safety with the thrill of the ride by fitting your pet with goggles, available in some pet supply stores.

If your pet was sprayed by a skunk—this is one symptom you won't have any problem recognizing—you will want to use a lot of saline solution and repeat the flushing several times a day. Skunk or chemical sprays can damage the eyes, Dr. Gigliotti adds, so don't take chances. "If the eyes are still red the next day, take your pet to the vet for an eye exam," he advises.

After flushing the eyes, you can wait a few hours before taking another look. When a foreign object is causing the problem, the irritation won't go away until you get rid of the object. Hold her eye open and take a look inside. If you see something, you may be able to snag it using the corner of a clean tissue. "But never use tweezers to remove a foreign body from the eye," warns Dr. Faber. "This is especially true if the foreign object is stuck under that third lid."

To remove a foreign object from your pet's eye, gently hold the eye open and use the corner of a clean tissue to swab the object out. You don't want to press too hard, which will irritate the eye further.

WHAT YOUR VET WILL DO

Even though bloodshot eyes usually aren't a sign of serious problems, they do mean that *something* is causing irritation. Don't take chances by ignoring the problem, especially if your pet keeps pawing at her eyes or the eyes look very irritated, says Dr. Faber. If the red doesn't disappear fairly quickly, you will want to take your pet to the vet for a thorough eye exam.

"If your vet suspects that a foreign body is the cause of the red, irritated eye, he may numb the eye with special anesthetic eyedrops," says Dr. Faber. This will allow him to examine the eye and remove the object without causing pain.

Or your vet may decide to put in staining drops that are often used to help identify different eye problems. One type of drop, for example, will reveal scratches on the surface (the cornea) of the eye. Another drop is used to numb the eye so that your vet can use an instrument called a tonometer to measure pressure beneath the eyeball. This will help reveal problems such as glaucoma.

Glaucoma can be serious and is nearly always treated with medications. A scratch on the cornea, however, usually isn't a big deal. Scratches will probably clear up on their own, although your vet may recommend using an ointment to help them heal faster and reduce the risk of infection. For tumors, the treatments vary widely but may include radiation, chemotherapy, or surgery.

BLUE EYES

Clues

- One or both eyes are bloodshot or irritated.
- Your pet is getting up in years.

Regardless of the breed or the color of their coats, most dogs and cats are born with dark-colored eyes. Sometimes, however, the eyes begin to change, taking on a distinctly bluish hue.

A shift toward blue is rare in young pets but often occurs as dogs and cats get older, says Nick A. Faber, D.V.M., a veterinary ophthalmology resident at the University of California School of Veterinary Medicine, Davis. The eyes are very efficient at creating new cells, but they aren't so good at getting rid of old ones. "As the old cells build up in the lens, the lens becomes quite dense," he says. This condition, called nuclear sclerosis, has little effect on vision, but it does cause the pupils to become slightly blue.

Another condition that may change the color of the eye—and which can have a serious effect on vision, sometimes causing blindness—is cataracts. Caused by a hardening of the lens, cataracts may result in blue, bluish white, gray, or even cloudy eyes. Pets with diabetes are particularly prone to cataracts, although they are common in healthy older pets as well.

A condition called glaucoma, which increases pressure within the eyeball, can also cause the eyes to turn blue. Glaucoma is often painful and can damage your pet's vision if it is not treated quickly, says Dr. Faber. One clue to look for is a layer of blue across the surface of the eye that obscures the pupil underneath, he explains.

The color of your pet's eyes is also influenced by the amount of tears they produce. It is common for the eyes to become somewhat drier with the passing years. Declining tear production may cause the eyes to reflect light differently, resulting in a bluish color in the cornea (the surface of the eye), says Dr. Faber.

If one eye has turned slightly blue, and your pet is also squinting or has bloodshot eyes, there is a good chance that he has a scratch on the cornea, says Nancy Willerton, D.V.M., a veterinarian in private practice in Denver.

WHAT YOU CAN DO

Eye problems can be difficult to diagnose on your own, and you don't want to take chances with your pet's sight. So it is important to see your vet if there is suddenly a sign of blue. Most of the time, however, there won't be anything to worry about.

Even if there is a problem, dogs and cats don't depend on vision to the same extent that people do because they compensate with their other senses. "Pets with dimming or even lost vision do remarkably well," says Dr. Willerton.

Pets with failing vision may get disoriented, however. That is why vets recommend trying to keep their surroundings as constant as you possibly can—by not moving the furniture too often, for example, and being sure to pick things up off the floor before they stumble into them. It is especially important to keep objects off the stairs, which could cause your pet to take a hard fall.

The eyes are surprisingly hardy, and corneal scratches will usually heal nicely on their own, says Dr. Willerton. But scratches can make the eye sore and sensitive to light, so you may want to pick up a sun-blocking visor at the pet supply store. Visors tend to work better for dogs, she adds, simply because cats will usually refuse to wear them. "If the eye seems no better in a day, take your pet to the vet," she adds.

WHAT YOUR VET WILL DO

It probably won't take your vet more than a few minutes to figure out what is making your pet's eyes blue. Eye exams can be somewhat uncomfortable, however, so she may put in anesthetic drops to keep your pet more comfortable. She may also use drops that stain the surface of the eye, which will show if a scratch is present. If your pet does have a corneal scratch, your vet may use antibiotic drops to prevent infection.

To test for glaucoma, your vet will use an instrument called a tonometer, which measures pressure in the eyes. When glaucoma is caught early and treated—with oral medications as well as medicated eyedrops—your pet's vision will probably be fine.

Pets with cataracts usually do fine without treatment. But if your pet is having trouble getting around, your vet may recommend surgery to remove them. "This can help your pet maintain the ability to see shadows or at least the outline of objects, which will make life a little safer for him," says Dr. Willerton.

BROWN STAINS ON FUR

Clues

- Stains are visible even on dark fur.
- Your pet is pawing at his eyes.
- There is a thick, cloudy discharge.
- The discharge doesn't dry quickly.

If you have white carpet at home, you know how important it is to remove stains quickly to prevent them from becoming permanent, although you may have to live with the occasional spot. The same is true of light-colored pets, like some poodles, pugs, or Persian cats. They occasionally develop brown stains that begin at the inner corners of the eyes and streak down the sides of their faces.

"Brown stains are almost always just a normal feature in these white-faced dogs," says Terri McGinnis, D.V.M., a veterinarian in private practice in the San Francisco area and author of *The Well Cat Book* and *The Well Dog Book*.

Tears contain iron, Dr. McGinnis explains. When they leave the tear ducts and are exposed to air, their iron turns an unsightly brown. "This is the same rusting process that occurs when iron-containing metal is exposed to moisture and air," she says.

This process occurs in all pets, not only those with white fur, she adds. But it is hard to see the stains in pets with darker coats. The one exception is when a pet has an eye infection, which can cause a copious discharge.

You should suspect an eye infection if the discharge around the eyes doesn't dry quickly but lingers for hours or days. The discharge may be thick or cloudy, and your pet may be pawing at his eyes as well, Dr. McGinnis says.

WHAT YOU CAN DO

If your pet is otherwise healthy, you really don't have to worry about the stains. But if you would like to keep his coat as pristine as your new carpet, a little daily maintenance is required. "It is as simple as washing his face every morning, just as a matter of routine," says Dr. McGinnis. "Wiping the area with a water-moistened washcloth effectively cleans away the rusting tear material, eliminating or significantly reducing the brown stains."

Changing his facial hairstyle can also reduce the rusting. Keep hair around the eyes trimmed short, which will allow the tears to dry as they leave the duct rather than soaking into and staining the longer fur. This

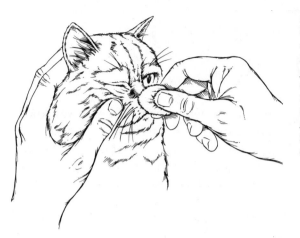

Brown stains around the eyes aren't dangerous, but they aren't beautiful either. To remove or lighten the stains, gently rub them daily with a cotton ball moistened with water. Eye-stain removers, which are available in pet supply stores, may help, but there is no substitute for daily cleaning.

works well for dogs, but is a bit tricky for cats since they usually won't hold still for styling, Dr. McGinnis adds. If your cat won't cooperate, you may want to have a cat groomer trim the hair for you with blunt-nosed scissors.

Some pet owners try to prevent brown stains by applying an antibiotic ointment every day. This may be effective, but it is also dangerous, says Dr. McGinnis. "Eye ointments are very specific to the pet's eye condition, and using the wrong one can damage the eyes," she says. If you suspect that your pet has an eye infection, you really have to see your vet.

WHAT YOUR VET WILL DO

Since brown stains are occasionally caused by infections or by painful objects in the eye, your vet will want to do a thorough eye exam. The exams may be somewhat painful, so she will probably begin by numbing the eye with anesthetic drops to make your pet more comfortable. In addition, she may apply specialized eyedrops that make it possible to discover other eye problems, such as scratches on the cornea (the surface of the eye), which can also cause stains to form.

If your pet does have an eye infection, your vet will clean the eye thoroughly and then send you home with antibiotics and possibly anti-inflammatory eyedrops. In most cases, the infection will clear up within a week or two.

See also Chapter 8: Discharge

BULGING EYES

Clues

- You have a Persian cat, Pekingese dog, or another short-faced breed.
- Her eye is red, dilated, or teary.
- Your pet has been fighting or roughhousing.

Just as some pets have white fur, long lashes, or a short chin, others have distinctly bulging eyes. In fact, Persian cats, Pekingese dogs, and other short-faced types of cats and dogs are bred specifically to have this appearance.

"While bulgy eyes are normal for these breeds, owners have to keep in mind that they really are a slight abnormality that can predispose the pet to eye problems, such as dry eyes," adds Terri McGinnis, D.V.M., a veterinarian in private practice in the San Francisco area and author of *The Well Cat Book* and *The Well Dog Book.*

For dogs and cats with "normal" eyes, there are several conditions that can cause the eyes to bulge. When pets get into scuffles or play too vigorously, for instance, pressure behind the eye can rise, forcing the eye partially out of the socket. Also known as a prolapsed eyeball, this condition is most likely to occur following a whack on the head or a hard bite on the neck. "Once the eyeball pops out, the eyelid clamps down behind it, trapping the protruding eyeball," explains Christopher J. Murphy, D.V.M., associate professor of ophthalmology at the University of Wisconsin School of Veterinary Medicine in Madison.

Anything that exerts pressure behind the eyes can cause them to bulge outward. Tumors or infections, for example, will sometimes cause bulgy eyes. So can an inflammation of the chewing muscle, which runs next to and under the eye, says Dr. Murphy.

A potentially serious condition called glaucoma, in which pressure builds up in the eyes, is a common cause of bulging eyes. Glaucoma sometimes comes on very quickly. If your pet's eyes are normal one day and bulging the next, glaucoma is a likely suspect. (Cocker spaniels, basset hounds, and older pets are especially prone to "fast" glaucoma.) Other signs of glaucoma include tearing, a dilated pupil, or redness in the eyes, says Dr. Murphy.

WHAT YOU CAN DO

When you first notice that your pet's eyes are bulging, it is essential to get her to a vet right away. There is not a lot that you can do at home, and every minute is important if you are going to save her sight, says Dr. Murphy.

One thing you can do at home if there is no way to get to a vet in a

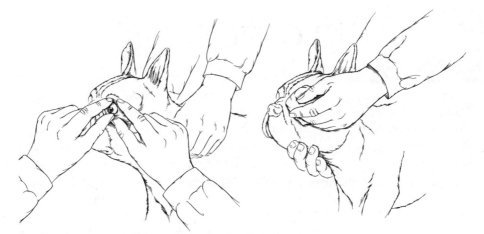

If an eyeball pops out, you only have about 10 minutes to save your pet's sight. If you can't get to a vet immediately, you can try to replace the eye yourself. With one hand, spread the eyelids open as far as you can. With the other hand, push the eyeball back into the socket in one firm motion. Once the eye is back in place, soak some sterile gauze or a clean cloth in saline solution and hold the moistened pad over the eye to moisturize it. Then get your pet to a vet as soon as possible.

hurry is to replace an eye that has popped out. It sounds scary, but it is fairly easy to do, says L. R. Danny Daniel, D.V.M., a veterinarian in private practice in Covington, Louisiana. "It is worth trying because you only have about 10 minutes to put the eye back before vision is lost," he says.

With one hand, spread the eyelids open as wide as possible. "With the other hand, put your fingers together and push the eyeball back into place quickly and firmly," says Dr. Daniel. It will be painful, so enlist a helper and don't be surprised when your pet cries or struggles, he adds. Once the eye is back in place, get your pet to the vet as soon as possible.

Incidentally, if your pet's eyes are naturally bulgy, it is worth taking a little time to keep them moist. "Just as if you had dry eyes, get in the practice of moisturizing your pet's eyes at least once daily," says Dr. McGinnis. You can buy artificial tears for dry eyes at the drugstore. Just be sure to avoid artificial tears that also contain ingredients for relieving red eyes since they may be harmful for pets. Saline solution also works well.

WHAT YOUR VET WILL DO

Before doing an eye exam, your vet will put anesthetic drops in your pet's eyes. This will make the exam easier, safer, and less painful, says Dr. Murphy.

To test for glaucoma, your vet will use an instrument called a tonometer, which measures pressure in the eyes. He will also remove fluids and possibly tissue from the eyes in order to check for infections or cancerous cells.

After a general checkup, your vet may recommend x-rays—another tool for finding tumors. He will also feel along the chewing muscle to see if it is sore or inflamed.

For glaucoma, your pet will need pills and possibly eyedrops to reduce pressure in the eye. Caught early, glaucoma can be cured, saving your pet's sight, Dr. Murphy says.

Eye infections are usually treated with antibiotics, says Dr. Murphy. An inflamed chewing muscle may also be treated with antibiotics as well as anti-inflammatory medications to reduce the swelling. Antibiotics work quickly, and your pet will start feeling better within a day.

If your pet's eyeball has popped out, you will have performed the most important sight-saving action by slipping it back into place. "But your vet will still have some work to do to save the pet's vision entirely," says Dr. Murphy. After cleaning the eye, he may need to add a few stitches to the eyelids, which will help it hold the eye in place in the future.

CLOUDY EYES

Clues

- Your pet's eye is gray, blue, or bluish white.
- His eye is red or teary.
- Your pet also has diabetes or high blood pressure.
- He is bumping into things.

The best camera in the world will take murky pictures if the lens has a cloudy coating of fingerprints or dust. Your pet's eyes, which are superior to the best lens ever designed, will also lose sharpness if they start getting cloudy.

The eyes are covered by a layer of cells called the cornea, which allows light to pass through to the lens beneath. Normally, both the cornea and the lens are transparent. But there are a number of conditions that can cause these complex layers of cells to get cloudy or even opaque.

Among the most serious causes of cloudy eyes is glaucoma. This is a condition in which fluid accumulates inside the eye, increasing pressure within the eyeball and impairing your pet's ability to see, says Christopher J. Murphy, D.V.M., associate professor of ophthalmology at the University of Wisconsin School of Veterinary Medicine in Madison. Glaucoma may occur on its own or following an injury to the eye. Besides cloudiness, other signs of glaucoma include teariness, a dilated pupil, or redness in the eye, says Dr. Murphy.

As pets get older, the lens of the eye often hardens a bit and begins preventing small amounts of light from getting through. This condition, called cataracts, causes the eye to get cloudy, possibly with a gray, blue, or bluish-white color. Pets with diabetes are particularly prone to cataracts, adds Dr. Murphy.

An eye infection may also cause cloudiness. So can internal problems such as high blood pressure or even cancer, says David A. Wilkie, D.V.M., associate professor and head of ophthalmology at the Ohio State College of Veterinary Medicine in Columbus.

WHAT YOU CAN DO

Because their other senses are so sharp, dogs and cats really don't need perfect vision in order to get along just fine. In fact, it is not uncommon for pets to have cataracts (or other minor vision problems) for years before their owners even notice that there is a problem.

Apart from surgery, there isn't a cure for cataracts. What you can do, however, is make it easier for your pet to find his way around. "Pets with poor eyesight memorize the layout of your home, so it is better not to rearrange the furniture too often," says Nancy Willerton, D.V.M., a veterinarian in private practice in Denver. It is also helpful to keep the floors clear of unexpected objects. A pile of books is easy for you to avoid, but pets with failing vision may walk right into them, possibly causing further injury to the eyes, she says.

Even though cataracts aren't always a serious problem, conditions such as glaucoma are. "You should always consider a cloudy eye to be an emergency situation and see your vet right away," says Dr. Murphy. In some cases, waiting even a day or two could result in permanent blindness for your pet, he warns.

WHAT YOUR VET WILL DO

Since glaucoma is so serious, it is probably the first thing your vet will look for, by measuring the internal pressure of the eye. When glaucoma is caught early and treated—with oral medications as well as medicated eyedrops—your pet's vision will probably be fine.

Glaucoma can hurt, so your vet may recommend giving medications to ease the pain. For dogs, aspirin works well, says Lori A. Wise, D.V.M., a veterinarian in private practice in Wheat Ridge, Colorado. Aspirin is dangerous for cats, however, so your vet will probably recommend using prescription medicines instead.

If glaucoma isn't the problem, your vet will need to do a thorough checkup to look for things such as diabetes, high blood pressure, poisoning, hereditary problems, or infection. Once the underlying problem has been diagnosed and taken care of, the cloudiness will usually go away fairly quickly.

Pets with cataracts don't always need further treatment. If the cloudiness is extreme, however, your vet may recommend surgery to remove the damaged lenses. Your pet's vision won't be perfect afterward, but he will be able to get around a little easier. "And that makes life a little safer for him," Dr. Murphy says.

See also Chapter 8: Blue Eyes

DILATED PUPILS

Clues

- You suspect that your pet has gotten into poisonous substances like antifreeze.
- Her eyes are red, cloudy, or teary.
- Your cat eats raw fish or is on a vegetarian diet.

Your pet's eyes are very sensitive to changes in light. The middle part of the eye, called the pupil, is constantly in motion, opening and closing to let in the correct amount of light.

Sometimes, however, the pupils stay open regardless of the amount of light they are receiving. This condition, called dilated pupils, nearly always means that something is seriously wrong. "When one or both eyes dilate in good light, your pet could have something wrong with the nerves connected to the eyes or in the brain or the eye itself," says Erika de Papp, D.V.M., a veterinarian at the University of Pennsylvania School of Veterinary Medicine in Philadelphia.

Nerves are responsible for sensing how much light is reaching the eye and for relaying the message to (and from) the brain, which instructs the eye to make the proper adjustments. When a nerve is damaged or under pressure because of an infection, for instance, or a growing tumor, the eye may not receive the necessary messages and may fail to work properly, explains Dr. de Papp. A swelling in the brain, which can happen following a blow to the head, can also press on the nerves controlling the pupil.

A fairly common condition called glaucoma, in which fluids accumulate in the eye, can also cause the pupil to stay dilated. (Other symptoms of glaucoma may include teariness, redness, or cloudiness of the eye.)

Pets that eat toxic substances such as antifreeze can also develop dilated eyes. If you suspect that your pet has swallowed poison, get her to the vet right away.

In cats, dilated pupils may be caused by a diet of raw fish. Fish contains

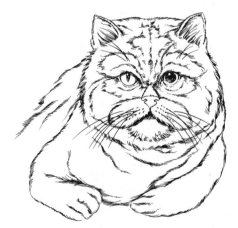

When one or both of your pet's pupils stay dilated, there could be a nerve or brain problem, and you need to call your vet right away.

an enzyme called thiaminase that destroys thiamin, a vitamin necessary for good vision, says Paul M. Gigliotti, D.V.M., a veterinarian in private practice in Mayfield Village, Ohio. In addition, cats given mainly milk or vegetarian diets may become deficient in an amino acid called taurine, which is essential for keeping the retinas healthy. When taurine levels fall, the eyes may dilate.

WHAT YOU CAN DO

Dilated pupils are a serious warning sign that should always be examined by a veterinarian right away. If it turns out that your pet has glaucoma, she is going to need medications to reduce the dangerous buildup of pressure. Until the medications take effect, your vet may recommend keeping your pet away from bright lights by closing blinds in the house, for example, or by fitting her with a visor, available in pet supply stores.

"If your pet has already lost part of her vision from glaucoma, you can help her adapt and live safely by keeping her surroundings constant," adds Dr. de Papp. This means not moving the furniture too often and being careful not to leave belongings where your pet might trip over them.

Cats with nutritional deficiencies are easily cared for by switching to name-brand, commercially prepared foods, all of which contain taurine and thiamin. If your cat simply loves fish, give her fish-flavored cat food. Or at least cook fish thoroughly before putting it in her bowl, which will deactivate the harmful substances it contains, says Dr. Gigliotti.

WHAT YOUR VET WILL DO

Since dilated pupils can signal brain or nerve problems, you won't have to wait long to see your vet. In fact, he will probably recommend that you come in right away.

Following an eye exam, your vet may recommend x-rays or blood tests to detect internal problems that could be putting pressure on the nerve. He will also measure the pressure inside your pet's eyes, which is a test for glaucoma.

"Don't be discouraged if the diagnosis is glaucoma," says Dr. de Papp, "because today we treat the disease with great success." Pets with glaucoma are usually treated with pills or eyedrops that reduce pressure in the eye.

If your pet has swallowed a toxic substance, your vet may induce vomiting to remove the poison. If she is showing other symptoms of poisoning, like seizures, your vet may give her medication to control the spasms.

If an infection is causing the problem, there is a good chance that antibiotics—and possibly medications to reduce swelling—will clear it up. But if the problem is a brain tumor or fluids accumulating near the eye, your pet may need surgery to relieve pressure on the nerve. After that, her eyes should quickly return to normal.

SYMPTOM) DISCHARGE

Clues

- Your pet has an eye infection.
- You have a bulgy-eyed breed like a Persian cat or Pekingese dog, or a giant breed of dog like a mastiff.
- Your pet is scratching a lot and has bloodshot eyes.

Like their human owners, dogs and cats sometimes wake up with "sleepers" in their eyes—a crusty discharge that results from the eye's natural self-cleaning efforts. All pets will occasionally have some discharge, although bulgy-eyed breeds such as pugs, Pekingese, and Persian cats are much more prone to it than others.

"If you can wipe away the sleepers in the morning with a damp tissue and they don't accumulate to any extent during the day, then you generally don't have to worry about it," says Nancy Willerton, D.V.M., a veterinarian in private practice in Denver. "But when the discharge continues throughout the day, your pet may have an infection."

Eye infections are fairly common, Dr. Willerton adds. They can crop up on their own or when something lodges in the eye. They can also occur when the surface of the eye, called the cornea, gets scratched. A telltale sign of infection is the appearance of the discharge: It will often be thick, yellow, gray, or green. It may form a crust on the eyelids as well.

Pets with viral infections such as feline respiratory disease in cats and canine adenovirus in dogs will often develop runny eyes. "It may start out as a watery discharge but then become thicker as the infection progresses," says Terri McGinnis, D.V.M., a veterinarian in private practice in the San Francisco area and author of *The Well Cat Book* and *The Well Dog Book*.

"Dogs and cats are prone to seasonal allergies, and the only sign may be a sticky eye discharge," adds Craig N. Carter, D.V.M., Ph.D., head of epidemiology at Texas Veterinary Medical Diagnostic Laboratory at Texas A&M University in College Station. Unlike bacterial or viral infections, allergies usually result in a clear discharge, he adds. Your pet may be scratching himself and have bloodshot eyes as well.

A problem in older pets is that the eyes naturally become drier. This makes it easy for the outer portion of the eye to get irritated and inflamed, which can result in a sticky, yellow discharge on the surface of the eyeball.

Finally, some pets have a slight genetic defect called entropion, in which the eyelid turns inward and causes the lashes to brush against the surface of the eye. In cats and some breeds of dogs, like golden and Labrador retrievers, entropion often affects the lower eyelid. In dogs with big heads and loose facial skin, such as Saint Bernards, shar-peis, and Chow Chows, both lids can be affected. Over time entropion can cause irritation and infection, resulting in a discharge.

What You Can Do

If your pet is prone to eye infections, it is a good idea to clean the eyes every day, which will make it harder for bacteria to thrive. "First thing in the morning, gently wipe away sleepers with a moistened tissue," says Dr. Willerton. You can moisten the tissue with saline solution, although tap water is fine, she adds.

If your pet has a discharge and is also pawing his eye, there may be something stuck inside. Prop his eye open by putting the thumb of one hand just above the eye and the thumb of the other hand just below it. "This helps to pull back the eyelids from the eye, giving you a better look inside," says Dr. McGinnis. "You can use a moistened tissue to remove foreign objects that aren't lodged in."

Even if you don't see anything in the eye, it is a good idea to give it a thorough flushing, adds Dr. Willerton. "That may be enough to wash out an undetectable but bothersome object," she says. She recommends washing the eye once or twice a day for two days. "As long as you start to see some improvement in the discharge after 48 hours, continue the eye-washes," she says. "Otherwise, it is time to see the vet."

Vets often recommend applying an antibiotic ointment made especially for the eye. Antibiotics only work against bacteria, however. There is not a lot you can do if your pet has a viral infection. "The disease will have to run its course, but bathing the eyes with saline solution can at least keep the discharge under control and help prevent a secondary bacterial infection from developing," says Dr. Willerton. In addition, keeping your pet's shots up-to-date will help prevent viral infections before they take hold.

Most pets with hay fever won't have serious problems with their eyes. If yours is the exception, however, you may want to keep him inside

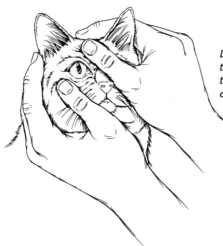

Dogs and cats don't like eye exams any more than people do. The only way to see if something is stuck inside is to hold his head firmly and use your thumbs to hold the eye open.

during the early morning and evening hours, when pollen counts tend to be highest.

For pets with dry eyes, an easy solution is to apply artificial tears, available from drugstores and pet supply stores, several times a day. These will keep the eyes lubricated and moist, reducing irritation that can lead to discharges or infections. Just be sure to avoid artificial tears that also contain ingredients for relieving red eyes since they may be harmful for pets.

WHAT YOUR VET WILL DO

Eye discharges may be ugly, but they are a valuable warning sign that something is wrong. This is important because infections can progress very quickly and even in some cases cause permanent eye damage. "Any off-colored eye discharge that persists for longer than 48 hours without improvement should be seen by a vet," says Dr. Willerton.

To find out what is causing the discharge, your vet will take a swab of the material and examine it under a microscope. In addition, she will probably look inside the eye with a specialized instrument called an ophthalmoscope, which makes it easy to spot (and remove) small objects that may be causing the problem. If your pet is uncommonly nervous, she may put a few drops of anesthetic in the eye to make the exam more comfortable, says Dr. Willerton.

If it turns out that your pet has a bacterial eye infection, your vet will probably apply an antibiotic ointment made especially for the eyes and give you pills to take home. For infections caused by allergies, she may use an ointment that also contains steroids, which will help reduce the inflammation, says Dr. Carter.

If your pet gets frequent eye infections due to allergies, your vet may recommend giving him allergy shots, which will make him less sensitive. "This may save the pet repeated aggravation—and save the pet owner money," says Merry Crimi, D.V.M., a veterinarian in private practice in Milwaukie, Oregon.

Vets usually advise that pets with dry eyes be given artificial tears once or twice a day. If the dryness is causing serious problems, however, your vet may recommend surgery to restore the normal flow of tears.

Surgery is often recommended to correct entropion as well. The surgeon will remove some of the loose skin from around the eyes, then reattach the remaining skin, pulling it tighter. This helps prevent the lids from rolling under and usually takes care of the problem.

See also Chapter 8: Squinting

SYMPTOM) EYELID GROWTH

Clues

- **Your pet is pawing his eyes.**
- **The eyes seem sore or irritated.**
- **There is loose skin on the edge of the eyelid.**

Your pet's eyelids act like windshield wipers set on automatic delay. All day long they periodically swipe a thin layer of moisturizing tears across the surface of the eyes, keeping them clean, moist, and free of irritating debris. But sometimes those wipers get a little ragged looking.

It is common for dogs and cats to develop tiny growths on the edges of the eyelids, which look like little bits of loose skin, says Terri McGinnis, D.V.M., a veterinarian in private practice in the San Francisco area and author of *The Well Cat Book* and *The Well Dog Book*. "In the overwhelming majority of cases, the little growths are benign, or noncancerous," she says.

In some cases, however, the growths can be bothersome, especially if they drop into your pet's line of sight or scrape against the eye when he blinks.

WHAT YOU CAN DO

When you detect eyelid growths that aren't causing problems, the best approach is usually to leave them alone. Still, you may want your vet to check the growths out, just to be safe. If your pet is squinting or pawing at his eye, however, or the eye looks red and irritated, you will need to call your vet right away.

"Pet owners have to be aware that a small percentage of these growths

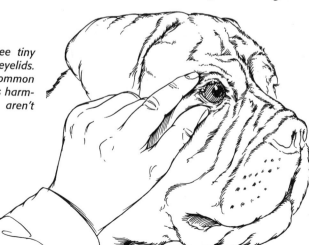

Don't worry if you see tiny growths on your pet's eyelids. They are extremely common and are almost always harmless as long as they aren't touching the eye.

are indeed cancerous," says Dr. McGinnis. "The only sure way to be safe is to have the growth removed by your vet and analyzed for the presence of cancer."

WHAT YOUR VET WILL DO

If your vet suspects an eyelid growth may be cancerous, she will begin by numbing the area with a local anesthetic. (When the growth is larger than average or your pet won't hold still, your vet may recommend putting him under general anesthetic.) Then she will remove the growth, being careful that none of it remains beneath the surface, and send the tissue to a laboratory so it can be tested for cancer.

In most cases, it will prove to be a false alarm. If it does turn out to be cancer, there are many treatments, including more surgery or radiation, that will help keep it from coming back.

EYELID IRRITATION

Clues

- Your pet's eyes are red or teary.
- She is squinting or avoiding the light.

Few things are more annoying than having the feeling that something is scratching your eye, and yet when you look, there is nothing there. Fortunately, this unpleasant sensation usually doesn't last very long—in humans. But some dogs and cats aren't so lucky. They always have that irritating feeling, and their eyes are red and teary. No matter how hard you look, however, you can't see what the problem is.

Take a closer look. The eyelids are designed to shield the surface of the eye without actually rubbing against it. But some pets have a condition called entropion, in which the eyelids turn under and the lashes brush against the eyes. "It feels like someone is brushing the surface of the eyes with a fairly coarse paintbrush," explains J. Pat Mims, D.V.M., a veterinarian in private practice in San Antonio.

Some pets have a genetic tendency to have loose skin around the eyes. This allows the lids to move around more than they should, and sometimes they turn under. In dogs, with big heads and loose facial skin, such as Saint Bernards, shar-peis, Chow Chows, both lids can be affected by entropion. In cats and some breeds of dogs like golden and Labrador retrievers, entropion often affects the lower eyelids.

The main symptoms of entropion are irritated, watery eyes. Pets may squint or shy away from light as well, says Robert L. Rooks, D.V.M., a veterinarian in private practice in Fountain Valley, California. Without treatment, entropion will never go away.

WHAT YOU CAN DO

The only treatment for entropion is to have surgery. To keep your pet comfortable in the meantime, it is a good idea to rinse the eyes once or twice a day with a soothing solution. You can choose either saline solution or a veterinary eyewash, which you can get in pet supply stores and drugstores, says Craig N. Carter, D.V.M., Ph.D., head of epidemiology at the Texas Veterinary Medical Diagnostic Laboratory at Texas A&M University in College Station. To apply, gently tilt your pet's head back, holding her muzzle firmly. Place the heel of the hand holding the dispenser above her eye. From the outside corner of her eye, direct the stream of solution onto the eye and let it wash over the surface. Take care not to touch the eye with the dispenser to avoid further injury.

"We also ask pet owners to watch for signs of infection," says Dr.

Rooks. The constant friction from the eyelids can scratch the surface of the eye, making it easy for bacteria or other organisms to get in. Eye infections usually cause a thick green or yellowish discharge. They can be quite serious, so you should call your vet if you suspect that an infection is starting.

WHAT YOUR VET WILL DO

The surgery for entropion is quite simple. The surgeon will remove some of the loose skin from around the eyes, then reattach the remaining skin, pulling it tighter. This prevents the lids from rolling under. Pets that have had such "face-lifts" get better very quickly, and the problem hardly ever comes back, says Dr. Mims.

The one drawback to surgery is that it is designed mainly for older pets that have finished growing. For young pets with entropion, vets often prescribe antibiotic or steroid drops, which will help keep the eye comfortable as the pet gets older. In some cases, the lid will correct itself and surgery won't be needed at all.

See also Chapter 8: Discharge, Squinting, Watery Eyes

EYELID SWELLING

Clues

- Your pet is taking a new medication.
- She has been stung by an insect.
- Your pet is pawing at her eyes.
- Her eye has a yellow or green discharge.

When one or both of your pet's eyelids puff up, she is probably having an allergic reaction—to an insect bite, a medication that she is taking, or simply seasonal pollen. Swelling may also occur when something gets stuck under the eyelid.

If the swelling comes on gradually and there is also a yellow or green discharge or crusting around the eyes, your pet could have an infection, either in the eyelid itself or in the tear-producing glands nearby.

Cats and some breeds of dogs like golden and Labrador retrievers are sometimes born with a defect in the eyelid known as entropion, which causes the lashes to brush against the eye. The constant irritation may cause the eyelids to swell. This usually affects the lower lid, although in dogs with big heads and loose facial skin, such as Saint Bernards, sharpeis, and Chow Chows, both lids can be affected.

WHAT YOU CAN DO

"Eyelid swelling that comes on very suddenly can be frightening, but it usually isn't serious," says E. Ann Lystrup, D.V.M., a veterinarian in private practice in Eau Claire, Wisconsin. And it generally clears up fast. Ask yourself if you are doing anything different that could be causing it. If you just started giving your pet a medication, for example, she could be having side effects, and your vet may recommend a different drug.

It is also a good idea to look inside your pet's eye to see if something is stuck inside an eyelid. Even if you can't see anything, take a moment to flush the eye with water or saline solution. This will wash away small particles that may be causing the problem, says Lori A. Wise, D.V.M., a veterinarian in private practice in Wheat Ridge, Colorado.

For dogs, vets sometimes recommend giving antihistamines containing diphenhydramine, such as Benadryl, to relieve swelling caused by insect bites and stings. The usual dose is one milligram for every pound of dog, three times a day, says Karen L. Campbell, D.V.M., associate professor of dermatology and small animal internal medicine at the University of Illinois College of Veterinary Medicine at Urbana–Champaign.

Cats can also take antihistamines. Vets recommend using Chlor-Trimeton, which contains an active ingredient called chlorpheniramine that is safer for cats than Benadryl. You can give half of a four-milligram tablet for every 10 pounds of cat, twice a day, says Dr. Campbell.

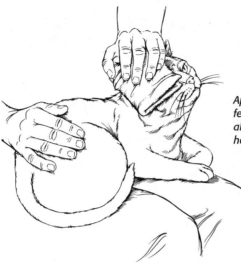

Applying a warm, moist compress to an infected eye will help it heal more quickly. It also feels good, and most pets won't mind holding still for it.

For dogs and cats, antihistamines "often relieve the swelling and also keep your pet from pawing at the eye, which makes her even more uncomfortable," says Dr. Wise. To be safe, check with your vet before giving antihistamines or other human medications to pets.

If the eyelid looks sore and infected, apply a warm, moist compress for about 10 minutes, three or four times a day, suggests Dr. Lystrup. This will relieve the discomfort, and often the infection will clear up on its own.

Since it is not always easy to tell what is causing the swelling, don't wait too long before calling your vet. "If you don't see some improvement after 24 to 36 hours, your pet's eyes need expert care," Dr. Lystrup says. You should take faster action if the swelling is accompanied by other symptoms, such as swelling of the tongue or difficulty breathing. These are signs of a serious allergic reaction and should be considered an emergency.

WHAT YOUR VET WILL DO

Some allergies can't be controlled with over-the-counter medications, so your vet may recommend giving your pet prescription antihistamines. Some prescription anti-inflammatory medications can help reduce the swelling.

When there is an infection in the eye that isn't relieved by warm compresses, your vet will probably give your pet antibiotics, either pills, an eye ointment, or both.

While medications can soothe the irritation, pets with entropion often need surgery to correct it. The surgeon will remove some of the loose skin from around the eyes, then reattach the remaining skin, pulling it tighter. This helps prevent the lids from rolling under and usually takes care of the problem. The surgery works best in older pets, however.

Red Lump in Eye

Clues

- Your pet's eyes look dry and irritated.
- You have a cocker spaniel, beagle, or a short-faced breed.

Your pet's eyes should be smooth, clear and bright, without any blemishes or bumps on the pristine surface. A red lump on the inside corner of the eye is definitely a problem—although not one you should panic about.

Dogs and cats have a unique structure called the third eyelid, a thin membrane that protrudes from the lower inside portion of the eye and swipes tears across the surface. Behind the third eyelid are tear and lymphatic glands. Periodically one of these glands may protrude over the top of the third eyelid, forming a red bulge. Vets call this condition cherry eye, and it can cause heavy tearing and frequent blinking, says Mark Nasisse, D.V.M., a veterinary ophthalmologist in private practice in Greensboro, North Carolina.

Cherry eye usually occurs when tissues that hold the gland in place are weaker than they should be. It is quite common in young dogs, especially Saint Bernards, German shepherds, Great Danes, cocker spaniels, beagles, and some of the short-faced breeds. Burmese cats will occasionally get cherry eye, but generally, it is more of a dog problem, says Jane Brunt, D.V.M., a veterinarian in private practice in Towson, Maryland.

Red lumps can also be caused by problems with the third eyelid itself. The eyelid contains a "spine" of cartilage. If this cartilage is somewhat misformed—a condition that vets call eversion—it will stick out slightly and irritate the surface of the eye.

Both cherry eye and third-eyelid eversion are quite rare in older pets, says Dr. Nasisse. Eye cancers, however, do develop later in life and sometimes they cause an irritated-looking red lump somewhere in the eye.

What You Can Do

Serious eye problems should always be treated by a vet, but sometimes you have to act quickly at home to protect your pet from further damage. If your pet gets cherry eye, for example, and for some reason you can't get to a vet, you may have to readjust the popped-out gland yourself, says Virginia Garrison, D.V.M., a veterinarian in private practice in Lexington, Kentucky.

It sounds scary, but it is often easy to do. Sliding the eyelids up over the "cherry" will usually cause the gland to pop back into place. Put your finger or thumb at the edge of the lower eyelid near the nose, says Dr. Garrison. Applying gentle pressure, slide both the outer and inner eyelids over the swelling. "This only works if you do it the very same day it popped out," she adds. If the lump doesn't pop back into place easily or if your pet seems to be in a lot of pain, give up right away and do your best to get to a vet.

Sometimes putting the gland back in place will correct the problem for good. But in many cases, pets will need surgery to eliminate the underlying cause. "The sooner we see a pet with this type of eye problem, the more quickly we can help him," says Dr. Nasisse.

WHAT YOUR VET WILL DO

Eye cancer isn't very common, but it is the first thing that your vet will want to check for if your pet is six years or older. Testing for cancer means putting your pet under anesthesia and taking a biopsy of the lump, says Dr. Nasisse.

Your vet will probably give you anti-inflammatory eyedrops to use at home. The drops will partially shrink the gland, which may help prevent it from popping out again. The vet may have to reposition the gland several times before it finally stays put for good—if indeed it ever does.

"The vast majority of cherry eyes—and all third-eyelid eversions—are going to need surgery," says Dr. Nasisse. For cherry eye, the surgeon will "tack" the gland into place with sutures that hold it more firmly than the eye tissues did. Eversions can also be easy to correct. The surgeon will trim away the excess cartilage that is causing the bulge. After the surgery, the eyelid will lie flat the way it is supposed to, and the lump will be gone, he says.

SQUINTING

Clues

- Your pet is elderly.
- Her eyes look irritated and painful.

When dogs and cats walk into sunlight after spending time in a darkened room, they will naturally clamp down their eyelids to as narrow a slit as possible. Squinting is the body's way of reducing the intensity of light while the eyes are adjusting to the change.

When squinting lasts more than a second or two, however, you can be pretty sure that something other than light is irritating her eyes, says L. R. Danny Daniel, D.V.M., a veterinarian in private practice in Covington, Louisiana. A small piece of debris, like dust or a grass seed, can be very painful when it lodges in the eye, he says. Even a blast of wind from riding in the car with her head out the window can irritate your pet's eyes and cause squinting later on.

As pets age, they may develop iris atrophy, in which the iris—the part of the eye that controls the amount of light getting in—begins to shrink. As the iris gets smaller, an uncomfortable amount of light may begin striking nerve fibers in the eyes, and pets will squint to reduce the glare.

Pets with glaucoma, a serious condition in which pressure builds up inside the eye, will often squint, says Nick A. Faber, D.V.M., a veterinary ophthalmology resident at the University of California School of Veterinary Medicine, Davis.

Another eye condition, called anterior uveitis, also causes painful pressure in the eyes, he adds. Often caused by infection, parasites, tumors, injuries, or internal problems such as high blood pressure, it can make the eyes intensely sensitive to light.

WHAT YOU CAN DO

If you discover that your pet has iris atrophy, about the only thing you can do is keep her away from bright light. One strategy is to plan her outdoor excursions for early morning and later in the evening, when the light isn't so bright. You may even want to feed her later (or earlier) in the day so that she won't have take trips outside during the brightest times.

"Keep her out of direct light inside the house, too," says E. Ann Lystrup, D.V.M., a veterinarian in private practice in Eau Claire, Wisconsin. This may mean keeping curtains and blinds slightly closed, at least in the rooms where your pet spends most of her time.

One way to protect her eyes without making your whole house dark is to give her a visor. Available in pet supply stores, visors are an excellent way to prevent direct light from hitting her eyes—if you can get her to wear it. "You

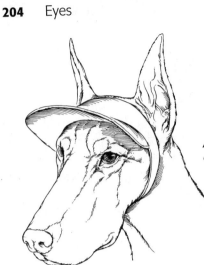

A visor can help protect your pet's eyes from direct light—and it looks rather sporty, too.

will just have to try it to determine if she has the personality to leave it on," says Beverly J. Scott, D.V.M., a veterinarian in private practice in Gilbert, Arizona.

If you are pretty sure that your pet is squinting because something is irritating her eyes—after a romp through tall grass, for example—try flooding the eyes with saline solution, says Dr. Daniel. This will help float away debris and will lubricate the eyes so that they are less dry and painful.

"If your pet is in a lot of pain, she may not allow you to rinse her eyes," adds Dr. Daniel. "That's a pretty good sign that she needs to get to a vet for immediate attention. If the cause is something serious, every minute counts when it comes to saving your pet's vision."

WHAT YOUR VET WILL DO

Eye exams can be painful, so your vet will begin by applying anesthetic drops, which numb the eye, says Dr. Faber.

He may follow that with additional drops that reveal certain kinds of injuries. "With a type of staining drop known as fluorescein dye, we can determine if the surface of the eyeball is scratched," says Dr. Daniel.

To test for glaucoma, your vet will measure the amount of pressure inside the eye. He will also check your pet's overall health since anterior uveitis can be caused by high blood pressure, infections, or even cancer.

"We can do just about anything for a pet's eyes that we can for a human's eyes," Dr. Faber adds. For instance, if your pet has glaucoma, taking medications will help reduce pressure in the eyes and relieve the discomfort. For anterior uveitis, treating the underlying condition, such as high blood pressure, will clear up the eye problem as well.

See also Chapter 8: Discharge

WATERY EYES

Clues

- Your pet is squinting.
- He has been riding with his head out the car window.
- Your pet has bloodshot eyes and itchy ears.

You are not aware of them, but tears are always present on the surface of your pet's eyes. They act as a lubricating fluid, keeping the eyes moist and protecting them from dirt and scratches. They also contain enzymes that help to prevent the growth of bacteria.

Sometimes the tear ducts open wide, producing torrents of water. This usually occurs when something lodges in the eye and irritates the surface. Copious tears are the body's attempt to flush it out. "When tearing comes on suddenly, the tears are clear, and just one eye is affected, you can be pretty sure that the cause is a foreign object," says Nancy Willerton, D.V.M., a veterinarian in private practice in Denver.

Dogs such as basset hounds, bloodhounds, and Newfoundlands are especially prone to problems because they have a large space between the eyelids and the surface of the eye, which allows grit to get inside.

Watering sometimes occurs if the conjunctiva, a thin layer of tissue covering the inside of the eyelids, gets irritated. A speck of grass or dust can irritate the conjuctiva, sometimes causing the eye to water for days. Too much sun or wind—from riding in the car with the windows open, for example—can also cause the conjunctiva to get red and inflamed.

A more serious cause of watery eyes is when the cornea, the surface of the eye, gets scratched. "Corneal scratches are painful, and your pet may squint to shut out painful light," says Dr. Willerton.

When both eyes are tearing and the liquid is clear, there is a good chance that your pet has allergies that are similar to hay fever in humans. "If the tearing starts at a change of season, you will have good reason to suspect an allergy," says Merry Crimi, D.V.M., a veterinarian in private practice in Milwaukie, Oregon. Other signs of allergies include red eyes and itchy ears, she adds.

Pets with glaucoma, a serious condition in which fluids accumulate inside the eye, will often have watery eyes. The eyes may also be dilated as well, causing the pet to squint to block out the excess light that his wide-open pupils are letting in.

In cats, watery eyes may be caused by viral infections such as feline respiratory disease. If the infection is serious, watery eyes may be accompanied by other symptoms, like sneezing, drooling, or a loss of appetite. In addition, the eye discharge may change from clear to yellow, sticky, and puslike.

Watery eyes aren't always a problem. Certain short-faced breeds like miniature poodles and Persian cats have bulgy eyes, and they need the extra tears to keep their eyes moist. In fact, some breeds only *appear* to produce a lot of tears. Because of the way their heads are constructed, the tears may run down their faces instead of along the tear canals, making the moisture more visible.

What You Can Do

When only one eye is watery, prop it open and take a look inside. There may be a bit of dirt or grass that is causing irritation. "Try to snag it with the edge of a clean tissue, but don't use tweezers or any other instrument in your pet's eye," says Dr. Willerton.

If you can't see anything, try flooding the eye with saline solution or plain water. If the eye continues tearing for 48 hours, you will want to call your vet. Occasionally, grit gets trapped out of sight, and you will need help from your vet to get it out, says Dr. Willerton.

If you suspect that your pet's eyes are simply sun- or windburned, bathe them with saline solution or warm water, Dr. Willerton suggests. Then keep him out of the sun and wind for a few days.

Hay fever isn't all that difficult to recognize, but it can be very tricky to prevent. About all you can do on your own is try to keep your pet away from whatever is making his eyes water. This might mean staying indoors during the early morning and evening hours, when pollen counts tend to be highest. You will also want to keep him off freshly mowed lawns since mowing spews clouds of allergy-causing molds into the air.

Most minor eye problems will clear up within a few days. But if the eye is still watering after two days, play it safe and take your pet to the vet. "You won't want to wait even that long if your pet seems to be in a lot of pain, or if an off-colored discharge develops in the injured eye," says Dr. Willerton.

What Your Vet Will Do

Eye exams can be painful, so your vet will probably start the checkup by putting a few drops of anesthetic in your pet's eyes. After that, she will take a look inside—and, if you are lucky, she will quickly spot whatever is causing the problem and fish it out.

If there is a scratch on the cornea, your vet may give you an antibiotic ointment to apply every day to help heal the injury and prevent infection. "If your pet paws excessively at the eye, your vet may bandage it for several days to speed healing," says Dr. Willerton.

Allergies aren't always a problem. If your pet simply has watery eyes

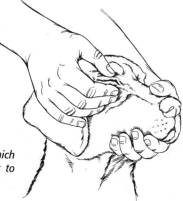

When applying an antibiotic eye ointment, hold your pet's head securely and apply a thin line of ointment along the lower inside eyelid or directly on the eye, making sure that the tip of the tube doesn't touch his eye.

Hold his eye closed for a few seconds, which will warm the ointment and cause it to spread evenly over the eye.

and doesn't seem uncomfortable, your vet will probably recommend leaving them alone. If the eyes are also red and inflamed, however, she may recommend giving your pet a skin test to identify what he is sensitive to. If your pet does have allergies, he might need antihistamines to relieve the discomfort. In more serious cases, your pet may need a series of anti-allergy shots.

Glaucoma is always a serious problem, which is usually treated with eyedrops or oral medications to reduce pressure inside the eye. "In days gone by, there wasn't much we could do for glaucoma, but today things are very different," says Dr. Willerton. Since glaucoma can make the eyes very sensitive, your vet may recommend keeping your pet away from bright light until the condition is under control.

Pets with viral respiratory infections—and the resulting watery eyes—often don't need medical treatment, says Dr. Willerton. This type of infection usually clears up in a short time. If the original infection is serious, however, your vet may give him antibiotics to treat (or prevent) bacterial infections that may have taken hold. Your pet may also need fluids, sometimes given intravenously, to reverse dehydration.

The best treatment for respiratory infections is prevention: Vaccinating your cat on schedule will help prevent the most common infections from getting started.

COMMON EYE CONDITIONS

Cataracts. Something different is going on if your pet's eyes develop a gray, bluish, or whitish cast or form little silver specks. These changes, known as cataracts, occur when the lens (the part of the eye that focuses light rays) gets slightly hard and loses its transparency. The change of eye color is caused by the light rays bouncing off the lens rather than passing through.

Almost all dogs and cats will have cataracts to some degree by their eighth birthdays. The condition is especially common in pets that have diabetes or have had eye injuries in the past. But the way that cataracts affect your pet are not at all comparable to the way they affect humans. Most dogs and cats will adapt nicely. For one thing, cataracts are rarely severe enough to cause blindness. In addition, dogs and cats can compensate for the loss of vision by depending more on their other senses—especially their senses of smell and hearing. It is only when cataracts are severe or pets are having trouble coping that vets recommend surgery to remove them.

Conjunctivitis. The surface of the eye is exceedingly delicate, which is why it has a tough, but nearly invisible layer of protection called the conjunctiva. The conjunctiva's job is to protect the eye from wind, grit, and other foreign objects.

If something gets lodged inside the conjunctiva, the eye will get sore, red, and watery. This condition, called conjunctivitis, can be very painful. "If the inflammation doesn't heal within a few days, an infection may crop up," says Nick A. Faber, D.V.M., a veterinary ophthalmology resident at the University of California School of Veterinary Medicine, Davis. You will know there is an infection because the discharge from the eye, rather than being clear and runny, may turn a nasty yellow or green color, and there may be a thick, crusty material on the eyelids.

You can often treat conjunctivitis at home by flooding the eye with saline solution or artificial tears. Just be sure to avoid artificial tears that also contain ingredients for relieving red eyes since they may be harmful for pets. If something is stuck inside an eyelid, you can swab out the speck with the tip of a handkerchief or tissue. If an infection has already taken hold, however, your vet will need to treat it—usually with an antibiotic ointment made especially for the eyes or with oral medications.

Corneal scratches. The transparent tissue that forms the front of the eye is called the cornea. When the cornea gets scratched—by a bit of dust or a low-hanging branch, for example—the eye can get red, watery, and very sore.

Corneal scratches are common in dogs and cats simply because they tend to run first and look where they are going afterward. "It doesn't take much for an injury to scratch the cornea," says Nancy Willerton, D.V.M., a veterinarian in private practice in Denver.

Corneal scratches usually aren't serious and will heal on their own. If the eye is still sore after 48 hours or if your pet is blinking repeatedly or squinting to block out the light, you should call your vet right away.

Entropion. Some pets are born with a slight deformity in which the eyelid rolls inward, causing the eyelashes to constantly brush against the surface of the eye. This condition, called entropion, can affect both eyelids in dogs with big heads and loose facial skin such as Saint Bernards, shar-peis, and Chow Chows. In cats and some breeds of dogs like golden and Labrador retrievers, entropion often affects the lower lids only. "This is a very irritating condition, causing eyelid swelling, tearing, and even corneal scratches," says Dr. Willerton.

Your vet may suggest that you keep your pet's eyes lubricated by putting in drops of saline solution. For older pets who have finished growing, veterinarians sometimes recommend surgery, which will prevent the lids from rolling under.

Glaucoma. The eyes are naturally filled with fluids, which create just enough internal pressure for the eyeball to hold its shape. But in pets with glaucoma, pressure inside the eyes rises to dangerous levels, causing pain and possibly blindness, says Christopher J. Murphy, D.V.M., associate professor of ophthalmology at the University of Wisconsin School of Veterinary Medicine in Madison.

Glaucoma occurs more often in dogs than in cats, and in some breeds of dogs more than others. Cocker spaniels and basset hounds have an especially high risk of glaucoma. In both cats and dogs, it is much more common as they get older, says Dr. Murphy.

You can't diagnose glaucoma at home, but warning signs include red or cloudy eyes, teariness, a dilated pupil, a blue layer across the surface of the eyes, and possibly bulging eyes. Since glaucoma is painful, your pet may be squinting or pawing his eyes as well.

You need to see your vet immediately if you suspect that your pet has glaucoma. Once it is diagnosed, it can easily be treated with medications that help bring the pressure down.

Nuclear sclerosis. The eyes normally shed and replace cells at a roughly the same rate. As the eyes get older, however, they become less efficient at discarding old cells. Instead of being washed away, discarded cells accumulate, thickening the eyes and causing them turn slightly blue. Vets refer to this condition as nuclear sclerosis.

Nuclear sclerosis usually isn't serious. Some pets will lose a little vision, but in most cases it doesn't cause any problems at all, says Dr. Faber.

Prolapsed eyeball. It is scary to think about, but an accident or a hit on the head can cause the eyeball to literally pop out of its socket, a condition called prolapsed eyeball, or proptosis. "While this can occur in any breed of dog or cat, pets with bulgier eyes, like pugs, Pekingese, and Persians, are at greater risk simply because their eyes stick out farther to begin with," says L. R. Danny Daniel, D.V.M., a veterinarian in private practice in Covington, Louisiana.

This prolapsed eyeball is obviously quite serious. Once the eyeball pops out, the eyelid clamps down behind it, trapping the eyeball outside the socket and possibly cutting off the supply of blood. It is essential to get the eye back into its socket within about 10 minutes in order to preserve your pet's sight, says Dr. Daniel. If you can't get to your vet's office immediately, it is possible to replace the eye yourself, but it is best to get to a veterinarian immediately, he adds. (For more information on how to perform this procedure, see Bulging Eyes on page 185.)

Hindquarters

Your pet's back end is a busy place. This is the area where the urinary, digestive, and reproductive systems all come together in a complex, intertwined series of tubes, valves, storage vessels, and openings. A problem in any one part can cause problems all the way up the line—which is why hindquarter symptoms can be so confusing. Blood in the urine, for example, could be a sign of a urinary tract infection—or it could mean that something is wrong with the uterus. Pets with prostate problems often have abdominal tenderness, as you might expect, but another symptom might be flattened stools. It is tricky even for vets to figure out what is causing the symptoms.

There are dozens of problems that can affect this area. Infections are common simply because the hindquarters includes a number of openings to the body, including the anus, urethra, and the vagina.

Pets with hindquarter problems often need antibiotics or other medications. Just as often, simple lifestyle changes, like getting more exercise or a change in diet, will help keep them healthy.

See Your Vet If:

- Your pet's tail is limp.
- A discharge from the anus, penis, or vagina has lasted two days or more.
- Your pet is constantly licking his back end.
- The vagina or anal area is red and swollen.
- There is a growth on the anus or genitals.
- Urine is dribbling while your pet sleeps.

- There has been a change in your pet's urinating habits, or he is unable to urinate.
- There is blood in the urine.
- He's lost fur on the top or base of the tail.
- The tail is greasy or infected, or it is getting thicker.
- The anal opening stays open.
- Your pet has been scooting for two days or more.

ANAL SECRETIONS

Clues

- There is a discharge, bleeding, or a foul smell in the anal area.
- Your pet is frequently scooting or licking her bottom.

It is not as elegant as a bouquet of roses or a handwritten note, but dogs and cats have their own method for communicating: They sniff each other's bottoms. Every pet releases a fluid that contains unique scent signals, which they use for marking territory, establishing status, and simply identifying themselves.

Most of the time, these pet-to-pet signals are invisible, and you will never see them. When you can actually see a discharge, however, there is probably something wrong.

In dogs (but usually not cats), an anal discharge may occur when tissues in the anus and rectum get inflamed and ulcerated, a condition called a perianal fistula. Vets aren't sure what causes this, although it may begin when bacteria invade hair follicles around the anus, causing a painful and potentially serious infection. In addition to a foul-smelling discharge, there may be bleeding. This condition can occur in any dog but is most common in large breeds such as German shepherds and English and Irish setters.

An anal discharge can also occur when the anal sacs—one on either side of the anus—don't drain properly. The buildup of fluids can lead to an infection, possibly followed by an abscess, an open sore that can ooze and bleed, says Lori A. Wise, D.V.M., a veterinarian in private practice in Wheat Ridge, Colorado. Since an anal abscess can be extremely uncomfortable, dogs and cats will often scoot on their bottoms to relieve the irritation. In fact, scooting is one of the main signs of anal problems.

WHAT YOU CAN DO

An anal discharge almost always means that your pet has an infection, and you will need to get her to the vet right away. Even if you don't see a discharge, watch out for other warning signs, like frequent scooting or licking the rear end for long periods of time. The anal sacs are probably blocked and need to be drained of their excess fluid. "Doing this quickly can prevent a painful infection that will be even more difficult to treat," says Dr. Wise. (For more on draining anal sacs, see Licking Hind End on page 220.)

Even when your pet is being treated for an infection, it may take a week or more to stop the discharge. In the meantime, you may want to buy little protective panties at the pet supply store. Made for dogs and cats, they have a small cotton panel that will help keep the house and fur-

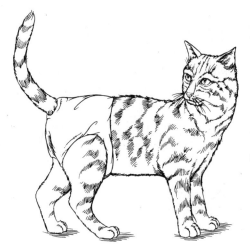

Diapers aren't very dignified, but when your pet has an anal infection, they will help keep the house clean.

niture clean, says Paul Gigliotti, D.V.M., a veterinarian in private practice in Mayfield Village, Ohio. You will need to change them several times a day to prevent the secretions from irritating tender tissues.

WHAT YOUR VET WILL DO

When the anal sacs are infected, your vet will begin by cleaning out the infected material. It sounds unpleasant—and it is—but it usually takes just a few minutes to do. Once the sacs are empty, your pet will be given antibiotics to knock out the infection. In addition, your vet may apply an anti-inflammatory cream to relieve the swelling.

A perianal fistula is much more serious than a simple abscess. Medications alone won't help. In most cases, your vet will need to do surgery to remove the damaged tissues and possibly to repair or strengthen the area around the anus.

BLOOD IN URINE

Clues

- The urine is red.
- Your pet is urinating more than usual.
- Your female dog or cat has recently had a heat cycle or has given birth.
- The penis or testicles are swollen.

Few things are more alarming than seeing blood in your pet's urine. Even though the causes of bleeding are usually easy to treat, fast action is essential. "The tissues of the urinary tract are very fragile, and any changes in your pet's health can cause bleeding," says Beverly J. Scott, D.V.M., a veterinarian in private practice in Gilbert, Arizona.

Urinary tract infections are the most common cause of blood in the urine. The infection may be in the kidneys, bladder, or urethra (the tube through which urine flows). Dogs and cats with urinary tract infections will usually urinate much more often than usual, and they may have fevers as well.

In male dogs (but usually not cats), blood in the urine may mean that the prostate gland, which produces semen, has become infected. Dogs with an infected prostate gland typically have a swollen penis and testicles, says Paul Gigliotti, D.V.M., a veterinarian in private practice in Mayfield Village, Ohio.

In female dogs and cats, blood may be a sign of a uterine infection, which typically occurs a month or two after a heat cycle or soon after giving birth. The blood comes from the vagina rather than through the urethra, but you are most likely to see it when they urinate.

Sharp little stones will occasionally form in the urinary tract, scraping the urethra and causing bleeding. "When the stones are tiny, like bits of gravel, some pets pass them without pain, but you may notice bloody urine," says Dr. Gigliotti.

Pets that have gotten into harmful substances such as rat poison will sometimes have bloody urine. (Other signs of poisoning include vomiting, diarrhea, or restlessness.) In addition, a bite from an infected tick can cause an infection called babesiosis, which destroys red blood cells. The body gets rid of the damaged blood cells by filtering them through the kidneys, which turns the urine red or brown.

Injuries can also cause urine to change color. Pets that have taken a hard fall or been hit by a car, for example, may look fine, but blood in the urine is a telltale sign that they have had internal injuries.

WHAT YOU CAN DO

"Bloody urine is a symptom that needs urgent veterinary care," says Dr. Scott. While some conditions such as minor bladder infections aren't emergencies, there is no way for you to know what is causing the problem or whether it is serious. So it is essential to call your vet right away, especially if you suspect that your pet has gotten into something poisonous.

Dogs and cats that have had urinary stones or urinary tract infections usually get them more than once, so prevention is important. "Keep her water bowl full of clean water, which will encourage her to drink more. This helps flush out the system and will help prevent both stones and infections," says Dr. Scott. Your vet may recommend feeding your pet foods that are low in magnesium, which will help prevent urinary stones, she adds. Any good diet designed to reduce the formation of stones in dogs and cats will have reduced magnesium.

Infections in the reproductive system aren't common, but they can be quite serious. You can prevent them entirely by neutering your pet. "The best time to neuter a pet is when he's around six months old," says Dr. Gigliotti.

WHAT YOUR VET WILL DO

Bloody urine is a symptom vets see all too often because there are more than 50 conditions that can cause it. Even so, it is usually not a difficult problem to diagnose. Your vet can tell a lot about the cause by testing a urine sample. If there is pus in the urine, he will know for sure that there is an infection somewhere in the urinary tract. He can also tell where the infection is by the type of blood cells that are present. "Depending on what these tests reveal, your vet may do x-rays and possibly an ultrasound of the urinary tract, especially when stones are suspected," says Dr. Scott.

Most infections can be cured with oral antibiotics. "When the infection is serious, your vet may give antibiotics intravenously, and your pet may have to stay at the clinic for a night or two," says Dr. Gigliotti. For uterine infections, which can be life-threatening, your vet may recommend spaying your pet immediately.

Stones in the urinary tract will often come out on their own. When they are large, however, your vet may recommend surgery to remove them. In addition, he may give your pet medications that will help prevent stones from forming there in the future.

If your pet has gotten into a rodent poison that causes bleeding, she will probably be given an injection of vitamin K_1, which can reverse the effects, says Dan M. Jordan, D.V.M., a veterinarian in private practice in Houston.

See also Chapter 9: Genital Discharge

SYMPTOM) GENITAL DISCHARGE

Clues

- The discharge is bloody or has a foul odor.
- Your dog or cat has a fever or diminished appetite.
- Your pet is spending a lot of time licking the backside.

It is normal for dogs and cats to have a slight discharge at certain times, such as when they are in heat. Most of the time, however, a genital discharge is a sure sign of infection, and you will need to take care of it right away.

In males, a yellowish or blood-tinged discharge usually means that they have an infection in the urethra (the tube through which urine flows) or in the prostate gland. Pets with a prostate infection are often quite sick, with abdominal pain and a loss of appetite, says L. R. Danny Daniel, D.V.M., a veterinarian in private practice in Covington, Louisiana. Less often, a bloody discharge in males may be caused by an injury to the penis.

Female dogs and cats are much more likely than males to have a genital discharge. Female pets that haven't been spayed will sometimes get a serious uterine infection called pyometra. This can result in a bloody, pus-filled discharge. "It commonly occurs about 45 to 60 days after the pet was in heat and wasn't bred," says Dr. Daniel.

Discharges will sometimes occur in pregnant dogs and cats when they are about to have a miscarriage. "This is nature's way of taking care of abnormal fetuses or an infection in the womb that would otherwise threaten the mother's life," says Dr. Daniel. This type of discharge will usually be bloody, possibly with a little pus mixed in.

Females that have recently had a litter are also prone to uterine infections. What sometimes happens is that part of the placenta stays behind after delivery, providing a fertile breeding ground for bacteria.

"You should suspect that something is wrong if the new mother, who is generally overprotective, ignores her offspring or refuses to eat," says Dr. Daniel. This type of infection usually causes a foul-smelling vaginal discharge that starts out watery and a little red, and then gets thicker and turns dark brown and contains pus as the infection progresses.

It doesn't happen often, but an infection and discharge may occur after dogs and cats are spayed if a little bit of the uterus was left behind, says Dr. Daniel. "If your pet is listless, lacks an appetite, drinks a lot of water, and is paying a lot of attention to her backside—such as excessive licking—check under her tail for a discharge." If you see a discharge, take her back to the vet immediately, he advises.

WHAT YOU CAN DO

By the time a genital discharge appears, the underlying infection is probably well-advanced and needs quick treatment. "These infections can be life-threatening, so get your pet to the vet as soon as possible," says Dr. Daniel. In males, it is a good idea to apply an ice pack to the penis until you can get him to the vet. This will help reduce swelling that can be caused by a prostate infection.

Even though you can't treat internal infections at home, they are often easy to prevent. Having your pet neutered will guard against almost all the problems that can cause a genital discharge in males as well as females, says Dr. Daniel.

WHAT YOUR VET WILL DO

Uterine infections are serious because there is a chance that the infection will spread to other parts of the body. "Your vet will probably keep a pet with a uterine infection at the hospital and give her intravenous antibiotics," says Dr. Daniel.

Infections in males are generally less serious. Your vet will probably give you a prescription for oral antibiotics, which will clear up the condition in a week or two. For problems with the prostate gland, the simplest solution is to neuter your pet. During the procedure the prostate gland—as well as the testicles—are removed.

SYMPTOM) INCONTINENCE

Clues

- Your pet urinates without being aware of it.
- Your female pet has been spayed.
- Your pet is having difficulty walking.

It is not a problem with kittens, but when you have a puppy in the house, it sometimes seems as though every square foot of carpet, tile, or hardwood floor has a bull's-eye on it—one that he can hit every time. With patience, however, accidents become much less common.

That can change as your pets get older. Both dogs and cats will sometimes lose bladder control—not because they have forgotten their lessons, but because they are not even aware that they are urinating when (or where) they shouldn't, says Paul Gigliotti, D.V.M., a veterinarian in private practice in Mayfield Village, Ohio.

This problem, called incontinence, tends to occur in older female pets that have been spayed. After spaying, estrogen levels decline. Since estrogen helps maintain muscle tone in the urinary tract, low levels of this hormone may cause these muscles to lose some of their holding power. The muscles will gradually become so weak that small amounts of urine will occasionally leak out, says Dr. Gigliotti. This problem is most common in Doberman pinschers, springer spaniels, and Old English sheepdogs, he adds.

In males, incontinence may occur when the prostate gland gets larger due to infections or natural changes that occur with age. If the prostate begins pressing on the bladder, urine can be forced out. Even when there is nothing physically wrong with your pet, muscles in the urinary tract tend to get weaker with age, Dr. Gigliotti adds. That is why incontinence is much more common in older dogs and cats than in their younger and stronger friends.

"When incontinence occurs in a younger animal, you should suspect a different type of problem," says Dr. Gigliotti. Some pets are born with physical abnormalities that make incontinence much more likely to occur, such as an oddly positioned bladder that gets pressed by the pelvic bones. Another problem that can cause incontinence in young dogs and cats is called persistent urachus. This occurs when a small tube connecting the bladder with the umbilical cord doesn't close after birth.

Dogs and cats with urinary tract infections will often leak a little urine because the infection causes a sudden urge to go—so sudden, in fact, that they don't have time to get to the litter box or to wait by the door. They may have an awkward walk because of pain in the abdomen as well.

Injuries that damage spinal nerves can also result in incontinence—

not just of urine, but of stool as well. And in rare cases, pets with tumors may have trouble controlling these basic functions.

WHAT YOU CAN DO

"The first thing that many people want to do when their pet becomes incontinent is to withhold water," says E. Ann Lystrup, D.V.M., a veterinarian in private practice in Eau Claire, Wisconsin. But cutting back on water won't cure the problem and may make the pet sick, she says. The one exception to this rule is at bedtime. Dogs and cats don't need to be drinking at night, and it is fine to pick up the water bowl when you go to bed. "You can take your pet out last thing at night, and then he won't have as much urine to lose during the night," she says.

You should always check with your vet if your pet has a sudden loss of bowel or bladder control. In the meantime, be sure to take your pet outside frequently or, for cats, put an extra litter box in the house so that they always have a place nearby. This won't prevent incontinence, but by reducing the amount of urine in the bladder, it can relieve the pressure that can lead to leaks at the wrong times.

WHAT YOUR VET WILL DO

Even though incontinence usually occurs in older pets, it is not an inevitable part of aging, says Dr. Lystrup. There is usually an underlying problem, and that is what your vet can treat.

Your vet will probably begin by taking a urine sample, which will reveal whether or not your pet has an infection that can be treated with antibiotics. She may draw blood to check for hormonal imbalances. And, if she suspects that there could be a spinal injury, she may recommend x-rays or a myelogram, a test in which dye is injected into the spinal canal to reveal whether or not any nerves are being damaged.

Female dogs and cats may need estrogen supplements and that will stop the problem, says Dr. Lystrup. For males, antibiotics are often used to knock out a prostate infection. "When they are troubled repeatedly by prostate infections or inflammation, we often recommend neutering them, which will clear up the problem," she says. In both males and females that have lost some of their "holding" ability, your vet may recommend medications that will help make the muscles stronger.

In rare cases, dogs and cats may need surgery to repair physical deformities that are causing the problem. If the bladder is in the wrong place, for example, your vet may recommend surgery to reposition it. Surgery may also be needed for a back problem, although it often will heal on its own within a few weeks if your pet is kept indoors and quiet.

LICKING HIND END

Clues

- Your pet is scooting across the floor.
- She spends more than a few seconds licking her bottom.
- She has had constipation or diarrhea.
- There are white specks in the stool or around the anus.

Even the best-trained dogs and cats don't use washcloths. But they are still a pretty clean crowd as long as they use their tongues. When they are feeling dirty, such as after using the litter box, they lick their backsides. It is just their way of keeping clean. "This grooming should take only a few licks," explains Bonnie V. Beaver, D.V.M., an animal behaviorist and chief of medicine in the department of small animal medicine and surgery at Texas A&M University College of Veterinary Medicine in College Station.

But some pets don't quit with a lick and polish. They keep licking long after they are clean. When you see this happening, you can be pretty sure that something is wrong.

The skin surrounding the anus is very fragile. A spell of diarrhea or the passing of a hard stool can irritate the skin, and dogs and cats will lick to ease the soreness. This is especially common when something hard in the stool, like a bit of bone, has scraped the anal area. This usually occurs in dogs because they are less careful than cats about what they eat.

Another common cause of licking is full anal sacs. These two sacs, which are located on either side of the anus, contain a strong-smelling liquid that gets released with every bowel movement. Sometimes, however, the sacs get blocked and the fluid can't get out. "When this happens, the fluid accumulates, and your pet becomes quite uncomfortable. This can cause her to lick excessively at the area to relieve the discomfort," says Dr. Beaver. In addition to licking, pets with blocked anal sacs will often scoot their bottoms across the ground.

Pets with tapeworms will often spend hours licking their bottoms. These lengthy parasites, which occasionally take up residence in the digestive tract, are made up of many little segments that are continually breaking off. As they leave the body in a stool, the clingy segments sometimes attach themselves with little tentacles to the anus, causing intense itching. You can spot tapeworms by lifting the tail and looking for what appear to be grains of white rice.

WHAT YOU CAN DO

"Many pets will get diarrhea or become constipated with even slight changes in their diets," says L. R. Danny Daniel, D.V.M., a veterinarian in private practice in Covington, Louisiana. His recommendation? Give your pet a high-quality food and stick with one brand. Don't give her leftovers from the dinner table because they may be too rich for her to comfortably digest.

It is also important to keep the water bowl full because pets that don't drink enough will often have hard stools. If your pet does get constipated, you can put a little Metamucil in her food, which will help keep her regular, says Lori A. Wise, D.V.M., a veterinarian in private practice in Wheat Ridge, Colorado.

For cats and small dogs, give about a half-teaspoon of Metamucil twice a day. For larger pets, give one to two teaspoons twice a day until they pass a normal stool, advises Karen Mateyak, D.V.M., a veterinarian in private practice in Brooklyn, New York. To be safe, ask your vet what dose is right for your pet.

It's not exactly fun to do, but applying a little petroleum jelly or an over-the-counter hemorrhoid ointment while wearing latex gloves can ease irritation and help the anal area heal, says Dr. Wise.

The only cure for blocked anal sacs is to unblock them. Most people have their vets do this, but it is not difficult to do at home, says Dr. Wise. You may, however, want to have someone hold the pet to help keep her calm. Put on a pair of latex gloves. Using a tissue, feel around the outside of the anus for the sacs. With your thumb and forefinger, press on one sac at a time until fluid comes out. The amount of fluid can vary from a few drops to as much as a quarter-teaspoon. In most cases, that will clear up the problem, says Dr. Wise.

When the licking is caused by tapeworms, you will have to do two things: get rid of the worms and launch an attack on fleas, since fleas can transmit tapeworms. Pet supply stores sell a number of deworming products, although the ones available from your vet may be more effective. "If

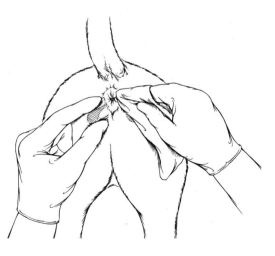

Blocked anal sacs are a common problem, but they are easy to treat. Feel around your pet's backside until you find two hard lumps on either side of the anus, at about the four- and eight-o'clock positions. The lumps can be as small as peas or as large as grapes. Using your thumb and forefinger, gently press each sac while pulling it toward the anal opening. This will release the fluid and relieve the uncomfortable pressure.

your pet spends a lot of time outdoors, she may benefit from a monthly flea treatment during the warm months," Dr. Wise adds.

"In addition to treating your pet, don't forget to treat your home for fleas," says Dr. Daniel. He recommends vacuuming very thoroughly, then treating the carpets with a flea powder. It is also a good idea to wash your pet's bedding in hot water and run it through the dryer. The combination of hot water and high heat will kill fleas as well as their eggs.

What Your Vet Will Do

While blocked anal sacs will often clear up on their own, other problems that cause pets to lick their backsides will need some professional help. This is especially true if your dog has swallowed bits of bone. Sometimes your vet will use an enema to flush away the irritating particles, but if the object is large and in deep, your vet may need to reach inside in order to remove it.

Vets are experts at unblocking anal sacs, and you may decide to have your vet do this procedure. In most cases, it takes just a few seconds to empty the sacs. To prevent infection, your vet may dab on a little antibiotic ointment as well.

Many pets will have blocked anal sacs once and never be bothered again. Others, however, are prone to blockages. If the problem keeps occurring, your vet may recommend surgically removing the sacs. "Cats and dogs get along just fine without anal sacs, so don't hesitate if your vet recommends this," says Dr. Daniel.

Take along a stool sample when you go to see your vet so that he can check for intestinal parasites. If your vet finds tapeworm evidence in the stool, he will prescribe oral medications that will clear out the parasite right away.

If everything appears normal but your pet won't quit licking, your vet is going to want to do a more thorough checkup, which may include some x-rays or blood tests. It is not common, but irritation of the anal area may be caused by intestinal infections or even tumors, which will need prompt treatment.

See also Chapter 9: Scooting, Specks around Anus

RASH

Clues

- Your pet has diarrhea or constipation.
- There are white specks in the stool.
- She has been noshing on bones.
- Your cat is licking her backside more frequently than usual.

It is not always easy to tell when dogs and cats have a rear-end rash because their tails can get in the way. But if your dog is sitting a little funny or if your cat keeps sitting down to lick her backside, it is worth lifting the tail to take a look.

When rashes result in sore, broken skin, bacteria may take up residence, resulting in a nasty infection, says Terri McGinnis, D.V.M., a veterinarian in private practice in the San Francisco area and author of *The Well Cat Book* and *The Well Dog Book*.

In cats, rashes sometimes occur because they are a little too conscientious about keeping themselves clean. It is normal for cats to lick their backsides after using the litter box, but generally it is a "lick, lick—I'm done" routine. "Some cats, though, get a little carried away, which can break down the skin," says Dr. McGinnis.

Both cats and dogs will sometimes get rashes after a spell of diarrhea or when they have had a hard bowel movement. This is especially common in dogs because of their penchant for chomping bones. When bone fragments pass out in their stools, the pieces can scrape the anal area, setting the stage for rash and possible infection.

Insect bites and stings are a common cause of under-the-tail rashes. So are tapeworms, unpleasant parasites that can irritate the anal area. Any irritation can induce dogs and cats to lick and scratch themselves, and this can lead to a painful rash.

WHAT YOU CAN DO

Regardless of what is causing the rash, applying a little over-the-counter hemorrhoid cream twice a day can be very soothing. "Choose the type with cortisone in it, which helps stop the itch," says Lori A. Wise, D.V.M., a veterinarian in private practice in Wheat Ridge, Colorado. And use latex gloves when you apply it.

Helping your pet stay regular will increase your chances of keeping her backside rash-free. Many dogs and cats have sensitive digestive systems that don't take well to new foods or even to tasty leftovers. It is a good idea to keep them on their regular diets and to make sure that they are getting plenty of water since this helps prevent hard bowel movements and will also keep them regular. It is especially important not to give them bones, which can irritate or even damage their digestive tracts as well as skin around the anus, explains Dr. Wise.

You can tell if your pet has tapeworms by looking at her stool or the area around the anus. Little specks that look like rice are the telltale sign of tapeworms. While tapeworms are creepy, they are not too difficult to get rid of. Pet supply stores stock a variety of tapeworm medications. Or your vet may give you a stronger type that is likely to be more effective, says Dr. Wise.

In addition, it is important to rid your house of fleas, since fleas can transmit tapeworms. Thoroughly clean the areas where your pet spends time and run her bedding through a hot wash. Then give her a bath with a medicated flea shampoo and spray or powder her with a flea-stopping product, says Dr. Wise. Once you get rid of the fleas, the risk for tapeworms will also drop.

What Your Vet Will Do

Most rashes will begin clearing up in about a week, especially when treated with a hemorrhoid cream. If a rash hangs on longer than that or starts getting worse, you need to see the vet because your pet is probably getting an infection.

Applying an antibiotic ointment is the easiest way to clear up skin infections. The problem is that pets often lick off the ointment before it has a chance to work. So your vet may recommend oral medications instead.

It isn't normal for dogs and cats to have frequent constipation or diarrhea. If you suspect that one or both of these conditions is causing the rash, your vet will probably want to do a variety of tests, including x-rays and blood evaluations, to see if there is an internal problem. Take a little of your pet's stool with you when you go to the vet so that he can examine it under a microscope to see if tapeworms or other parasites are present. Make sure that the stool is no more than 24 hours old.

Intestinal parasites aren't that hard to treat, but it is tricky to rid the house and pet area of fleas that transmit tapeworms. Your vet may recommend giving your pet oral medications that stop fleas from reproducing. Over time, this may help prevent rashes from occurring.

See also Chapter 6: Constipation, Diarrhea

SCOOTING

Clues

- Your pet is scooting at least once a day.
- There are white specks in his stool or around his anus.
- Your pet scoots only after using the litter box or making a pit stop in the yard.

It is a silly sight, but it serves a practical purpose. "Most often, a pet scooting along on his bottom is trying to relieve an itch," says Terri McGinnis, D.V.M., a veterinarian in private practice in the San Francisco area and author of *The Well Cat Book* and *The Well Dog Book*.

An itch where your pet sits is usually caused by blocked anal sacs, Dr. McGinnis says. These two sacs, which are located on either side of the anus, contain a strong-smelling fluid that dogs and cats use to mark where they have been. The scent is unique, which is why pets—especially dogs—sniff rear ends when they meet.

When the sacs are functioning normally, a little bit of the fluid is released during each bowel movement. But sometimes the opening to one or both sacs gets blocked. When the fluid can't get out, the sacs swell, becoming itchy and uncomfortable, says Dr. McGinnis.

Blocked anal sacs aren't the only cause of scooting. Tapeworms, intestinal parasites that sometimes attach themselves to the anal area, can also cause that region to be very itchy, says Lori A. Wise, D.V.M., a veterinarian in private practice in Wheat Ridge, Colorado. Tapeworms are easy to spot, she adds. Just lift your pet's tail. If you see white particles around the anus that resemble white rice, your pet has tapeworms and will need medications to knock them out. You can also see tapeworm segments in the stool, she adds.

Scooting isn't always a sign of problems, especially when your pet only does it now and then, adds Dr. McGinnis. After using the litter box or making a stop in the yard, for example, some pets will scoot simply to clean themselves. In addition, dogs that have recently chomped bones and then passed hard little fragments in their stools may rub their bottoms to relieve the irritation. "Fairly large bone fragments can pass all the way through the intestine without too much trouble but then become lodged in the rectum," says Dr. McGinnis.

WHAT YOU CAN DO

Blocked anal sacs are a nuisance because they are so common. Some pets, in fact, get them all the time. While your vet can unblock them in just a few seconds, it is easy to do it yourself if you have a strong stomach and are willing to give it a try. (For instructions on unblocking the anal sacs, see Licking Hind End on page 220.) Once the sacs have been emptied, the discomfort will fade, and your pet won't need to scoot anymore, says Dr. Wise.

Tapeworms are a little more difficult to treat, just because there are so many places where they hide. To get rid of worms that are already in the digestive tract, you need to give your pet medications, which are available from vets as well as pet supply stores. While you are at it, you should treat your pet for fleas since they are the main reason that dogs and cats get worms in the first place. If your pet spends time outdoors, don't let him scavenge or hunt since eating birds or rodents can cause tapeworms in pets, especially dogs, says Dr. Wise.

What Your Vet Will Do

Scooting usually isn't a serious problem, although your vet may recommend removing the anal sacs if they are constantly getting blocked. The surgery is easy to do, and pets do well without the sacs once they are gone, says Dr. Wise.

If you suspect that your pet has tapeworms, but you are not sure, your vet will probably recommend that you take in a recent stool sample to check for intestinal parasites. Tapeworms are easy to find, and you will have an answer within a few minutes. If there are worms, medications from a pet supply store or from your vet will quickly get rid of them, says Dr. McGinnis. Your vet will also examine the anal area to see if a bone or anything else is causing the irritation.

See also Chapter 9: Specks around Anus

SPECKS AROUND ANUS

Clues

- There are white specks around your pet's anal area or in the stool.
- Your pet is licking her bottom or scooting across the floor.
- Your pet has been having problems with fleas.

Tapeworms can spend their entire lives in the digestive tracts of dogs and cats. Despite their size (adults can be more than 20 inches long), tapeworms are essentially harmless. But they are continually shedding rice-size segments of their bodies. As these segments leave the body in the stool, they will sometimes attach themselves to the anal area, causing intense itching.

Tapeworms are easy to recognize. Pets will often scoot their bottoms along the floor to relieve the itching. You will also see small, white specks in your pet's stool and around the anal area.

It is almost impossible to prevent tapeworms entirely. They are often transmitted by fleas. Pets also get tapeworms from eating prey such as birds or rodents, says Merry Crimi, D.V.M., a veterinarian in private practice in Milwaukie, Oregon.

WHAT YOU CAN DO

It is not that hard to get rid of tapeworms by using oral medications, which you can get from your vet or from pet supply stores. The hard part is preventing them from coming back. The only way to succeed is to stop tapeworms at the source—by getting rid of the fleas that cause them.

Take a little time to thoroughly vacuum the carpets and to run your pet's bedding through the wash. This will eliminate many of the fleas as well as their eggs. Also, periodically bathe your pet using a flea shampoo and treat her monthly with a topical flea medication, says Dr. Crimi. Your vet may recommend using medications such as Program or Advantage. Used once a month, these products provide very effective flea control.

WHAT YOUR VET WILL DO

Even though you can't treat tapeworms at home, you will want to see your vet if your pet is intensely itchy. Be sure to take along a stool sample, which your vet will examine to see for sure if tapeworms are causing the problem. If they are, he will give your pet oral medications and possibly something to relieve discomfort in the anal area.

See also Chapter 9: Licking Hind End, Scooting

TAIL LIMPNESS

Clues

- Your pet's tail isn't moving normally.
- One or more legs seem unsteady, or your pet has an odd walk.

Just as people use their hands to communicate, dogs and cats use their tails. The position of their tails lets you know they are jaunty or sad, scared or aggressive. It can also tell you if they have recently put their tails where they shouldn't—in the path of a closing door, for instance, or underneath the rocker of a rocking chair.

"When the tail is broken below where it connects at the base, your pet may have just half a wag," says Joan E. Antle, D.V.M., a veterinarian in private practice in Cleveland. "It will be limp just below the point of the break."

If the break is higher up, right at the base, your pet may not be able to move her tail at all, even when using the litter box or making a pit stop in the yard. This type of break is fairly serious and can cause a lot of pain, and your pet will let you know quite loudly that it hurts.

"Back trouble can also give your pet a limp tail," says Lori A. Wise, D.V.M., a veterinarian in private practice in Wheat Ridge, Colorado. Pets will occasionally get a herniated disk, which means that one of the protective cushions between vertebrae in the spine has cracked and ruptured.

This can result in pressure on a nerve, causing the tail to go limp. Pets with herniated disks may develop weakness or even paralysis in one of their legs as well. Dogs with long backs and short legs like corgis and dachshunds are especially prone to herniated disks.

WHAT YOU CAN DO

"When the break in the tail is below the base, pet owners can generally manage the problem at home just fine," says Dr. Antle. Here's what you need to do.

If the skin was broken, begin by washing the area with soap and water, then apply a sterile gauze pad. Using white cloth first-aid tape, wrap the entire tail snugly, but not so tightly that you cut off circulation. That will protect the tail and help the broken area heal. Change the dressing weekly and check for signs of infection. A broken tail will take about a month to heal, so see your vet if it takes longer or the area becomes infected.

Breaks at the base of the tail are much more serious and always need to be treated by a vet. This is also the case if your pet is having trouble walking, which could be a sign of nerve damage or spinal disk problems. These are emergency situations, so you should see a vet immediately, Dr. Antle warns.

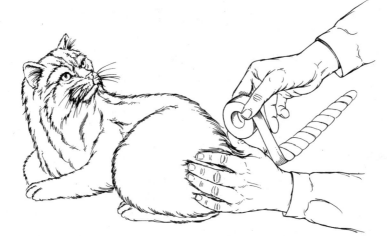

To stabilize a broken tail, wrap it first with gauze, then with cloth first-aid tape, starting at the tip and working down toward the body. Don't wrap it so tightly that you cut off circulation. Leave a little slack in each end of the tape. Then get your pet to the vet right away.

WHAT YOUR VET WILL DO

When the tail is broken right at the base, your vet may need to remove the entire tail. This sounds frightening, but most pets get along just fine after the surgery, says Dr. Antle.

Problems with the spine often require a number of tests. Your vet may recommend a test called a myelogram, in which a dye is injected into the spinal canal in order to reveal what's inside. In combination with x-rays, this test will show if your pet has a herniated disk, and, if so, whether it is pressing on spinal nerves.

Pets with disk problems will often recover on their own if they spend about two weeks in a confined area, moving as little as necessary. This gives the spine time to heal. In some cases, however, surgery may be needed to repair the damage.

SYMPTOM) TAIL SECRETIONS

Clues

- Your pet is an unneutered male.
- There is a brown discharge on the skin.
- You are seeing oily spots on furniture.

In people, the forehead and nose are the major oily zones. Your pets also have oil slicks—although theirs are farther south.

Dogs and cats have large, oil-producing glands on the upper sides of their tails, a few inches from where the tail meets the body. Normally these glands produce just enough oil to keep the skin healthy. But sometimes they get overly active and produce so much oil that the fur gets greasy. "If you part the fur, you will see that there is an oily, brown discharge on the skin," says Beverly J. Scott, D.V.M., a veterinarian in private practice in Gilbert, Arizona.

Both males and females can secrete excess oil, but it is much more common in unneutered males. In fact, this condition in cats is commonly referred to as stud tail.

WHAT YOU CAN DO

On rare occasions, the skin gets irritated or infected from tail secretions. That is really the only health concern. But there is still the cosmetic problem: Oil on the fur has a way of becoming oil on the couch or on your lap. So you may want to clean off the excess oil on the tail now and then.

Vets recommend washing the area two to three times a week with a medicated shampoo. (If your cat won't get in the tub, you can perch him on the bathroom counter and let his tail drop in the sink.) Ask your vet for a pet shampoo that contains benzoyl peroxide—the same ingredient that is in human acne medications, says Dr. Scott.

If the shampoo doesn't seem to help, you can soak a cotton ball in rubbing alcohol and rub the greasy area, parting the fur as you go. You can also brush on a little cornstarch, which will absorb some of the oil.

WHAT YOUR VET WILL DO

The only way to prevent tail secretions is to neuter male pets. "This generally eliminates the problem," says Dr. Scott.

Undescended Testicles

Clues

- One or both testicles haven't appeared by the time your pet is six months to a year old.

Even though the testicles spend most of their lives hanging free from the body, they actually start out inside the abdomen and remain there during much of the gestational period. By the time pets are born, the testicles have descended into the scrotum, the loose skin behind the penis.

But in some dogs and cats, one or both of the testicles stay inside the abdomen. "This can be a temporary condition or permanent," says Merry Crimi, D.V.M., a veterinarian in private practice in Milwaukie, Oregon. Most of the time, the laggard will drop into its proper place within six months to a year after birth. But sometimes it doesn't, and that can be a problem because an undescended testicle can be painful, she says. It also has a high risk for developing a tumor, she says.

What You Can Do

In young pets, it is worth checking now and then to make sure that both testicles are hanging where they should. You can't tell just by looking at the scrotum—you need to feel the loose skin to make sure that there are two firm, smooth, oval shapes inside. If there is only one—or none—it is time to call your vet for advice.

What Your Vet Will Do

In dogs, undescended testicles will sometimes drop on their own in six to eight months. In cats, it can take a bit longer—up to a year in some cases. When this doesn't happen, vets will sometimes use hormone shots to facilitate the testicle's descent. In most cases, however, this treatment is needlessly complicated and unnecessary for the simple reason that removing the testicles and neutering your pet is the better choice. Testicles that don't descend can be a hereditary problem, and pets with this condition that are allowed to breed will pass it on to future generations.

SYMPTOM) # URINATING DIFFICULTY

Clues

- Your pet is straining or taking a long time to urinate.
- The litter box is dry after your cat has used it.
- There is blood or sludge coming from your pet's penis.
- Your dog's stools are flat.

If dogs and cats went to the theater, you would never see a waiting line at the rest rooms during intermission. Whether they are making a pit stop in the yard or perching in the litter box, they can usually finish their business in just a few seconds.

But what if your dog or cat is taking a long time to urinate—or is straining but not getting results? Difficulty urinating usually means that something is blocking the flow of urine, and it can be extremely serious if you don't take care of it right away. (Pets that are urinating less often, but aren't straining, may still have serious problems. See Urinating Less Often on page 237 for more information.)

In cats, minerals in the urine may compact into hard little stones, which can block the urethra, the narrow tube through which urine flows. This usually occurs in male cats because their urethras are much narrower than a female's, explains L. R. Danny Daniel, D.V.M., a veterinarian in private practice in Covington, Louisiana. Cats with urinary stones will often have tenderness in the abdomen as well as difficulty urinating. In males, there may be blood or even bits of sandlike sludge coming from the end of the penis. Another telltale sign is spots of blood in the litter box.

Dogs can also develop stones in the urinary tract, but not as often as cats do. The main problems in dogs—and only in unneutered males—is prostate problems. As dogs get older, the prostate gland, which wraps around the urethra, sometimes gets larger. Eventually, it may press against the urethra, slowing or even stopping the flow of urine. An infection in the prostate, which also causes the gland to swell, can cause a similar problem.

Difficulty urinating is just one sign of prostate problems. They can also cause the stools to be flat because the swollen gland may press against the rectum. "Your dog may have swollen testicles, pain in his belly, and a fever," Dr. Daniel adds.

Both dogs and cats may have trouble urinating when they have a urinary tract infection, which can cause spasms in the urethra, narrowing the opening. And in rare cases, difficulty urinating may be caused by tumors in the urinary tract or by a lack of muscular strength in the bladder walls.

What You Can Do

If you don't take care of a urinary problem right away, the bladder can literally burst, warns Dr. Daniel. As soon as you notice problems, it is essential to get your pet to the vet immediately.

Even though you can't treat urinary blockages at home, there are ways to help prevent them. This is important after a first treatment because a pet that has had one blockage has a high risk of getting another, says E. Ann Lystrup, D.V.M., a veterinarian in private practice in Eau Claire, Wisconsin.

Since urinary stones are made from magnesium, switch your pet to a high-quality canned food that is low in magnesium, suggests Dr. Lystrup. Or use a dry food that has been specially formulated for pets with stone problems.

And keep your pet's water bowl full, says Dr. Daniel. Water dilutes urine, so stones are less likely to form if your pet's thirst is satisfied. One way to boost your pet's fluid intake is to add a pinch of salt to his food, he says. The salt will make him thirstier, so he will naturally drink more water. Salt is quite safe, although you shouldn't use it if your pet is elderly or has high blood pressure, he adds. It is a good idea to talk to your vet before adding salt to your pet's diet.

The more your pet drinks, the more he will urinate, and this is a good thing, notes Dr. Lystrup. "Pets that hold their urine tend to form stones more readily." Getting regular exercise will also help pets urinate more frequently, she adds.

What Your Vet Will Do

Urinary problems are generally easy to diagnose. Your vet will take a sample of urine for testing and may also recommend x-rays or ultrasound to identify where the problem is occurring.

In some cases, your vet will be able to release pent-up urine by pressing on the bladder right through the abdomen. If the blockage is in tight, however, she may need to insert a catheter through the urethra and into the bladder to help the urine drain. This can be an uncomfortable procedure, and most pets are given a general anesthetic first.

The catheter may be used only until all the urine is out. Or your vet may stitch the catheter in place and leave it there for a few days to allow stones and other sludge in the urinary tract to flow out. In the meantime, your pet will probably be given intravenous fluids to help flush the urinary tract.

Removing the obstruction may be all that is necessary. Some pets, however, will be given medications that make the urine more acidic, which helps prevent stones. In addition, your pet may need antibiotics if a urinary tract infection has taken hold.

In dogs with prostate problems, medications are sometimes used to reduce swelling of the prostate gland. More often, the best treatment is simply to surgically remove the testicles. "Neutering your pet eliminates this problem, so we often recommend it when pets have repeated prostate troubles," says Dr. Daniel.

See also Chapter 5: Crying While Using the Litter Box

URINATING FREQUENTLY

Clues

- There is blood in the urine.
- Your cat has started spraying.
- Your pet is drinking a lot more water than usual.

Maybe you have just finished a walk, and 10 minutes later your dog is waiting at the door again. Or perhaps your cat is using the litter box so often that you are thinking about charging a toll. What is making them urinate so often?

It is common for pets to urinate more on some days than others, but a long-lasting increase in bathroom activity means that it is time to call your vet.

In females, especially, the most common explanation is a bladder infection. "A bladder infection causes a painful burning in the bladder and the urethra, which makes the pet feel as though she has to urinate all the time, even when there isn't much urine in the bladder," says E. Ann Lystrup, D.V.M., a veterinarian in private practice in Eau Claire, Wisconsin. Pets with bladder infections may have blood in their urine and, because of pain in the abdomen, an unusual walk, she adds.

Urinary tract troubles—not just infections but also stones in the bladder or urethra—are much more common in cats than dogs. If your cat is urinating more and has also started spraying, you should suspect this is the cause.

A more serious condition that can cause frequent urination is diabetes. This is an illness in which sugar levels in the bloodstream gradually increase, damaging tissues throughout the body. In an attempt to remove excess sugars, pets will drink a lot of water and urinate much more frequently than normal.

Unspayed female pets that have a uterine infection or whose kidneys aren't working the way they should will also drink and urinate more. Thyroid problems or a tumor in the urinary tract can also cause frequent urination.

Dogs are legendary for stopping to water every tree or fire hydrant on their daily walks. This doesn't count as frequent urination because they are just doing what they are programmed to do, observes Merry Crimi, D.V.M., a veterinarian in private practice in Milwaukie, Oregon. "Most likely, your dog is just trying to mark the same trees that every other dog did."

WHAT YOU CAN DO

Since many urinating conditions are potentially serious, you should call your vet within a day or two. "This isn't the emergency situation that straining to urinate is, but you should definitely seek veterinarian care as soon as possible," says Dr. Crimi.

For prevention, make sure that your pet's water bowl is kept full. Although drinking water will naturally cause her to urinate more, it can help prevent bladder infections or bladder stones that could cause problems later, says Dr. Crimi.

WHAT YOUR VET WILL DO

Most urinary problems are easy to diagnose by testing a urine sample in the laboratory. If your vet needs "uncontaminated" urine for the tests, she will take it directly from the bladder by inserting a needle through the abdomen. This procedure sounds painful, but it really is not, says Dr. Lystrup. The needle used to remove urine is extremely fine and it zips right in even before your pet knows what is going on.

Your vet will probably give your pet an anti-inflammatory medication that will stop painful irritation in the urethra and bladder, often within a day, says Dr. Lystrup. Additional treatments will depend on what the tests reveal.

For a urinary tract infection, the usual treatment is to give antibiotics, says Dr. Crimi. For stones in the urinary tract, your vet may put your pet on a prescription diet that will help dissolve the stones as well as prevent them. When the stones are very large or there are a lot of them, the only solution may be surgery to remove them, she says.

Dogs and cats with diabetes will often need insulin to prevent sugars in the bloodstream from rising to dangerous levels, says Dr. Crimi. They will also be put on a high-fiber diet that is designed to keep blood sugar levels steady.

If kidney or liver conditions are causing frequent urination, they can be complicated to treat. Your vet will need to perform a variety of tests, possibly including ultrasound, to find out where the problem is and what is causing it. Your pet will almost certainly need medications to keep the problems under control. Changes in her diet may also be required, says Dr. Crimi.

SYMPTOM

URINATING LESS OFTEN

Clues

- The urine is either very clear or very dark.
- Your pet has a fever or is feeling sick.

Dogs and cats are very predictable in their habits, especially when it comes to asking to be let outside or using the litter box. If your pet suddenly starts urinating less often than usual, there is almost certainly something wrong. (Straining to urinate, rather than merely doing it less often, is an emergency that needs to be treated by a vet right away. See Urinating Difficulty on page 232 for more information.)

One of the most serious conditions that causes dogs and cats to urinate less is kidney disease. The kidneys are responsible for filtering many of the body wastes and eliminating them in the urine. When your pet isn't urinating as often as usual, it could be because the kidneys aren't working the way that they should and have lost some of their filtering ability. "Pets with kidney disease can get quite sick as fluids and wastes build up," says L. R. Danny Daniel, D.V.M., a veterinarian in private practice in Covington, Louisiana.

One of the telltale signs of kidney disease is very clear urine. It turns clear because when the kidneys aren't working properly, wastes stay in the body instead of being concentrated in the urine, Dr. Daniel explains.

Urinary tract infections usually cause pets to urinate more rather than less. In some cases, however, an infection may weaken the bladder, making it less able to push urine out. A similar problem can occur if spinal nerves get damaged or compressed—by an injured spinal disk, for example. Pressure on the nerves can block the impulses that tell the body when it is time to urinate.

Finally, dogs and cats that have a fever will often urinate less simply because they are burning up more fluids internally, says Dr. Daniel. "Or the problem may be as simple as a little dehydration from hotter weather moving in, and you may not be filling her water bowl often enough," he adds.

WHAT YOU CAN DO

Any change in your pet's urinating habits is potentially serious and should be checked out by a vet. To prevent problems, however, there are things that you can do at home.

For starters, make sure that there is always water in her bowl. Dogs and cats can get dehydrated very quickly, even in the cooler months. Giving them plenty of water to drink will help keep the entire urinary tract working well, says Dr. Daniel.

If your pet is urinating less than usual and seems to be under the weather, it is worth taking a few minutes to check her temperature, says Beverly J. Scott, D.V.M., a veterinarian in private practice in Gilbert, Arizona. The normal temperature for dogs and cats is between 100.5° and 102.5°F. If her temperature is 103°F or higher, your pet has a fever and you need to call your vet.

What Your Vet Will Do

Since one of the main symptoms of kidney disease is urinating less often, your vet will want to do a very thorough checkup. He will get a lot of answers simply by checking your pet's urine in the laboratory. When urine is dark and concentrated, your pet may not be getting enough fluids. If the urine is extremely watery, there is probably something wrong with the kidneys.

In some cases, kidney problems are temporary—caused by poisoning, for example. Vets can treat this type of problem by giving dogs and cats dialysis, which removes harmful toxins from the body. This can help the kidneys work properly again.

When the kidneys are damaged, your vet may recommend putting your pet on a low-protein diet. Part of the kidneys' job is filtering protein by-products. Giving your pet foods that are low in protein will put less strain on the kidneys, explains Dr. Daniel.

Your vet may also check your pet's bladder by feeling it through the abdomen. If the bladder has lost muscular strength, it may be distended and have thin walls, says Dr. Scott. Your vet may also check the spine—either by feeling along the spinal column or by doing x-rays or other tests—to see if there are nerve problems that could be interfering with your pet's ability to urinate.

If it turns out that the bladder is weak, there are a number of medications that can help restore its ability to contract the way it should. For nerve problems, however, pets usually need surgery to repair the damage, Dr. Daniel says.

COMMON HINDQUARTER CONDITIONS

Blocked or infected anal sacs. Dogs and cats depend on their sense of smell to identify territory and recognize other pets. Unlike humans, who may introduce themselves by handing out calling cards, dogs and cats say "Hi" by releasing a strong-smelling liquid from the anal sacs—two small pouches on either side of the anus. When other pets smell this liquid, either on the ground or by sniffing rear ends, they are able to tell who they are talking to.

The openings to the anal sacs are quite small. They often get impacted, which prevents fluids from draining. Pets with blocked anal glands get very itchy and sore. They may develop infections as well.

"Once the fluid accumulates, your pet will have a sore backside," says Terri McGinnis, D.V.M., a veterinarian in the San Francisco area and author of *The Well Cat Book* and *The Well Dog Book*. To relieve the discomfort, dogs and cats will often lick their behinds or scoot them along the ground.

Anal sac problems are very common and, in most cases, easy to treat. Veterinarians can usually unblock the openings and ease the pressure simply by pressing on the glands. If there is an infection, your pet will probably need antibiotics as well.

Herniated disk. Dogs and cats walk on all fours, so they don't do a lot of bending, which is why spinal problems in pets are quite rare. As they get older, however, the protective cushions between the vertebrae, called spinal disks, will occasionally weaken. (This is particularly common in dachshunds because their long bodies puts additional stress on the disks.) If a disk breaks or ruptures, the material inside will ooze out, possibly putting pressure on a spinal nerve. This condition, called a herniated disk, may cause dogs and cats to lose control of their bowels or bladder, or to have an unstiff tail or a limp, says Joan E. Antle, D.V.M., a veterinarian in private practice in Cleveland. If there is enough pressure on their spinal cords, pets may become paralyzed.

A herniated spinal disk is potentially serious and should always be treated by a vet right away—especially if your pet is in a lot of pain or is reluctant to move. Most of the time, however, keeping dogs and cats confined, such as in a crate, for two weeks will allow the disk to heal on its own. If it doesn't get better, your pet may need surgery to remove it. Removing the disk will relieve pressure on the spinal nerves, and the symptoms will start to improve right away.

Kidney failure. The kidneys are responsible for filtering wastes from your pet's body and eliminating them in the urine. When the kidneys aren't working properly as a result of infections, for example, wastes begin to accumulate, often rising to dangerous levels. Kidney disease is an emergency that always requires quick attention.

There are several warning signs when the kidneys aren't working the way they should. Your pet's urine is normally yellow or amber. If it suddenly turns clear, it could mean that the kidneys have stopped filtering wastes. Over time, pets with kidney disease will start producing less and less urine, which means that the kidneys have essentially shut down.

Because kidney disease is so serious, it is critical to call your vet as soon as you notice *any* change in your pet's urine or urinating habits.

Perianal fistula. The tissues of the anus and rectum are very fragile. When they get inflamed and irritated because of an infected hair follicle, for example, or because mucus-producing glands have become blocked by stool, they can break down and bleed, forming painful sores. These sores, called perianal fistulas, can make having a bowel movement extremely painful and may cause a foul-smelling discharge as well. They are most common in German shepherds, Irish setters, and other large dogs.

Dogs with perianal fistulas will often need antibiotics to treat and prevent dangerous infections. In addition, surgery is usually needed to remove damaged tissue and to "rearrange" your pet's anatomy so that the area drains better in the future.

Prostate problems. The prostate gland is responsible for producing much of the liquid that makes up your pet's semen. Due to the influence of male hormones, the prostate gland often gets larger as dogs and cats get older. It may get so large, in fact, that it begins pressing on the urethra, blocking the flow of urine. It can also get irritated and infected, causing intense abdominal pain.

You should suspect your pet is having prostate problems if the penis and testicles are swollen or if there is a bloody discharge in the urine. In some cases, prostate problems will cause the stools to be flat instead of round because the gland is pressing against the rectum, says Paul M. Gigliotti, D.V.M., a veterinarian in private practice in Mayfield Village, Ohio.

Prostate problems are often treated with antibiotics, which will stop infection and help reduce the swelling. Most of the time, however, vets recommend neutering male pets in order to reduce the amount of male hormones in the body. Once the testicles are removed, there will be no further problems, says Dr. Gigliotti.

Tapeworms. They are extremely creepy, but tapeworms usually aren't a serious problem. Most dogs and cats will get them at some time in their lives—often from eating birds, mice, or other rodents, or from swallowing infected fleas. Tapeworms spend their entire lives in the digestive tract. You only discover them because they periodically shed small segments of their bodies, which look like bits of white rice and appear in the stool or around the anus.

Tapeworms will occasionally cause fever or fatigue. More often, the main symptom is itching, which occurs when tapeworm fragments irritate the anal area. Dogs and cats with tapeworms will often scoot their bottoms on the ground or spend a lot of time licking their backsides.

Tapeworms are very easy to treat with medications that you can get from your vet or pet supply stores. The problem is that the worms often come back; most people will treat their pets for tapeworms more than a few times. One of the best ways to prevent tapeworms is to go after the fleas that often cause them. When you control the flea population, you will automatically reduce the risk for tapeworms.

Urinary stones. The urine looks like it is all liquid, but it actually consists of dissolved chemicals, minerals, and other wastes. Most of the time, these wastes stay in a liquid form. In some dogs and cats, however, the minerals will bond together to form hard little stones, usually the size of fine gravel but sometimes as big as a pea. As you would expect, passing these stones in the urine can be extraordinarily painful, says L. R. Danny Daniel, D.V.M., a veterinarian in private practice in Covington, Louisiana. Pets with stones will often cry when they urinate, and there may be blood in the urine as well.

Urinary stones are more of a problem for male pets simply because the tubes in their urinary tracts are narrower than in females. The usual treatment is to give pets medications to make their urine more acidic, which helps prevent stones from forming. In addition, many pets will be put on special diets so that they get less of the stone-causing minerals in their systems. When the stones are large, however, the only solution may be surgery to remove them.

Pets that have had one attack of urinary stones will invariably get another. To reduce the risk, vets recommend giving pets plenty of water. This helps dilute the urine, making it harder for stones to form.

Urinary tract infections. Bacteria can make themselves at home anywhere in the urinary tract—in the bladder, kidneys, or urethra (the tube through which urine flows). Most of the time, these bacteria don't cause problems. But when they multiply to large enough numbers, they can cause painful infections. Pets with urinary tract infections will often urinate more often than usual because the lining in their urinary tracts is sore and irritated. There may be blood in the urine as well.

Most urinary tract infections aren't too serious, although they always need prompt treatment to prevent the infection from getting worse. Your vet will probably give your pet oral antibiotics, which will relieve the infection in a week or two, says Beverly J. Scott, D.V.M., a veterinarian in private practice in Gilbert, Arizona. Your vet will also recommend that you encourage your pet to drink water as often as possible. Getting more fluids will help wash bacteria out of the urinary tract before they are able to cause an infection.

Uterine infection. Dogs and cats get mild infections all the time, and their immune systems usually clear things up even before you notice that there is a problem. Not so with uterine infections. Pets with this condition—usually new mothers or pets that are pregnant—can get extremely sick very quickly. There may be a strong-smelling, pus-filled, or bloody discharge. Your pet will probably have a fever as well, and she won't feel like eating or exercising. Uterine infections are always an emergency. Call your vet immediately if you even suspect that this could be the problem.

CHAPTER 10

Legs, Hips, and Paws

Your pet's legs, hips, and paws are made up of more than 100 bones and more than 50 joints. Each joint is tied together with one or more ligaments. The whole package is fleshed out with muscles, veins, nerves, and skin, supported by the pad of the paw and tipped with 10 fast-growing nails.

It is a very efficient system that normally works smoothly, propelling your pet where he wants to go. But as you would expect from a machine with this many parts, problems sometimes develop. Most of the time, the problems are minor: a pulled ligament or everyday bumps and bruises. These are the same types of aches and pains that people get when they overdo things or aren't as careful as they should be. A bruise or a pulled muscle or ligament will hurt for a few days or weeks, then gradually get better. They slow dogs and cats down for a while, but hardly put them out of business.

Less often, your pet may develop more serious symptoms in the paws, legs, or hips, like nonstop itching or pain from Lyme disease. One of the most serious conditions that affects dogs (but usually not cats) is hip dysplasia. This is usually an inherited condition in which the bones that form the hips don't fit together as tightly as they should. Pets that have had serious injuries, such as from a car accident, can also develop hip dysplasia. Whether it is caused by genetics or bad luck, the results are the same. The poorly formed hip joints have a lot of wobble. Whenever your pet moves, the bones (and their protective coverings) slap together instead of gliding smoothly back and forth. This causes the joints to wear prematurely, often causing a painful form arthritis. Hip dysplasia is most common in large breeds of dogs, and it needs a lot of hands-on care to reduce inflammation and pain.

Both dogs and cats often get a little gimpy because of problems with the paw pads. Covered with a leathery-looking layer of skin, the pads look pretty tough. But they take quite a pounding on hot concrete in the summer and on road salt and hard ice in the winter. And in all seasons, the pads undergo a lot of friction for the simple reason that dogs and cats go barefoot all the time. The pads can get cracked, dry, and sore, and it can take a long time for them to heal.

Another common source of discomfort is the nails. They grow quite quickly, and unless you keep them trimmed, they are always slapping against the ground. It is common for the nails to crack or splinter. Sometimes a long or cracked nail snags on a rough carpet or a crack in the sidewalk, pulling it loose. This can be enormously painful as well as messy; torn nails can bleed copiously. Even though they usually don't cause long-term problems, torn nails are a scary sight. They require fast first-aid and, in some cases, a trip to the vet to stop the bleeding and prevent further damage.

When you think of their tremendous energy and the sheer number of miles pets travel (they take about 10 steps for every one of yours), it is surprising that they don't get injured more seriously more often.

It is often difficult for owners to know what to make of leg, hip, or paw problems. Minor conditions, such as a cut pad, can cause big symptoms, while more serious conditions will often look minor. It may take a trip to the vet to figure out what the problem is.

But once you know what's wrong, many leg, hip, and paw problems can be controlled at home. What's more, they can often be prevented with a little daily care: exercise to keep the joints limber, a good-quality food to feed the muscles, and regular nail trimming to keep the claws neat and safe.

See Your Vet If:

- Your pet has begun having trouble walking, getting up, or climbing stairs.
- One or more legs is dragging.
- He has a limp that doesn't go away.
- One or more legs is in an awkward position.
- There is swelling in the toes, feet, or legs.
- Your pet can't get up.

- Your pet is constantly licking or biting his feet.
- The nails are broken, cracked, or bleeding.
- There are cuts, blisters, growths, or burns on his paw pads.
- Your pet is lame first in one leg and then another.
- He has pain when jumping off a bed or changing position.

SYMPTOM

CLAWS WON'T RETRACT

Clues

- Only one claw won't retract.
- Your cat is a Burmese.
- Your cat is in his senior years.
- The toe is swollen or tender.

Unlike dogs, whose claws are out all the time, cats only extend their claws when they are playing, fighting, or scratching. When they are done using them, they retract their claws, sheathing them like a sword into a scabbard.

When the claws won't retract, it is probably because they have gotten too long or too thick to fit back in the paw, says Margie Scherk, D.V.M., a veterinarian in private practice in Vancouver, British Columbia. Older cats are particularly likely to develop thicker nails, she adds. Even young cats can have fat, long claws, especially if they don't spend enough time grooming them by scratching trees or carpets.

Daily scratching by cats is essential for keeping their claws neat and short, but it requires a certain amount of work. If your cat has an underlying illness like arthritis, diabetes, or kidney disease, he may not be up to the job, says Dr. Scherk.

Cats with hyperthyroidism, a condition in which the thyroid gland is overactive, have the opposite problem. They have plenty of energy, but their claws will grow unusually fast—too fast for these cats to keep them suitably short.

If your cat is able to sheath all but one of his claws, he could have an infection, a broken bone, or a tumor on that particular toe, says Grant Nisson, D.V.M., a veterinarian in private practice in West River, Maryland. Each of these problems will probably be accompanied by pain and swelling, he adds.

It is rare, but occasionally cats will have trouble retracting their claws because of a nervous system disorder or feline leukemia, which can cause a loss of muscular control, says Dr. Nisson. They want to retract their claws, but the muscles simply won't respond. In addition, some cats, particularly the Burmese breed, may develop a potassium deficiency called hypokalemia, which also causes a loss of muscular control.

WHAT YOU CAN DO

Trimming your cat's claws will usually make it easier for him to put them away when he is done using them. You don't need specialized equipment—inexpensive human nail trimmers will do the job nicely. "I hate the guillotine-type pet nail trimmers," says Dr. Scherk. "They tend to crush the claws instead of clip them." Dogs and cats dislike having their nails trimmed, but it is not that hard to do, she adds.

When you are ready to do a "*pet*-acure," here is what vets advise.

- Hold your cat in your lap with a towel wrapped around his chest and back. This will prevent your feisty feline from putting his claws to work on you.
- Press on the first knuckle of the paw to push the nail outward. Clip off the sharp tip of the nail. Don't clip farther down and into the pink area, which will be painful and may cause bleeding. When you're done, move on to the next nail. If your cat doesn't struggle too much, you can do all the nails in a few minutes.
- A cat's claws grow in layers from the center out, like an onion. After you trim the tip of a nail, gently flake away the loose outer layers. Some people file the nails afterward, but this isn't necessary.
- If you accidentally clip too far down and the claw bleeds, pressing flour on the cut will help stop the bleeding. (Or you can rub the cut place with nail-trimming powders that you can buy from a pet supply store.)

What Your Vet Will Do

Unless it is obvious that your cat simply needs his nails trimmed, your vet will examine the toes very carefully for signs of infection or swelling. If only one claw won't go back in, your vet will probably recommend x-rays to see if a fracture, arthritis, or a tumor is causing the problem. If more than one claw is affected, she may do blood tests to check for internal conditions, such as thyroid disease or diabetes.

In some cases your pet may need surgery or long-term medications— or, in the case of a potassium deficiency, potassium supplements—to clear up the problem. Most of the time, however, he will just need more-frequent trims.

DIFFICULTY GETTING UP

Clues

- Your pet is elderly or overweight.
- The stiffness is mainly in her hips.
- The discomfort came on suddenly.
- Your pet hasn't been eating well and appears to be ill.

Puppies and kittens play like athletes. They chase toys, tunnel through briars, and leap up each morning ready to start a new day.

As pets get older, however, their joints get a little creaky, and their backs stiffen up a bit. Plus, they have probably put on a little weight, which puts additional stress on tired joints. Eventually, some older pets begin having trouble moving or even getting up.

If your pet is generally in good health, difficulty getting up is probably caused by arthritis, says Joanne Hibbs, D.V.M., a veterinarian in private practice in Powell, Tennessee. Years of chasing Frisbees or climbing trees can cause joints to break down, a condition that vets call osteoarthritis or degenerative joint disease. Dogs and cats can also get rheumatoid arthritis, though not as often as people do.

Since pets do a lot of twisting and turning, both of which put a lot of stress on the back, arthritis of the spine is especially common. "A lot of dogs hurt their knees when they twist around at a full run," adds Grant Nisson, D.V.M., a veterinarian in private practice in West River, Maryland. "Injured joints can show signs of arthritis within a month."

Another condition that makes getting up difficult is hip dysplasia, a hereditary problem that literally means "badly made hips," says Dr. Nisson. When the hipbones don't fit together the way they should, pets can get sore and stiff. Any dog can get hip dysplasia, but it is more common in certain breeds of large dogs like German shepherds and Labrador and golden retrievers. Cats can get hip dysplasia, too. Persians are particularly prone to it. But because cats are well-muscled and relatively light, it usually doesn't bother them as much as it does dogs.

Finally, dogs and cats with internal illnesses like diabetes or cancer may have trouble getting up. To tell the difference between joint problems and more serious conditions, take a look at how well your pet is feeling, says Dr. Nisson. If she is eating well and seems happy and the stiffness has been coming on gradually, she probably has joint problems. But if the stiffness came on all at once, or she is losing her appetite or feeling under the weather, something more serious may be going on, and you should call your vet right away.

WHAT YOU CAN DO

It is easy to give cats or small dogs a little boost when they need help getting up. For larger pets, however, lifting them up can be a challenge. Dr. Nisson recommends slipping a towel beneath your pet's belly and giving a gentle lift. Most pets with arthritis can move fairly well once they get their stiff hind legs off the ground, he says.

Dogs that have arthritis will sometimes have trouble raising their hind feet high enough to get over curbs or up a few steps. You can give a helping hand simply by using her tail as a handle, Dr. Nisson says. Grip the tail close to her body and gently lift her while she moves. As long as her tail is in good condition and you do this gently, she will appreciate the extra help.

Dogs and cats that are overweight are much more likely to have joint problems than their thinner friends. If your pet is getting pudgy, helping her shed a little weight will make it easier for her to jump out of bed in the morning, says Dr. Hibbs. Here is what you need to do.

- Reduce the calories that she is taking in. Vets recommend switching to low-calorie foods, which are available from vets and pet supply stores, says John Fioramonti, D.V.M., a veterinarian in private practice in Towson, Maryland. You want to buy a food that contains about 35 percent fewer calories than her usual chow. Ask your vet which foods would be the best choices, he advises. The food should also contain more fiber, since fiber will help your pet feel full and satisfied even when she is getting fewer calories.
- Make changes gradually. If your pet is too attached to her current food to comfortably make the change, you will have to scale back the servings. Measure how much she usually eats in a day and then give her 10 percent less, says Dr. Fioramonti.

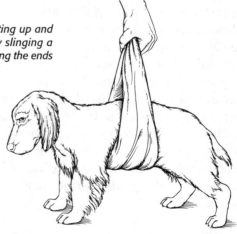

If your dog is having trouble getting up and around, you can help her out by slinging a towel beneath her belly and holding the ends to support her weight.

- Help keep her satisfied. Dogs and cats take mealtimes very seriously, so don't be surprised if your pet seems unhappy when she first begins her new diet. To keep her stomach satisfied, you may want to add a few green beans, carrots, or some canned pumpkin to her diet. These foods are low in calories and high in fiber, which means that she can eat a lot of them without gaining weight.
- Cut back on snacks. The best diet in the world can be destroyed by snacking, so crank up your willpower and quit doling out treats. At the very least, make sure that the snacks are healthy ones, like vegetables or small amounts of high-fiber dry cereal, says Dr. Fioramonti.
  Pet supply stores sell a variety of dog treats that are labeled "low-calorie." Unfortunately, they aren't as low in calories as you might think, so don't use a lot of them, Dr. Nisson says.
- Take it slowly. Losing too much weight too quickly can be dangerous, especially for cats, Dr. Fioramonti warns. Losing about ½ pound a month is a good rate for cats. Dogs can lose weight a little faster—about 2 percent of their weight per week. So if you have a 100-pound dog, she can safely lose 2 pounds a week.

Vets aren't sure why, but puppies that are given foods low in protein and fat are less likely to develop serious arthritis in their hips than dogs that are eating high-fat-and-protein foods. Look for foods labeled "for large-breed puppies," which are available from veterinarians and in pet supply stores. These foods are formulated to give at-risk dogs the best chance to grow correctly.

Regardless of what your pet eats, regular exercise—walking and swimming are particularly good—can be very helpful for easing the aches and helping her get up easily again, says Joanne Smith, D.V.M., a veterinarian in private practice in Edgewater, Maryland. Exercise strengthens muscles around the joints, helping them work more efficiently. At the same time, it causes the joints to produce more synovial fluid, a lubricating fluid that acts like oil on a rusty hinge, helping quiet creaks and squeaks. Even pets with advanced hip dysplasia often get better once they start exercising.

Vets recommend that most pets—including those with arthritis—get at least two exercise sessions a day for 10 to 15 minutes each, says Dr. Smith. If your pet has been hurting lately, however, be sure to start slowly. Dr. Smith recommends starting out by hiking on soft trails or simply walking around the yard. As she gets in better shape, you can increase the intensity of her workouts.

Applying warm, moist heat is an excellent strategy for relaxing stiff joints, says Dr. Nisson. He recommends giving dogs a 10-minute soak in a warm bath. An easier strategy for dogs and cats may be to wrap a hot-water bottle in a towel and lay it on the sore joints for 5 to 10 minutes, at which point they will usually be feeling a little better.

Don't use electric heating pads, Dr. Nisson adds. Not only do they dry the skin, they can also get very hot. If your pet is having trouble getting up, she may be unable to move away from the heat when she starts getting uncomfortable.

Massage can be very helpful because it improves circulation to arthritic joints, keeping the muscles limber, says Carvel Tiekert, D.V.M., a veterinarian in private practice in Bel Air, Maryland, and executive director of the American Holistic Veterinary Medical Association. When giving a massage, use firm, circular motions, putting pressure on the surrounding muscle and not on the bone itself. Squeeze the muscle gently between your thumb and fingers. If your pet squirms or pulls away, try using a little less pressure. When you have the right touch, she will relax and look happy.

One way to help your pet get up more easily—a way that she is sure to enjoy—is to give her a comfortable bed, says Dr. Tiekert. At the very least, you should provide a pile of thick, warm blankets to sleep on. Or you can buy an orthopedic bed that is made for pets. These beds have dense, foam padding, which cushions joints and helps retain body heat so that the joints stay warm and mobile.

If your pet is having a lot of pain, vets sometimes recommend giving over-the-counter pain relievers. "I usually start dogs on a coated aspirin (like Ascriptin)," says Dr. Hibbs. The usual dose is 10 milligrams per pound of pooch, given once or twice a day. Your vet will let you know if this is the right dose for your pet. Aspirin and other over-the-counter pain medicines can be dangerous for cats, however, and shouldn't be used without a veterinarian's supervision.

Finally, there are many nutritional supplements that veterinarians have found may help ease pain and inflammation caused by hip dysplasia and arthritis.

- A supplement called superoxide dismutase can be very helpful, particularly when given in combination with vitamins E and C and the mineral selenium, says Patricia Shema, V.M.D., a veterinarian in private practice in Glenn Dale, Maryland. This supplement is available in health food stores, but you will need to ask your vet for the correct dose for treating your pet.
- Other supplements that you may want to try include glucosamine and chondroitin sulfate. Glucosamine may be found alone or in combination with chondroitin sulfate. The usual daily dose is 10 milligrams of glucosamine per pound of weight; divide this daily dose in half and give it twice a day.

These and other nutritional supplements are safe, although you will want to check with your vet about the proper dose, says Dr. Hibbs. Don't expect dramatic results overnight, she adds. You will need to use them for two or three months before you notice a lot of improvement.

WHAT YOUR VET WILL DO

Since difficulty getting up may be a sign of serious illness, it is important to see your vet as soon as you start noticing problems.

In most cases, your vet will agree with your hunch that arthritis is the problem. He will probably recommend x-rays to find where the bad joints are and to see how serious the damage is. In addition, he may take a blood sample to test for kidney or liver damage, high blood sugar levels, or infections. He may draw a little fluid directly out of a joint for additional tests.

An increasing number of vets have started using acupuncture to relieve the pain of arthritis and hip dysplasia, says Dr. Tiekert. Most dogs and cats don't mind the treatments, and it can provide long-term relief, particularly when used in combination with prescription or over-the-counter medications.

If your pet reaches a point where she simply can't get up without assistance, your vet may recommend surgery to repair the joint. In some cases, surgeons can rearrange bones in the hips so that they fit together more precisely. They can also replace the original hip with a brand-new metal one.

| SYMPTOM | # FOOT LICKING

Clues

- Your pet's paws are always damp.
- He is limping, licking, or favoring one or more paws.
- Your cat's paws seem soft or puffy.
- His paw is red or has a bad smell.

Dogs and cats love to run—through fields, over lawns, and across grungy kitchen floors. Not surprisingly, their feet can get plenty dirty by the end of the day. Since they can't use a sink and washcloth, they lick their paws clean.

It is normal for dogs and cats to lick their feet from time to time. In some cases, however, they don't know when to quit. They can literally lick (and bite) their feet for hours on end, sometimes causing raw, irritated skin or even open sores called lick granulomas.

Pets that lick their feet all the time may have allergies, says Patricia Shema, V.M.D., a veterinarian in private practice in Glenn Dale, Maryland. Veterinarians aren't sure why, but pets that are allergic to certain foods or airborne particles like pollen often get itchy feet, while other kinds of allergies typically cause itching elsewhere on the body. Contact allergies, which occur when pets step on something that they are sensitive to, can also cause itchy feet, she says.

It is not only allergies that cause pets to lick their feet. When your pet has a sore paw—from a thorn, a cut pad, or a broken nail—he will lick until it gets better. In fact, any problem that makes the feet hurt, such as arthritis, Lyme disease, or infections from parasites, can result in licking.

Just as humans will sometimes bite their nails or twirl their hair when they are bored, pets may turn their attention to their feet, licking them for long periods of time. In addition, some dogs—especially Doberman pinschers and German shepherds—will get compulsive about their feet, licking them until they are raw and sore, says Steven A. Melman, V.M.D., a veterinary dermatologist in private practice in Potomac, Maryland, and author of *Skin Diseases of Dogs and Cats*.

A problem unique to the feline set is an infection called plasma cell pododermatitis, which causes the feet to get puffy, soft, and sensitive. Also, cats that have been declawed may lick and chew their feet until the cuts from the surgery have completely healed, says Margie Scherk, D.V.M., a veterinarian in private practice in Vancouver, British Columbia. Sometimes, in fact, the claws will start growing back, which can also cause cats to lick their feet.

WHAT YOU CAN DO

To find out why your pet is licking, take a good look at his feet—between the toes, under the fur, and on the pads. If the paw is red, swollen, or has a bad smell, he may be injured, and you will probably want to call your vet. If the paw looks completely normal, however, there is a good chance allergies are to blame. This is especially true if your pet has what vets call the gloves-and-socks syndrome, which means that he is not focusing just on one foot, but on two or four, says Dr. Melman.

The best way to treat allergies is to keep your pet away from whatever it is that is making him itch. Veterinarians sometimes recommend keeping a "feet-licking diary," in which you jot down everything that is happening when his tongue goes to work. Does he lick mainly in summer or winter? Does he lick only on weekends (after you have cleaned the house) or during the week. As you gather more details, you will start to see patterns that will help you identify the problem.

Suppose, for example, your pet always licks his feet after running in the field behind your house. It is possible, says Dr. Shema, that he is stepping on fertilizer or other chemicals that may be causing itchy feet. Other common culprits are household cleaners and carpet deodorizers. By keeping an eye on where he runs and plays, you may learn what is behind the problem—and what he needs to avoid to get better.

Since many dogs and cats suffer from allergies in the spring and summer, you may want to try keeping him indoors during the early morning and evening hours, when pollen counts are highest. In winter, you may want to clean your pet's paws well after walks since chemicals used to de-ice roads can irritate the feet and cause licking, says Dr. Shema. It is also a good idea to remove packed snow and ice from his paws since prolonged moisture can cause them to get tender.

Here is another winter tip: When snow and ice are on the ground, apply a light coating of petroleum jelly before he goes outside, says Joanne Howl, D.V.M., a veterinarian in private practice in West River, Maryland. This will help protect his paws from ice, snow, and road salt, while keeping the pads soft and moist. Wipe off the petroleum jelly before he comes back in the house, she adds.

Since food allergies are very common, a good starting place is with an elimination diet, says John Daugherty, D.V.M., a veterinarian in private practice in Poland, Ohio. This means putting your pet on a totally different diet, for 8 to 10 weeks, being careful not to slip him little extras like snacks or rawhide chews. (Even certain medications may skew the results, so it is a good idea to review all your pet's medications with your vet before starting this kind of diet.) If he starts leaving his feet alone during this time, you will have a pretty good idea what you need to avoid in the future.

Even when you can't figure out exactly the problem is, there are still ways to stop the licking. Cool baths can be a big help since the water assists in relieving itching. At the same time, it washes particles from his coat that may be causing an allergy, says Dr. Melman.

When you are giving a bath, it is a good idea to use shampoos that contain moisturizers, adds Dr. Daugherty. In addition, veterinarians sell shampoos that contain a mild anesthetic, which can stop itching fast. At the very least, you may want to add a little colloidal oatmeal (like Aveeno) to the bathwater, which can be very soothing. Just be sure to rinse your pet thoroughly after the bath since any soap that remains can make the itching worse.

Even though dogs may appreciate a cool dip, cats aren't so enthusiastic. Making the water lukewarm instead of cold will help them tolerate it better. Or if your cat would rather fight than get in the tub, wet a washcloth in warm water, wring it out, and wipe him gently from his ears to the tip of his tail.

You don't have to wash your pet's whole body for him to get the benefits, says Carvel Tiekert, D.V.M., a veterinarian in private practice in Bel Air, Maryland, and executive director of the American Holistic Veterinary Medical Association. Simply soaking his feet for 5 or 10 minutes, four times a day, in cool water can help control licking. For additional relief, add a sprinkling of Epsom salts to the water, he suggests.

Since a rash, cut, or mild infection can cause your pet to lick his feet, you may want to try soaking his feet in a mild mixture of Betadine Solution and water. (The mixture should be the color of weak tea.) Soak the feet for 10 minutes, three times a day, and repeat for about four days, says Grant Nisson, D.V.M., a veterinarian in private practice in West River, Maryland. A solution made by mixing equal parts white vinegar and water can also be helpful.

You can even try soaking his feet in a solution made from brewed tea, since tea contains chemicals called tannins, which help dry rashes and ease irritated skin, says Dr. Tiekert.

Chamomile tea is also good, says Dr. Scherk. You don't even have to soak his feet to get the benefits. Just brew a cup of tea as you normally would, then soak a clean towel in the cooled tea to make a compress and apply it directly to his paw for three to five minutes, up to five times a day, she says. Tea can discolor fur, so don't be surprised if your pet seems to be wearing socks when you are done.

It is always a good idea to wash your pet's feet after he has spent time outdoors, says Dr. Tiekert. This especially helps pets with allergies to grasses," he says. He recommends washing the feet in a very dilute bleach solution, mixing one teaspoon bleach in a quart of water.

Some vets recommend giving oral medications to control licking caused by allergies. For example, you can give dogs over-the-counter antihistamines containing diphenhydramine, such as Benadryl. Give one milligram for every pound of pooch, three times a day, says Karen L. Campbell, associate professor of dermatology and small animal internal medicine at the University of Illinois College of Veterinary Medicine at

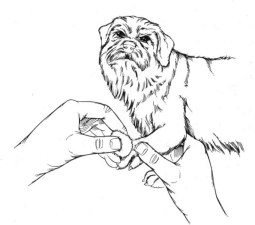

Your pet's furry feet are natural traps for pollen and other allergens. To prevent him from tracking allergy-causing particles indoors, you need to keep his feet clean. To get between the toes, hold the foot between your thumb and forefinger and apply gentle pressure to the top and bottom, which will cause the toes to spread.

Urbana–Champaign. For cats, a better choice is a product containing chlorpheniramine, such as Chlor-Trimeton. The usual dose is half of a four-milligram tablet for every 10 pounds of cat, twice a day, says Dr. Campbell.

In addition, fatty-acid supplements, which are available in pet supply stores, catalogs, and from veterinarians, can also help relieve itching. To be safe, however, always check with your vet before giving human medications to pets, says Dr. Melman.

One of the best remedies for stopping feet licking is also the most fun. Since pets often lick their feet when they are bored, keeping them entertained can make a big difference. Go to the park. Play a game of catch. Toss a catnip mouse. Drag some string. Take a walk. It doesn't really matter what you do as long as it is fun. When your pet's mind is on fun and games, he won't be thinking about his feet, says Dr. Shema.

Worried owners will sometimes try coating their pets' paws with hot spices or bitter-tasting sprays or ointments, such as Bitter Apple, to stop the licking. Or they will wrap the feet in bandages. But these remedies usually don't work. "Pets will chew themselves anyway because the itching is so intense," says Dr. Shema. "If a dog is determined to lick, nothing you put on the paw is going to stop it."

WHAT YOUR VET WILL DO

If your pet just won't quit licking his feet, or his feet are getting sore and tender, you are going to need some help from your veterinarian.

After examining the paws, your vet will probably test for fungus, bacteria, or parasites, all of which can cause feet licking. If your pet is infected or infested, your vet will probably prescribe antibiotics or other medications, which should clear up the problem.

When there doesn't appear to be an infection, your vet may take a tiny sample of skin to test for more serious problems, such as tumors or problems with the immune system.

Since allergies are so common and so difficult to identify, your vet may recommend that you see a veterinary dermatologist for specialized testing. In addition, she may prescribe medications such as steroids, which quickly relieve irritation and break the "lick cycle." These drugs have the added benefit of putting the brakes on the immune system, which produces the allergy symptoms. Finally, pets with severe allergies may undergo a series of shots to help desensitize them to whatever they are allergic to.

In some cases, your vet won't be able to find anything physically wrong. It may be, says Dr. Melman, that your pet simply is obsessing about his feet and won't leave them alone. When that's the case, your vet may give mood-changing drugs such as fluoxetine (Prozac), which can be very helpful for keeping his mind (and mouth) off his feet.

LEG DRAGGING

Clues

- Your pet's toes are cold or purple.
- He is dragging more than one leg.
- He has recently had an injection.

It is not unusual for pets to bump or bruise their legs. If one of the legs is actually dragging, however, he may have a serious problem.

"When I see a cat or dog dragging his leg, I think of nerve damage," says Joanne Hibbs, D.V.M., a veterinarian in private practice in Powell, Tennessee. Nerves are responsible for carrying messages to and from the legs, spinal cord, and brain. When nerves are damaged, the messages get blocked—and your pet may be unable to use his leg.

There are many possible causes of nerve damage. Pets that have been hit by cars may bruise or tear a group of nerves (the brachial plexus) under the armpit that controls the front leg. An injury to this area may cause pets to drop to their elbows and drag their wrists on the ground.

If one or both of the hind legs is dragging, there could be an injury to the sciatic nerve, which carries signals from the spinal cord all the way down the leg.

It is very rare, but nerve damage may occur during routine vaccinations or other shots. Injections are often given in the back of the thigh, where muscles wrap around the sciatic nerve. Hitting the nerve with the needle or bathing it in irritating medications may cause the leg to drag, says Dr. Hibbs. Fortunately, this doesn't happen often, and when it does, the leg usually heals within a month.

If your dog suddenly starts dragging both hind legs and he hasn't been in an accident, there is a good chance that he has ruptured a disk in his back, says Dr. Hibbs. Disks are the padding between the bones of the spine. They are designed like a jelly doughnut—firm on the outside with a softer gel inside. If the outer portion weakens, the gel can ooze out, possibly pressing on the spinal cord and preventing signals from reaching the legs, she says.

Cats don't get disk problems very often, but they are susceptible to a condition called aortic thromboembolism, in which a blood clot gets trapped in a vein serving the hind legs, says Dr. Hibbs. In addition to dragging their hind legs, cats with this condition may develop cold, painful, and slightly purple toes. This condition is usually caused by an underlying heart problem, she adds.

WHAT YOU CAN DO

Leg dragging is always serious and sometimes an emergency, so you will want to call your vet right away. Once you know what is causing the problem, however, there are things that you can do at home to help your pet recover more quickly.

Nerves that have been bruised, torn, or stretched (rather than cut completely) will usually start to heal within a month. It is very important to keep your pet quiet so that he doesn't do further damage to the nerve, says Grant Nisson, D.V.M., a veterinarian in private practice in West River, Maryland. Encourage him to lie comfortably in a crate or in small room and don't give him any vigorous exercise without checking with your vet.

For dogs, keep them on a leash when going outside and be sure to keep the pace slow. They won't enjoy the strict rest, but it is essential for healing, adds Dr. Hibbs.

Ice or cold packs can also be helpful, says Dr. Nisson. On the first day of the injury, apply a cold compress three or four times for 5 to 10 minutes each time to help reduce bruising and swelling. On the second day, apply a warm compress three times a day for 5 to 10 minutes each time. The compress should be warm, not hot.

Your vet may also recommend giving your pet some physical therapy by gently moving the leg through its full range of motion. Do this for five minutes at least four times a day to stimulate the nerve and help it recover more quickly, says Dr. Nisson. Every nerve injury is different, however, so it is important to do range-of-motion exercises only when your vet says it is safe to begin.

For cats with aortic thromboembolism, vets sometimes recommend massaging the lower leg for two to five minutes every two hours, which will help restore circulation, says Dr. Hibbs.

Finally, you may want to take steps to protect the paw and wrist while they are still dragging. Dr. Nisson recommends using booties, available from pet supply stores or catalogs, to protect the feet.

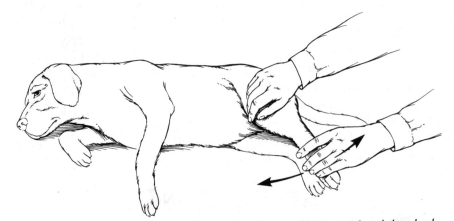

To help muscles in the legs recover, slowly move the hind leg forward and then back, stretching it about the same distance it would travel if he were walking. Then do the other leg.

WHAT YOUR VET WILL DO

Nerve damage can affect many parts of the body, so your vet will manipulate your pet—twisting his neck, squeezing his toes, and making him hop in odd positions—to see how well his nervous system is working and where the problems are.

If your vet suspects that he has a damaged spinal disk, she will recommend spinal x-rays. She may also recommend that your pet have a myelogram, specialized x-rays in which a dye is injected into the spinal column. Myelograms are the best way to tell exactly where the problem is and what treatments are likely to be needed.

Pets having myelograms are always given sedation, Dr. Hibbs adds. For x-rays, sedation isn't needed as long as your pet will hold still long enough for the films to be exposed.

Sudden injuries to the nerves or the spine are often treated with steroids to reduce swelling, followed by rest to help speed recovery. In some cases, surgery is needed to relieve pressure on the spinal cord or other nerves.

If your cat is dragging his hind legs, your vet will want to give him a thorough heart exam, which will include x-rays, an electrocardiogram, and other tests. If he does have a blood clot, he will need to spend several days in the hospital. Your cat will also be given drugs to help the clot dissolve, and he may need surgery as well.

SYMPTOM) **LIMPING**

Clues

- Your pet won't let you touch his paw.
- The leg is swollen and in an odd position.
- There is a bad odor around the paw.
- He had ticks before the limping began.

Dogs and cats don't get knee injuries playing football or sprain their ankles tripping over toys, but their lives—and limbs—aren't exactly risk-free. They race through gardens, leap on trees, and sprint after rabbits. Which is why they sometimes come limping home as if they had a hard day at the mine.

Limping usually means that they have hurt one of their paws, says Grant Nisson, D.V.M., a veterinarian in private practice in West River, Maryland. Pets that spend a lot of time outdoors will sometimes step on a thorn or pick up a splinter from a tree. Glass can also be a problem, especially for pets who spend time on beaches or city streets, he says.

Long toenails can be a limp ready to happen since dogs and cats sometimes snag them on carpets or other rough surfaces, causing painful tears. Even running on hard surfaces like sidewalks can cause nails to break or tear, which is why vets usually recommend cutting your pet's nails at least once a month.

If your cat is hobbling about on three legs and won't let you touch the fourth, there is a good chance that he has an abscess, an infected wound that can be excruciatingly painful, says John Fioramonti, D.V.M., a veterinarian in private practice in Towson, Maryland. While dogs occasionally get abscesses, they are much more common and, generally, much more painful in cats.

Dogs and cats aren't always the most graceful creatures, and sometimes they take painful tumbles. If your cat comes home with a limp, he may have slipped off a fence and landed on his rear (myths to the contrary, cats don't always land on their feet). In addition, dogs and cats often push their bodies harder than they were meant to go, pulling muscles or straining ligaments in the process. Dogs are particularly fond of running at full speed, then suddenly changing direction, which can tear the ligament in the knee, says Joanne Smith, D.V.M., a veterinarian in private practice in Edgewater, Maryland. Cats do plenty of swerving, too, but because they are more limber than dogs, they are less likely to damage their knees.

Finally, some limps are caused by broken bones, says Dr. Smith. It is usually easy to recognize a break because the area will be swollen and very tender, and the leg may not "fit" the way it is supposed to.

Not all limps are caused by injuries, however. Pets that have been bitten by ticks may develop Lyme disease or Rocky Mountain spotted fever, both of which can cause sore muscles and creaky, aching joints, says Dr. Nisson.

In addition, dogs under one year old may limp because of growing pains, says Dr. Fioramonti. In most cases, this is a minor (and short-lived) problem, which will clear up when your dog gets a little older.

WHAT YOU CAN DO

Before you can help your pet feel better, you have to figure out what is making him limp. Here are a few easy-to-follow guidelines: If you let him outside and he came back limping, he probably did something to injure himself. If, on the other hand, he was fine when he went to sleep, but woke up as creaky as an old war hero, he may have a more serious underlying problem.

If your pet simply has a cut pad, all you have to do is clean the area well. Most cuts aren't a problem since they are usually shallow and will heal quite quickly, says John Daugherty, D.V.M., a veterinarian in private practice in Poland, Ohio.

To clean the foot thoroughly, soak it in a mixture of Betadine Solution and warm water. (Add the Betadine to the water until it is the color of weak tea.) Soak the foot for 10 minutes, three times a day, and repeat for about four days, says Dr. Nisson.

If the area is already infected—signs of infection include pus, swelling, or a bad smell—call your vet since your pet will probably need antibiotics, Dr. Nisson says. The same is true if there has been a deep puncture wound, such as from a long thorn, since these often get infected. In the meantime, you can make him more comfortable by holding a damp, warm cloth against the infected area for about 10 minutes. This will help the infection drain.

If you can't see anything wrong, and your pet doesn't seem to be in a lot of pain, he is probably just bruised and needs a day or two to recover. To reduce swelling, put ice cubes in a plastic bag wrapped in a towel and hold it against the sore spot for about 10 minutes. Repeat this three to four times during the first 24 hours. On the second day, put the ice away and apply a warm compress for 5 to 10 minutes several times a day, which will provide quick relief, says Dr. Nisson.

Aspirin is another way to provide quick relief—but only for dogs since aspirin can be dangerous for cats, Dr. Nisson says. When your dog is limping, he recommends giving him a buffered or coated aspirin (like Ascriptin). The usual dose is 10 milligrams for every pound of dog, given once or twice a day, but be sure to check with your vet before giving your dog any medications.

There isn't much that you can do if you suspect a bone is broken—

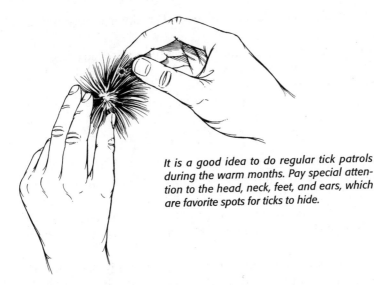

It is a good idea to do regular tick patrols during the warm months. Pay special attention to the head, neck, feet, and ears, which are favorite spots for ticks to hide.

except, of course, to get your pet to the vet right away, says Joanne Hibbs, D.V.M., a veterinarian in private practice in Powell, Tennessee. To prevent your pet from causing further injury, it is important to keep him as still as possible. Dr. Hibbs recommends keeping your pet in a crate or on a leash until you are able to get him to the vet. In some cases, you may need to splint the leg as well. (For instructions on making a splint, see "Fractures" on page 30.)

Even though you can't treat Lyme disease or Rocky Mountain spotted fever at home, there are ways to prevent your pet from getting sick in the first place. Since both diseases are caused by ticks, take a flea comb or a comb with closely spaced teeth and go through your pet's coat every day to remove ticks before they have a chance to latch on. Doing these daily tick patrols can vastly reduce the chances that he will get infected, says Dr. Fioramonti.

If your dog has growing pains, giving aspirin can be a big help. You can also try switching from a puppy food to a food for adults, Dr. Fioramonti suggests. Adult dog foods have less fat and protein, and appear to sometimes be helpful in reducing growing pains.

WHAT YOUR VET WILL DO

When limping doesn't go away or you suspect that the problem is too serious for you to handle at home, you will want to get in to see your vet right away. Don't be surprised if your vet, after giving your pet a thorough exam, walks to the end of the hall and watches as you and your pet stroll around. This will help her figure out what the problem is.

If your vet can't see the problem right away or if your pet appears to have a broken bone, your vet will probably take x-rays to show what is going on inside. She may also use a needle to take fluid from a joint. The fluid can then be analyzed to see if there is an infection or other serious problem happening inside.

Conditions such as Lyme disease and Rocky Mountain spotted fever are somewhat difficult to diagnose—blood tests are usually needed—but they are very easy to treat. Once your pet is given antibiotics, he will probably start feeling like his old self within a day or two.

If there is an abscess, your vet will drain the fluid and clean the area thoroughly. Because abscesses can be very painful, she may have to use a local or general anesthetic to get the job done. In addition, she will probably prescribe oral antibiotics to tackle the infection from the inside out.

Broken bones, of course, will have to be repaired, and your pet will probably come home wearing a cast. Everyone in the neighborhood will have time to sign it since he will be wearing it for about six weeks.

Some dogs with knee injuries are fortunate enough to recover after a few weeks of rest. If your dog severely damaged a ligament or the cartilage, however, he will need surgery to get the leg back into working order, says Dr. Nisson.

SYMPTOM   NAIL CRACKING

Clues

- More than one nail is cracked.
- Your pet's nails fell out and then grew back cracked.

Unlike human nails, which are good for trapping dirt and not much else, your pet's nails go to work nearly every day—digging holes, climbing trees, and scratching posts. They take quite a beating, and sometimes they crack and splinter. For a dog or cat, cracked nails are not only painful but also prone to hard-to-treat infections, which can cause even more cracking.

Nails usually crack for the simple reason that they got too long, says Nancy E. Wiswall, D.V.M., a veterinarian in private practice in Bethesda, Maryland. Since all of your pet's nails grow at roughly the same rate, more than one will often crack at one time, she adds.

Though they don't look or feel like skin, nails are really an extension of the skin layer. Anything that causes unhealthy skin, like dietary or immune system problems, can also cause cracked nails, says Dr. Wiswall. Pets eating low-quality food will sometimes develop cracked nails because they are not getting all the nutrients that they need, she adds.

In dogs, a condition called lupoid onchyodystrophy (also known as 20-nail disease) can cause all the nails to fall out. When they grow back, they will usually be brittle and prone to cracking, says Grant Nisson, D.V.M., a veterinarian in private practice in West River, Maryland. Vets aren't sure what causes this condition, although it may be related to the immune system, he says.

WHAT YOU CAN DO

Unless your pet has an underlying illness, keeping the nails trimmed will usually prevent them from cracking. Most pets need trimming about once a month, although older dogs and cats may need more frequent pedicures, says Dr. Wiswall.

Cracked nails tend to splinter during trimming, so be sure to use a sharp trimmer. For cats, a human fingernail clipper works fine. For dogs, you may want to use a heavier, side-to-side-style trimmer designed for their thicker nails or simply a nail file to slowly work the nails back. Don't use a guillotine-style trimmers because they tend to crush brittle nails. First, soak the nails for 15 minutes in warm water to make them easier to cut, suggests Dr. Wiswall.

If your pet won't sit still for soaking, you can use a wet dressing. Soak a cloth in warm water and wrap it around the foot for 10 to 15 minutes, says Charles McLeod, D.V.M., a veterinary pathologist at Antech Diagnostics in Carney, Maryland. If you don't want to hold the foot that long,

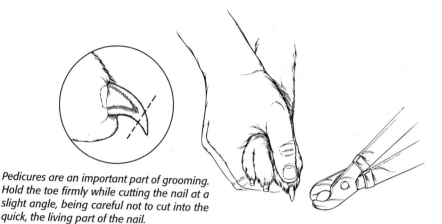

Pedicures are an important part of grooming. Hold the toe firmly while cutting the nail at a slight angle, being careful not to cut into the quick, the living part of the nail.

cover the cloth with a plastic bag and tape it on.

If you are using a cut-rate food, you may want to switch to a better-quality, name-brand food. In addition, your vet may recommend giving your pet dietary supplements containing fatty acids, which are good for the skin. These may be particularly helpful for dogs with 20-nail disease, says Dr. Nisson. You can buy fatty-acid supplements from veterinary offices, pet supply catalogs and stores, and health food stores. Ask your vet what dose will be right for your pet.

Dietary changes can be helpful, but don't expect fast improvements, says Dr. Wiswall. It can take more than six months for a nail to grow all the way out. If you are unsure that things are improving, ask your vet to take a look.

WHAT YOUR VET WILL DO

Cracked nails tend to keep cracking, so the first thing that your vet will do is trim the nails and remove damaged slivers before they get snagged in a carpet or on tree bark. She may even fill cracks in the nail with surgical glue to strengthen it while it heals.

If your vet suspects an infection has taken hold, she will take swabs from the nail and put them under a microscope to see what, if anything, is causing the problem. In addition, she will probably do blood work to check your pet's overall health.

If your pet does have an infection, be prepared to be patient. Nail infections are time-consuming to treat, and your pet will probably need to take antibiotics for at least a month, says Dr. Wiswall.

When one or more nails simply won't heal, your vet may recommend removing them. It is not a difficult procedure, but it does require general anesthetic and a day in the hospital. If your vet only removes the dead portion of the nail, it will gradually grow back. In some cases, however, it is necessary to remove the entire nail, including the bone that supports it.

SYMPTOM) PAD CALLUSES

Dogs and cats put a lot of miles on their feet, running and leaping just for the fun of it. Ordinary skin isn't built to withstand this pounding, which is why their paw pads are thick and springy.

The paws get additional protection from calluses—thick, dry skin that accumulates on the pads wherever there is a lot of pressure. Dogs that run on concrete, for example, normally have thicker paw pads than those that stroll on grass or carpet, says Patricia Ashley, D.V.M., a veterinary resident in dermatology at the University of Tennessee College of Veterinary Medicine in Knoxville. "Your pet's skin gets thicker with age, just like people's skin does," she adds.

In some cases, however, the pads accumulate too much callus or the callus forms unevenly. Heavily callused pads lose their flexibility and the ability to absorb shock. Your pet's feet may get sore and tender. She will feel as though she is walking on stones.

Heavy or uneven callus may be caused by the way your pet walks. "The feet can tell us if a pet has a problem with her elbow, for example, because of the wear pattern on the pad," says Dr. Ashley. In dogs particularly, being overweight can put a lot of pressure on the outsides of their feet, causing uneven calluses to form.

Calluses on all four feet may be a sign of internal problems such as liver disease. Even immune system diseases such as lupus can make the pads thick and painful, says Charles McLeod, D.V.M., a veterinary pathologist at Antech Diagnostics in Carney, Maryland.

Zinc is an important nutrient for healthy skin. A dog that isn't getting enough zinc in her diet may get very thick paw pads. (This problem doesn't occur in cats.) Siberian huskies and Alaskan malamutes often run low in zinc because they have a genetic defect that makes it hard for their bodies to absorb this important mineral, says Dr. McLeod. In addition, pets eating low-quality foods or taking calcium supplements can have problems getting enough zinc.

Another problem unique to dogs, called hard-pad disease, may occur after a bout with canine distemper, says Dr. Ashley. Cats that have feline leukemia sometimes develop thick, cone-shaped calluses on one or more feet, which look like unicorn horns and often stick out to the sides. These horn-shaped calluses usually don't cause discomfort, says Margie Scherk, D.V.M., a veterinarian in private practice in Vancouver, British Columbia.

WHAT YOU CAN DO

Unless you can figure out why your pet's feet are getting callused, it is very hard to get them back to normal. And because calluses may be a sign of internal problems, you will want your vet to take a look. Meanwhile, here are a few things that you can do to help your pet be more comfortable.

"I'm a firm believer in using plain warm-water soaks," says Dr. Ashley. She recommends soaking callused feet for 10 to 15 minutes to let the water work its way deep into the skin. Do this two to three times a day until the pads are soft. Then repeat the treatments whenever the calluses start getting bothersome again.

For pets that won't stand still for a soak, you can use a wet dressing. Soak a thick washcloth in warm water and wrap it around your pet's foot for 10 to 15 minutes, says Dr. McLeod. If you don't want to hold the foot the entire time, you can cover the washcloth with a plastic bag and tape it on.

Even though warm-water soaks get moisture into the pad, they won't keep it there. To prevent moisture from escaping, apply a moisturizer. "Kerasolv, which you can get from vets, is one of the best callus remedies you can use," says Dr. Ashley. Lanolin and petroleum jelly are also effective, although using petroleum jelly may result in greasy footprints around the house.

While moisture is good for calluses, you don't want the rest of the foot to stay wet, or it may get inflamed and itchy, says Dr. Ashley. She suggests using a dry towel to wipe between the toes after each soak to keep the toes healthy.

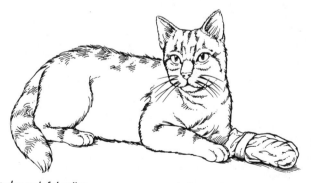

To moisturize dry, painful calluses, wrap a wet washcloth around your pet's paw and cover it with a plastic bag. Loosely tape the top of the bag to hold it in place.

WHAT YOUR VET WILL DO

In most cases, calluses are normal for your pet's age or way of walking, and your vet will show you how to keep the feet healthy. But since thick, callused pads may be a symptom of internal problems, your vet will take a careful look at your whole pet, not just her feet.

Your vet may take blood samples, which will give him an idea of your pet's general health. He may also order special blood tests for feline leukemia or autoimmune diseases, such as lupus or pemphigus. In addition, he may snip a small sample of the paw pad and send it to a laboratory for examination.

Problems with the immune system or liver can usually be controlled with medications and perhaps changes in your pet's diet. If it turns out that your pet isn't getting enough zinc, your vet may recommend giving her supplements. It is also important to use a high-quality, name-brand food, which will make it easier for your pet to absorb the zinc.

See also Chapter 10: Pad Cracks

PAD CRACKS

Unlike humans, who fill their closets with tennis shoes, high heels, and other forms of sole protection, dogs and cats prefer going barefoot. In hot weather and cold, on hard ground and soft, they pad about on tough, flexible pads that provide incredible protection.

When the paw pads take more of a beating than nature intended, however, they may form a thick layer of protective callus, which is much less flexible than the pad itself. And when the callus gets rough treatment, it may crack, says Patricia Ashley, D.V.M., a veterinary resident in dermatology at the University of Tennessee College of Veterinary Medicine in Knoxville. Cracks in the pads can be very painful and are prone to infection, she explains.

Most dogs and cats don't have a problem with callus, she adds. But dogs that work hard in harsh climates—sled dogs, for example—will often have problems with painful cracks.

Callus isn't the only thing that causes paw cracks. Allergies can also be a problem. Unlike humans, who often sneeze or scratch when allergies flare, pets tend to get itchy feet. They will lick and bite and chew at their feet, sometimes for hours at time. The pads can get wet, sore, and raw, causing cracks to form, says Nancy E. Wiswall, D.V.M., a veterinarian in private practice in Bethesda, Maryland.

Internal illnesses can also cause pad problems. Pets with liver disease, for example, may develop paw cracks. They are also related to zinc deficiency, which occurs in pets fed low-quality foods and in certain dog breeds with a genetic tendency to absorb too little zinc. Problems with the immune system can cause cracking as well, says Steve Young, D.V.M., a veterinarian in private practice in North Scituate, Rhode Island. So if your pet is feeling under the weather and is also having paw problems, there is a good chance that the problems are related. This is especially true if more than one pad is cracked.

In cats, pad cracks as well as swelling may be caused by an illness called plasma cell pododermatitis, in which the immune system doesn't work the way it should.

Cracks in your cat's pads aren't always easy to spot, adds Dr. Ashley. Unlike dogs, which tend to develop deep, ugly cracks, cats usually get cracks that appear as fine white lines or a bit of flaking skin.

WHAT YOU CAN DO

Regardless of what is causing the cracks, it is important to give them a chance to heal, but it won't happen overnight. Dr. Young recommends keeping your pet calm for a few weeks. Cats should be kept inside so that they don't run around too much. Dogs should be kept on a leash and walked only on grass or other soft surfaces.

If your dog spends most of his time outside, you may want to protect his feet with booties similar to those worn by Arctic sled dogs, says Dr. Ashley. You can find a selection of booties in large pet stores or pet supply catalogs.

A less expensive option is to cover his feet with baby socks, says Dr. Ashley. Tuck some cotton padding in the bottom of the sock, put his foot inside, and wrap a little masking tape around the top and to his skin to hold it on.

Most cats (and some dogs) won't tolerate the socks, she adds. But if your pet doesn't mind having his paws covered, the sock will protect the pad from further harm. You will need to change the sock at least once a day, or whenever it gets wet or dirty.

Since it is easy for bacteria to set up camp inside a crack in your pet's pad, you should clean the pad regularly to prevent infection. Mix two tablespoons of 2 percent chlorhexidine (an antiseptic available in drugstores) in a gallon of cool, clean water. Dr. Young recommends soaking the paw in the solution for 10 to 15 minutes, twice a day. If he won't hold still for soaking, you can soak a cloth in the solution and hold it on the pad for 5 to 10 minutes.

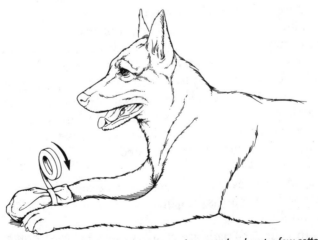

To protect cracked paw pads and give them a chance to heal, put a few cotton balls in the bottom of baby socks and put the socks on your pet's feet. Use a little tape around the top and on the skin to hold the socks in place, wrapping the feet loosely so that you don't cut off circulation.

Since cracked pads are usually dry pads, adding extra moisture will help them heal more quickly. Dr. Ashley recommends coating the pad with a light film of lanolin. Or you can coat your pet's feet with Humilac or Kerasolv, softeners that you can get from your vet.

Ointments that contain antibiotics and steroids will help cracked pads heal, especially if the pads are infected. Ointments aren't always effective, however, because pets will often lick them off before they have a chance to work, says Craig N. Carter, D.V.M., Ph.D., head of epidemiology at the Texas Veterinary Medical Diagnostic Laboratory at Texas A&M University in College Station.

WHAT YOUR VET WILL DO

Paws that won't heal on their own may be a telltale sign of internal problems. Your vet will probably take blood samples to check for problems with the liver or immune system or to see if there are nutritional deficiencies. She may recommend using ultrasound or x-rays as well. "Often, the only way to know the cause of a persistent problem is by taking small sample of the skin of your pet's cracked pad and submitting it to a laboratory for examination," says Dr. Ashley.

When cracked pads are caused by underlying illnesses or problems, your pet will probably need medications, such as drugs to control an overactive immune system or supplements for a nutritional deficiency. Once the underlying condition is taken care of, Dr. Ashley says, the paws will quickly return to normal.

Allergies can be tricky, or at least time-consuming, to diagnose. If the cracking is severe, your veterinarian may recommend that your pet undergo allergy tests to find out what's causing the problem.

See also Chapter 10: Pad Calluses

PAW SWELLING

Clues

- More than one foot is swollen.
- Your cat has recently been in a fight.
- The swelling is soft and spongy rather than firm.
- Your dog is developing patchy fur.

Dogs and cats don't always look before they leap. When they have a hard landing after jumping from a ledge, for example, their feet can get bruised and sore.

Paw swelling usually isn't serious and will clear up in a day or two. If a bone is broken, however, the paw can double or even triple in size, causing excruciating pain.

Cats are more agile than dogs, and lighter, so they are less likely to break bones in their paws. But they do tend to roam outdoors and get into fights. Fight wounds, which often get infected, can cause a very painful swelling called an abscess, says Chaim Litwin, D.V.M., a veterinarian in private practice in Fairfield, Connecticut. An abscessed foot can swell to twice its size overnight. This problem is much more common in cats than dogs, he adds.

Insect bites or stings can also cause your pet's paws to swell, says Valerie Fadok, D.V.M., Ph.D., a veterinary dermatologist and consultant in Denver. You should suspect an insect attack if the paw is sore and slightly firm to the touch. In most cases, the swelling will start to go down within a few hours, she says.

In dogs, swollen paws—along with patches of lost fur—may be a sign of red mange, which is caused by mites that burrow into the skin, making it sore and tender. (Cats, however, don't get this condition. The mites that cause swollen paws are called demodex mites, which are different from ear mites.) Infestations of the feet can be particularly hard to treat, says Patricia Ashley, D.V.M., a veterinary resident in dermatology at the University of Tennessee College of Veterinary Medicine in Knoxville.

Dogs naturally have these mites on their bodies, she adds. They only cause problems when the dog isn't eating properly, has a weak immune system, or is otherwise in poor health.

When more than one foot is swollen, your pet may have allergies. She may be allergic to her food or airborne particles such as pollen. Swollen feet can also be caused by an immune system disorder called lupus, says Dr. Litwin. When the swelling includes the leg as well as the paw, your pet could have a serious condition called pitting edema, in which fluids—due to hormone problems or heart disease—aren't draining the way that they should.

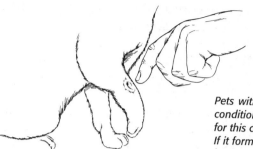

Pets with swollen feet may have a serious condition called pitting edema. An easy test for this condition is to press the swollen skin. If it forms an indentation and doesn't spring back, see your vet right away.

What You Can Do

Since swollen paws are potentially a sign of serious problems, you should call your vet if the swelling doesn't go down within a few days. An abscess requires even faster action. You should call your vet immediately if the paw is hot and infected. But if you are sure that the problem is minor—if, for example, you recently pulled a thorn from your pet's paw—you may want give the paw a thorough soaking.

Mix two tablespoons of 2 percent chlorhexidine (an antiseptic available in drugstores) in a gallon of cool, clean water. Dr. Litwin recommends soaking the paw for 10 to 15 minutes, two or three times a day. The soaks will ease the discomfort as well as help prevent infection.

For cats or dogs that won't stand still for a soak, you can drench a cloth in the solution and then hold it on the swollen paw for 5 to 10 minutes at a time, several times a day. Applying ice for five minutes after the swelling begins and then every few hours can also help, says Dr. Litwin.

Allergies can be difficult to prevent because it is not always clear exactly what your pet is allergic to. For quick relief, your vet may recommend giving your pet antihistamines. Every pet will need a different dose, so check with your vet for the proper amounts.

There isn't a lot that you can do at home to control red mange. What you can do, however, is make sure that your dog is eating well. She should be eating a high-quality, name-brand food, says Dr. Ashley. Some vets recommend giving dogs with red mange a super-premium food, such as Eukanuba, Nutro, or Science Diet, which will be higher in quality nutrients than other foods.

In addition, giving your pet fatty-acid supplements may be helpful, says Dr. Ashley. Available from veterinarians and pet supply stores and catalogs, the supplements can help make the skin healthier, especially in dogs with red mange. Your vet will tell you the proper dose for your pet. The supplements need to be given for at least 60 days, and they won't have a direct effect on the swelling itself, says Dr. Fadok.

Swollen paws will usually return to normal within a day or two. When the swelling doesn't go away or if more than one paw is swollen, you should call your vet, says Dr. Litwin.

WHAT YOUR VET WILL DO

If your vet doesn't see an obvious reason for the swelling, such as an infection on the paw, he will need to do a variety of tests. Skin swabs and scrapings of skin may be used to check for mites or infection-causing bacteria, says Dr. Litwin. In addition, your vet may take x-rays to check for broken bones.

If your cat has an abscessed paw, your vet will lance the wound to help it drain, then clean it thoroughly to remove pus and other debris. He will also give antibiotics to help clear up the infection, says Dr. Litwin.

While a broken toe will often heal on its own, broken bones in the foot usually require surgery, during which pins are inserted to hold the bones together.

Since demodex mites can be a challenge to treat at home, your vet will probably recommend bringing your pet into the office so that he can give her a medicated bath or dip. In addition, he may recommend oral medications that will fight the mites from the inside out.

TOE SORENESS

Clues

- The toe is swollen or crooked.
- Your cat has recently been declawed.
- The toe has a strong odor, or is discolored.
- There is more than one sore toe.

Dogs and cats have surprisingly strong toes that help them balance as they run, twist, and play. But because your pet runs barefoot all day—on asphalt, over rough ground, and through household obstacle courses—she will sometimes stub a toe, making it sore and bruised.

Hard knocks not only bruise toes, but can break them, too. A broken toe usually looks crooked, like the bones don't fit together in the way they should. As you would expect, can also be swollen and excruciatingly tender—so much so that many pets will lie around rather than attempt to walk.

Sore toes can also be caused by cuts or scrapes, especially if the cut gets infected, says Patricia Ashley, D.V.M., a veterinary resident in dermatology at the University of Tennessee College of Veterinary Medicine in Knoxville.

In cats that have recently been declawed, the claw will sometimes start growing back, says Dr. Ashley. When the new claw starts poking into healed skin, it can be very painful—just as an emerging wisdom tooth in humans is painful.

Both dogs and cats will occasionally have achy toes because of whole-body problems, such as arthritis or Lyme disease, says Chaim Litwin, D.V.M., a veterinarian in private practice in Fairfield, Connecticut. If your pet seems to have more than one sore toe or if the aches come and go repeatedly, you should suspect an internal problem and ask your vet to take a look, he says.

WHAT YOU CAN DO

If the toe is swollen, discolored, crooked, or has a bad smell (a sign of infection), you will want to call your vet. But if your pet is just a bit sore and limpy, here are a few easy ways to make her more comfortable while she recovers.

To speed healing for bumps and bruises, keep your pet indoors or on a leash for a few days so that she doesn't aggravate the injury, says Dr. Litwin. To decrease pain and swelling, you can apply ice or a cold pack to the paw for five minutes every few hours on the day of the injury. By the second day, your pet should be feeling better.

If your pet has an infection or simply a painful sore, a cool-water soak can be very soothing. You can use plain water or a solution made by mixing two tablepoons of 2 percent chlorhexidine (an antiseptic available in drugstores) in a gallon of water. Soak your pet's foot in the solution for 10 to 15 minutes, two or three times a day, says Valerie Fadok, D.V.M., Ph.D., a veterinary dermatologist and consultant in Denver. The medicated solution will help heal the sore and kill bacteria that may be causing the problem.

Most cats, of course, would rather fight than stick their feet in water. For water-shy pets, you can soak a cloth in the solution and hold it directly on the paw.

For dogs, an over-the-counter aspirin can be very helpful. "I usually

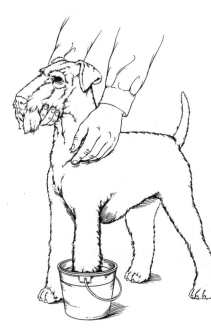

A paw soak is an effective remedy for cut or infected paws. For added protection, mix a little antiseptic into the water. It will kill bacteria and help the paw heal more quickly.

Some pets, especially cats, hate getting their paws wet. An alternative is to hold a damp compress on the sore paw for a few minutes several times a day. To prevent your cat from struggling, you may want to wrap her in a towel before you begin.

start dogs on a coated aspirin (like Ascriptin)," says Dr. Litwin. Give about 10 milligrams for every pound of pooch, no more than twice a day. (For a 15-pound dog, for example, you would give half of a 325-milligram tablet of aspirin.) While aspirin and other over-the-counter drugs may be helpful for dogs, they are extremely dangerous for cats. Never give your cat a pain pill without a veterinarian's supervision.

WHAT YOUR VET WILL DO

If the toes look healthy, but your pet is still in pain, your vet may use blood tests to check for internal problems such as arthritis or Lyme disease, as well as x-rays to check for broken bones. Most of the time, however, the cause of the pain will be easy to recognize and treat, and your pet should get better fairly quickly.

If a toe is hot or swollen, your vet will probably take a smear or a scraping of the skin and examine it for bacteria or other organisms that may be causing infection. Toe infections are usually treated with oral antibiotics or with antibiotic soaks.

If your cat has been declawed and the pain is caused by the claw trying to grow back in, your cat will need surgery to remove it. She will probably need to spend a night in the hospital, but will recover quite quickly, usually within a few days.

COMMON LEG, HIP, AND PAW CONDITIONS

Allergies. Pets suffer from allergies when their immune systems respond to common things like pollen or food in the same way that they respond to aggressive viruses or bacteria—by attacking.

People with allergies often have runny noses or digestive complaints, while pets tend to itch. The itching can affect the whole body, although certain kinds of allergies—especially allergies to food and pollen—tend to affect the paws. To get relief, dogs and cats will lick or bite their paws, sometimes for hours at a time. Eventually, the paws may become wet, red, and swollen. In severe cases, they will even develop painful sores that take a long time to heal.

There isn't a cure for allergies, but they can be controlled. The obvious solution, of course, is to help your pet avoid whatever it is that is making him itch. In the case of food allergies, for example, switching foods will resolve the problem. But it is almost impossible to avoid other common allergens, like pollen or house dust. That is why your vet will probably recommend ways to ease the symptoms, such as using cool soaks for itchy feet or giving your pet antihistamines. (Your vet will recommend a brand of antihistamines and dose that's right for your pet.)

When allergies are severe, your vet may recommend giving your pet a brief course of medications such as steroids, which suppress the immune system. Or he may advise that your pet undergo a series of shots that will make him less sensitive in the future.

Arthritis. Meaning "inflammation of a joint," arthritis is among the most common causes of pain in dogs and cats. There are many types of arthritis, but the kind that usually affects pets is osteoarthritis, or "wear-and-tear" arthritis.

Osteoarthritis occurs when soft cartilage inside a joint becomes inflamed, usually as a result of years of normal daily motion. The inflammation gradually damages bones in the joint, causing them to form ridges, grooves, or even bits of new bone called spurs. The spurs interfere with the joint's normal movements, causing pain and even more inflammation.

Other kinds of arthritis can be caused by infections or problems with the immune system, says Grant Nisson, D.V.M., a veterinarian in private practice in West River, Maryland. Pets with Lyme disease, for example, can develop very painful arthritis. So can dogs and cats with lupus, a serious immune system disorder.

If caught early, some forms of arthritis, such as those caused by infections, can be cured entirely by treating the underlying problem. In most cases, however, the only solution is to treat the symptoms. Your veterinarian has several good choices for pain control that are safer and more effective than over-the-counter drugs. (These include prescription pain relievers as well as alternative therapies such as acupuncture.) In addition, he may recommend medications that increase lubrication in the joints as well as drugs that can speed the repair of damaged cartilage, making it stronger and more flexible.

Cruciate ligament injuries. The knees are held together by tough muscular straps called cruciate ligaments. These ligaments are extremely strong and resilient, but they aren't invincible. Sometimes they get torn, which causes pain and allows the knee joint to slide back and forth like a dresser drawer.

This type of injury is rare in cats but is fairly common in dogs, particularly when they are having a good time playing with other dogs. "He might run and turn wrong or get a hard blow to the knee, just like in football," says Joanne Hibbs, D.V.M., a veterinarian in private practice in Powell, Tennessee. If your dog comes home limping after fun and games or he is unable to put any weight on one of legs, he could have this type of injury.

Minor tears in the ligaments will often heal with rest and perhaps physical therapy. When the tear is severe, however, your dog may need surgery to repair it. Unfortunately, he is unlikely to have the relatively easy kind of surgery, called arthroscopic surgery, that is commonly used on humans. Knee surgery in pets usually requires a long surgical incision and a day or two in the hospital. After the surgery, however, the knees usually heal completely and quickly.

Hip dysplasia. Many breeds of dogs have hip joints that don't fit together the way they should. This condition, called hip dysplasia, occurs when the ball of the hip doesn't smoothly match the opposing socket. As a result, the joint grinds and wobbles. Over time, this wobble causes wear and tear on the joint, eventually leading to painful arthritis that makes it difficult for pets to move.

Hip dysplasia is a genetic disease, meaning that it is passed from generation to generation. It is most common in large-breed dogs like German shepherds, golden retrievers, and Labrador retrievers. Cats can also get hip dysplasia, but because they are so small and light, they don't usually hurt because of it.

"Our main treatment for hip dysplasia is controlling pain because you can't cure the disease," says Dr. Hibbs. When the problem is severe, however, surgery may be needed to repair or even replace the hip. The procedure can be quite successful, she adds.

For young dogs that either have hip dysplasia or are likely to get it, vets recommend regular exercise because it tightens the joint by strengthening the surrounding muscles. In addition, vets sometimes give medications that increase the amount of lubricating fluid around the joint, which can help reduce the pain.

Immune system problems. The immune system is your pet's first line of defense against a variety of health threats, from bacteria and viruses to cancer cells. But sometimes it starts turning its formidable powers inward. "The immune system can get confused and think that part of its own body is a foreign invader," says Alice Wolf, D.V.M., professor in the department of small animal medicine and surgery at Texas A&M University College of Veterinary Medicine in College Station. "The attack begins and the body, which is really an innocent bystander, gets blasted."

There are a number of immune system problems, called autoimmune disorders, that affect the legs, hips, and paws. Pets with autoimmune disorders such as pemphigus and lupus may develop thick, split, or sore paw pads. The nails may get flaky or brittle, and the nail bed can get infected. In addition, pets with these problems often feel sick generally. They may have skin problems as well as painful joints.

Treatment for autoimmune disorders is aimed at getting the body's natural defenses to stand down, says Dr. Wolf. Medications such as steroids, gold salts, tetracycline, or niacinamide will partially suppress the immune system, making it less likely to attack its owner, she explains.

Lick granuloma. Dogs are a lot like people: Once they do something for long enough, it can be very hard for them to stop, even when the behavior is doing them harm.

People sometimes get in the habit of pulling their hair or smoking cigarettes. Dogs, on the other hand, may get in the habit of licking their feet. At first they do it for a good reason—because they have allergies, for example, or flea bites that itch. But even when the original problem is gone, they can't stop the habit and may continue chewing and licking. They will do it for so long that the skin can develop painful sores called granulomas. Cats can develop compulsive behaviors of their own, but they rarely get this condition.

To prevent your dog from getting "addicted" to licking, it is important to act quickly and stop whatever is making him itch. This might mean using flea collars, for example, or keeping him indoors when pollen counts outside are highest. If your pet is already itchy, cool-water soaks can be very soothing. So can moisturizers and anti-itch creams, which you can get from your vet or pet supply stores.

Once pets have developed lick granulomas, it can be a challenge to get rid of the sores. Dabbing moisturizers on them may be helpful. If the sores are infected, applying a triple-antibiotic cream can help them heal. (Pets will often lick ointments off before they have a chance to work, so your vet may recommend oral medications.) In addition, your vet may advise that you give your dog fluoxetine (Prozac) or other mood-altering medications, which will make him calmer and more secure—and less likely to lick himself excessively in the future.

Luxating patella. A luxating patella is simply a kneecap that regularly pops out of place. The thighbone and shinbone, which meet to form the knee, have deep grooves that allow the kneecap to slide smoothly back and forth. If the grooves aren't formed properly or have been damaged, the kneecap may periodically jump off its tracks. When this happens, your pet won't walk smoothly but will actually skip a few steps.

This condition normally doesn't hurt and is usually more of an annoyance than an immediately serious problem. In the long run, however, it can cause bone damage that leads to arthritis. And in some cases, the kneecap won't slip back into place. That is when surgery may be required.

Luxating patellas are most common in certain small-dog breeds, such as Chihuahuas and poodles, and in some breeds of cats. Since it is an inherited condition, vets usually recommend that pets that have it not be used for breeding.

CHAPTER 11

Mouth, Nose, and Teeth

Just as humans use their hands for nearly every activity, dogs and cats use their noses and mouths—for licking their coats, identifying strangers, and, of course, gobbling breakfast. It's hard for us to imagine how serious a problem in either one of these areas can be.

Consider your pet's nose: Dogs and cats have millions more scent receptors than people do. They can detect and identify smells that humans don't even know exist. It is quite a talent, and in the wild, it was necessary for their survival. Their sense of smell allowed them to recognize littermates, find their way home, and pick up the scents both of predators and prey.

Dogs and cats live calmer lives today, but they continue to identify their world largely through their sense of smell. They know when another pet has visited the yard—even that animal's sex and its status in the pet world—just by sniffing the grass where he walked. They can tell things about you as well—like whether you were paying attention to someone else's pet at lunch or if you had been at the doctor's office or, worse, at the veterinarian's. You might not think that the faint alcohol smell at the vet's office would stick to your clothes, but your pets can smell it.

So a stuffy nose can be big deal for pets, especially cats. Cats depend on their sense of smell to work up an appetite. (That's why pet food manufacturers make cat food so smelly.) When they can't smell, they often won't eat. And when cats don't eat, even for as little as one or two days, they can develop a liver problem that is potentially life-threatening.

It takes a lot to make dogs stop eating, and even having a stuffy nose won't slow a dog down too much. Since they know their world largely by the way it smells, however, problems with the nose can be almost like going blindfolded—life gets confusing in a hurry.

Humans don't worry too much when they learn they have gingivitis—a mild gum infection that's caused by bacteria that thrive in food particles and on the surfaces of the teeth. But in pets, the bacteria that cause gum disease will sometimes slip into the bloodstream and travel to the heart, kidneys, or other internal organs. In fact, whenever veterinarians see pets with certain kinds of heart disease, they automatically take a look in their mouths because that is where the problem probably began.

Because dogs and cats aren't always careful about the things they pick up and chew, cracked or broken teeth are extremely common. As you would expect, tooth damage can be excruciatingly painful since dogs and cats usually eat hard, dry food without a lot of give. Imagine biting on kibble when a tooth is sore: It's a wonder they don't go hungry more often.

Fortunately, it usually doesn't take long to notice when pets are having problems with their mouths, noses, or teeth, if only because they love putting their faces close to ours. Getting up close and personal is a great way to spot a broken tooth or a strange color on the tongue or a nose that has suddenly gone pale. It is also an opportunity—though not one you will always appreciate—to tell if their breath has taken a turn for the worse. Any one of these symptoms means that something has happened in this all-important area, and you will need to investigate to find out what it is.

So the next time you see that your pet has a runny nose or is pawing his mouth or drooling more than usual, you will know that you need to pay attention. It is worth doing because problems in this area tend to get worse in a hurry. The more quickly you spot them, the more quickly you will be able to take the necessary steps to keep your pets healthy.

See Your Vet If:

- Your pet can't open his mouth or is having trouble opening it.
- He can't close his mouth.
- He won't eat or has difficulty chewing or swallowing.
- His tongue, lips, or muzzle are swollen.
- There is a foreign object stuck in his mouth.
- His gums are red and swollen, or there is bleeding.
- Your pet is drooling or panting excessively.
- His tongue or gums are blue or pale.
- Your pet has ulcers on his tongue.
- He is gagging frequently.
- There is a lump anywhere on his face.
- He is pawing frequently at his mouth or face.
- There is a discharge from his mouth or nose that lasts two days or longer.
- His breath is consistently bad.
- Your pet's nose is dry, crusty, or bleeding.
- His mouth is foaming, or he's grinding his teeth.
- There is dried saliva around the mouth.

SYMPTOM) # BAD BREATH

Clues

- There is a broken tooth or a sore in your pet's mouth.
- Her breath has a sickly sweet or ammonia-like smell.
- There is something stuck in your pet's teeth.

You would be insulted if someone said that you have "dog breath." But then, your dog might be insulted, too. "The breath of healthy pets should be nearly odorless," says Ira Luskin, D.V.M., a veterinary dentist in private practice in Baltimore.

Dogs and cats with bad breath nearly always have periodontal disease, a condition in which bacteria in the mouth cause infections that lead to gum problems or tooth decay, says Dr. Luskin. Veterinarians estimate that 60 to 80 percent of cats and dogs have serious periodontal disease by the time they are five years old.

Bad breath can also occur if your pet has something stuck in her teeth or under the gums. Even a grass seed, if it stays there long enough, can cause an infection, giving her breath a potent punch. A broken tooth can cause smelly breath. So can tumors or ulcers in the mouth, says Stephen A. Smith, D.V.M., a veterinarian in private practice in Pasadena, Maryland.

If your pet's breath smells odd but not exactly awful, she could have an underlying illness that is causing it, says Dr. Smith.

- Diabetes can make the breath unpleasantly sweet.
- Pets with kidney disease may have breath with an ammonia-like smell.
- An intestinal blockage can make the breath smell like stool.

Bad breath isn't always caused by health problems. There is a big difference between a foul smell and a food smell. If your dog has been gnawing a meat-flavored chew toy, her breath will be a little musky. Your cat will have a pungent purr after polishing off a can of tuna. In addition, both dogs and cats will have terrible breath after licking their anal glands, which are filled with a thick liquid that has a room-clearing smell.

WHAT YOU CAN DO

A toothbrush is the best weapon against bad breath, says Dr. Luskin. Research suggests that brushing your pets' teeth twice a week is enough to keep the teeth clean and their breath fresh; however, your best bet is to set a goal for daily brushing. To get your pets used to brushing, here is what vets recommend.

- Begin by rubbing the gums once or twice a day with the tip of your finger. This will get them used to having their mouths handled.

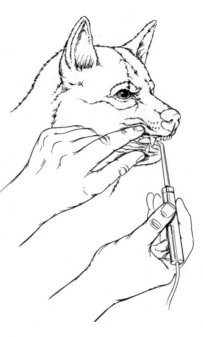

Oral irrigators such as Water Pik are very effective at removing food from your pet's teeth. Set it on low and aim the water jet where the teeth and gums meet.

- After a week or two, wrap a piece of gauze around your finger and rub the surfaces of the teeth and gums. When your pets get used to this, start using a toothbrush—a soft child's brush is ideal. Just use a little water on the brush, says Dr. Luskin. Or you can use a toothpaste made especially for pets. Avoid human toothpastes because they contain ingredients that can upset your pet's stomach.

Some dogs and cats have crooked teeth that trap food, making their breath smell like yesterday's dinner. You may want to use an oral irrigator, such as a Teledyne Water Pik, to clean away the crumbs.

No amount of brushing will freshen the breath of pets with periodontal disease or a buildup of tartar on the teeth, says Dr. Luskin. If her breath doesn't improve with home care, you should call your vet.

WHAT YOUR VET WILL DO

Since bad breath can be caused by a variety of illnesses, your vet will want to give your pet a complete exam. Dogs and cats can "hide" things in surprising places. Cats love to play with string, for example, and sometimes a strand will get tangled beneath the tongue, producing a bad smell.

Your vet may recommend x-rays to see if your pet has an abscessed tooth, a tumor, or a foreign object in the digestive tract. If he suspects an infection, he will give your pet antibiotics to clear it up.

In older pets especially, all that is needed may be a professional teeth cleaning. Once the teeth are cleaned, your pet's breath will improve.

BLUE TONGUE OR GUMS

Clues

- Your pet is having trouble breathing.
- He is gagging or choking.
- He has gotten into acetaminophen.

When your pet is feeling robust and hearty, you say that he is "in the pink of health." Taking a peek in his mouth will give a hint where the term comes from. Healthy dogs and cats usually have mouths that look like bubble gum—nice and pink.

"A pet with a blue tint in his mouth is a sick pet," says Paul D. Pion, D.V.M., a veterinary cardiologist in Davis, California, and founder of the Veterinary Information Network, an online service for veterinarians. The color of your pet's mouth reflects how much oxygen is circulating in the bloodstream. Tissue that's well-oxygenated will be a healthy pink. The bluer the mouth and gums, the less air he is getting.

Many things can cause pets to run low on oxygen. If he has a respiratory problem like asthma or pneumonia, he won't be able to breathe efficiently enough to get sufficient air into the lungs. Pets that have something stuck in their airways, like a small toy or a large piece of food, can also get blue in the mouth, says Chaim Litwin, D.V.M., a veterinarian in private practice in Fairfield, Connecticut.

Since the body's red blood cells are responsible for carrying oxygen, anything that damages the cells, like getting into the acetominophen bottle and swallowing a few pills, can also cause oxygen levels to drop, says Dr. Litwin. (While this medication is safe for humans, it should never be given to dogs and cats.)

Heart failure can also turn the mouth blue. When the heart isn't pumping blood properly, oxygen won't circulate, and tissues throughout the body may start running short of it. Without rapid attention, heart problems can be deadly.

Regardless of the cause, a blue tint in the mouth is a very dangerous warning sign, and you should call your vet immediately.

WHAT YOU CAN DO

Acetaminophen can be toxic for dogs and cats, and you should treat it as a serious poison. If you are unable to get to a vet right away, you can provide a quick antidote by giving your pet the ulcer drug ranitidine (Zantac), which is available with or without a prescription, depending on the strength. Research has shown that it can quickly help counteract the effects of acetaminophen. You want to give about 1.3 milligrams per pound of pet. For example, one Zantac pill (about 84 milligrams) could be given to a 64-pound dog. A sixth of pill is about right for a cat. "It's a very safe drug. You won't overdose the pet, and you might help save his life," says Robert Washabau, V.M.D., Ph.D., associate professor and section chief of medicine at the University of Pennsylvania School of Veterinary Medicine in Philadelphia. It is not a cure, however, and you will still need to get your pet to the vet as quickly as possible.

If your pet has something stuck in the windpipe, look inside his mouth to see if you can remove it. If the obstruction is out of sight or he is not breathing, you are going to have to do a Heimlich-type maneuver to get it out. (For specific instructions on this technique, see "Choking" on page 28.)

Regardless of what is causing it, a blue tint is always an emergency, and you need to see your vet. On the way there, it is a good idea to put your pet in front of the car's air-conditioning vent. This will make it easier for him to breathe.

WHAT YOUR VET WILL DO

Running low on oxygen can make your pet very sick. Your vet may begin by giving him oxygen—either by fitting him with a mask or by putting him in a special cage. Your vet may give him a sedative as well, which will help your pet breathe easier.

During the checkup, your vet will pay special attention to your pet's heart and lungs. She will listen to his chest, take his pulse, and press on his gums to see how fast blood flows back into his skin (about two seconds is normal). These tests will help show how well the heart is working. In addition, your vet will want to do blood tests to see if there are underlying problems, like infections or poisoning, that are causing the symptoms.

Because so many problems can cause a blue mouth, there are many possible treatments. For heart problems, dogs and cats may be given drugs such as digoxin (Cardoxin), which help the heart pump more strongly. Pets with asthma, on the other hand, are often treated with drugs to open up the airways as well as with anti-inflammatory drugs to prevent swelling that can interfere with breathing.

CHEWING PROBLEMS

Clues

- Your pet picks up food, then drops it again.
- There are sores on his gums or tongue.
- Your dog is having trouble opening his mouth.

Given half a chance, dogs and cats will chew just about anything—from dry kibble at breakfast to tennis balls, table legs, nubby sweaters, and anything else that they can get their teeth around. When they are having trouble chewing, you can be pretty sure that something is wrong.

Pain in the mouth is the most common cause of chewing troubles, says Ira Luskin, D.V.M., a veterinary dentist in private practice in Baltimore. Pets with gum disease, for example, may have infections or loose teeth that make chewing difficult. A tooth that is broken or abscessed or has a cavity can be extremely painful. If your pet excitedly grabs a treat, then drops it as if he had been burned, he probably has a sore tooth, says Dr. Luskin.

Sores on the tongue, which may be caused by internal illnesses as well as cuts or scrapes, can also be a problem. You should suspect that there is a tongue problem if your pet is drooling and having trouble chewing, says Mark Riehl, D.V.M., a veterinarian in private practice in Bristol, Tennessee.

Vets don't know why it occurs, but dogs—often German shepherds and weimaraners—will occasionally develop a condition called masticatory myositis, which temporarily damages the muscle fibers and nerves of the chewing muscles. Your dog may have trouble chewing or even opening his mouth. It is a scary sight, but dogs will usually be fine when given medications for a few months.

Rabies is extremely rare in household pets, but trouble chewing is one of the main symptoms, says Jack Casper, D.V.M., head of the Animal Health Diagnostic Laboratory in Frederick, Maryland, and president of the Maryland Veterinary Medical Association. Rabies isn't likely to be an issue if your pet's vaccinations are up-to-date. But if you have recently adopted a new pet or your pet has been bitten by another animal, you should call your vet immediately.

WHAT YOU CAN DO

Pets have to chew in order to eat, and any problem that interferes with eating should be given a vet's attention, says Dr. Casper. In the meantime, encourage your pet to drink plenty of water, which will help keep him hydrated. Sore teeth may be sensitive to water that is too hot or cold, so fill his bowl with body-temperature water, says Dr. Riehl. Adding a little chicken or beef bouillon to the water will encourage him to drink more.

Even if he can't eat regular food for a while, he will probably be able to suck up soup or food that has been pureed in a blender, Dr. Riehl adds. He recommends putting canned pet food in a blender, adding enough water to make it soupy when pureed.

WHAT YOUR VET WILL DO

Your vet will begin by looking under your pet's tongue for splinters, cuts, or even a bit of an object like thread or string, which could be causing irritation. She will also check the teeth to see if they are sensitive or if the gums are infected.

Dogs and cats with severe gum disease may need oral antibiotics to clear up the infection. Dog's with masticatory myositis will probably be given oral prednisone for a month or more. This powerful drug suppresses the immune system, which helps the nerves and muscles work properly again.

Finally, your vet may recommend having your pet's teeth professionally cleaned. It will eliminate plaque and bacteria from the surfaces of the teeth, which will relieve (and prevent) gum disease. Your pet may need additional dental work as well—anything from a root canal to removing a damaged tooth.

See also Chapter 11: Bad Breath, Drooling, Gum Bleeding, Mouth Lumps, Tongue Spots

SYMPTOM) # DROOLING

Clues

- Your pet is drooling after eating.
- She has a history of seizures.
- You suspect that she has eaten something bitter.
- Your pet is lethargic.

It is not exactly elegant, but dogs waiting for breakfast will often show their appreciation by getting a little moist around the mouth. And some breeds, like Saint Bernards and Newfoundlands, drool almost all the time. But if your pet is normally dry, yet suddenly starts flowing like a faucet, you can bet there is something wrong. This is especially true for cats, who generally drool less than dogs.

"As soon as I see a drooling cat, I'm thinking ulcers in the mouth or immune system disease," says Mark Riehl, D.V.M., a veterinarian in private practice in Bristol, Tennessee. Cats with feline AIDS, leukemia, or even the flu will sometimes get mouth sores that cause them to drool, he says. Kidney problems can also cause sores and drooling in cats as well as dogs.

While dogs often drool because of mealtime anticipation, cats may salivate for sheer pleasure, which is why you may feel a few drips when your friendly feline starts nuzzling your neck. Conversely, cats will also drool when they are afraid, like when it is time for a bath.

Some pets will drool after eating instead of before. In medium- and large-breed dogs, this is sometimes caused by a condition called bloat, in which the stomach twists and then expands, says Jim Hendrickson, V.M.D., a veterinarian in emergency private practice in Rockville, Maryland. Dogs with this condition usually appear restless and will try unsuccessfully to vomit. Bloat is an emergency that may require surgery, so you will need to see your vet right away.

Dogs and cats with epilepsy may drool before a seizure. And many pets will drool when they have digestive problems or even car sickness.

It is very common for pets to drool copiously when they have eaten something bitter, anything from a lemon wedge to drain cleaner. They will also drool when they have mouth pain due to dental problems, for example, or a splinter stuck in the gum.

WHAT YOU CAN DO

Depending on the breed and situation, drooling can be both natural and normal, which won't make you any happier when your best couch or the Oriental carpet are taking direct hits.

If your pet is naturally a little drippy, about all that you can do is to keep a towel handy to wipe off her mouth now and then. Or you can tie a

*Coating your dog's lower lip with petro-
leum jelly will help prevent drooling from
causing infections. Put the jelly on the tips
of your fingers and generously slather it
on. Don't worry about being too neat because she will just lick off the excess.*

bandanna around her neck to keep her coat (and the floor) from getting
sloppy. You may also want to coat your pet's lower lip with petroleum jelly
once or twice a day. This will protect it from the constant deluge and help
prevent infections, says Dr. Hendrickson.

When the drooling is a recent thing, however, you need to take a look in
your pet's mouth, Dr. Riehl advises. If there are sores or the gums are red
and swollen, you are going to need to see your vet. In the meantime, you
can dip a cotton swab in 3 percent hydrogen peroxide and swab the gums
several times a day. This will ease the irritation and possibly slow the
drooling. Don't use too much hydrogen peroxide, he adds, because it can
make dogs and cats throw up.

Another way to ease mouth sores is to give your pet foods that are easy
to eat. One of the easiest solutions is to use the blender. Add some
bouillon to her dry food and hit puree. A soft meal will be a lot easier for
her to eat, says Dr. Hendrickson.

WHAT YOUR VET WILL DO

When your pet keeps drooling and you can't tell why, it is important
to get her to the vet for a checkup. If she is having other symptoms as well
as drooling—she seems dizzy or is tired and lethargic—you should consider it an emergency and get her in right away.

Your vet will start with the obvious by looking in your pet's mouth. If
nothing is stuck inside but your pet has sores, your vet will probably take
blood to check for leukemia, liver disease, or other underlying problems
like poisoning, which are going to require serious medical care.

See also Chapter 6: Bloat; Chapter 11: Chewing Problems

SYMPTOM) # GAGGING

Clues

- Your pet gags only when he is on a leash.
- Your dog is coughing as well as gagging.
- Your cat is coughing up hair balls.
- Your dog or cat has a runny nose and scratches frequently.

There is a place at the back of your pet's throat called the pharynx that acts like a switching station. It is responsible for sending food to the stomach and air to the lungs. When confronted by something unexpected, such as a trickle of postnasal drip, the pharynx doesn't know where to send it. It responds by gagging.

For dogs and cats, an occasional gag is just business as usual, says J. M. Tibbs, D.V.M., a veterinarian in private practice in District Heights, Maryland. Older dogs are especially prone to it because they produce a lot of mucus and their pharynges get more sensitive over time. When your pet is gagging frequently, however, there may be an infection or another problem that is irritating the pharynx.

Dogs with kennel cough, for example, will often gag. "You will hear 'cough, cough, cough—ack,'" says Patricia Shema, V.M.D., a veterinarian in private practice in Glenn Dale, Maryland. "The *ack* is the gag. It sounds awful, but it is the cough that you have to worry about," she adds.

Anything that produces a lot of mucus, from viral infections to allergies, will often cause dogs to gag, says Dr. Shema. So can a more serious problem, like a weak esophagus or cancer of the throat.

Some pets have anatomical peculiarities that make them more prone to gagging, says Dr. Tibbs. English bulldogs and pugs, for example, often have extra tissue at the back of their throats that can be very irritating to them. In addition, cats sometimes develop polyps in their ear canals. If a polyp dangles into the pharynx, it can cause gagging.

In general, cats don't gag as often as dogs. The one exception is when an upcoming hair ball hits the throat. Cats will gag once or twice, then throw it up. Tonsillitis can also cause problems. "Cats have six tonsils, so imagine how it would feel if they were infected," says Margie Scherk, D.V.M., a veterinarian in private practice in Vancouver, British Columbia.

Pets will gag when their collars are too tight, says Dr. Shema. It might not happen when your pet is lying around, but you are sure to notice it during walks when the leash pulls the collar tighter against his throat.

WHAT YOU CAN DO

Dogs and cats with allergies—other symptoms of which may include runny eyes and frequent scratching—can be given antihistamines. For dogs, vets often recommend Benadryl. The usual dose is one milligram for

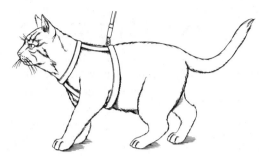

Dogs and especially cats will often pull on their leashes, causing their collars to press against the throat. An alternative is to use a harness, which keeps them under control without the painful pressure.

every pound of dog, three times a day, says Karen L. Campbell, D.V.M., associate professor of dermatology and small animal internal medicine at the University of Illinois College of Veterinary Medicine at Urbana–Champaign. For cats, vets recommend Chlor-Trimeton, which contains the antihistamine chlorpheniramine that is safer for cats. You can give half of a four-milligram tablet for every 10 pounds of cat, twice a day, she says. To be safe, check with your vet before giving pets antihistamines.

There are several tricks for stopping the tickle of hair balls. Pet supply stores stock a variety of hair-ball remedies. Better yet, brush your cat often. "It's the best remedy for hair balls that I know," says Dr. Tibbs.

If your pet is gagging because he swallowed something, it is probably in too deep for you to reach, so you are going to have to get him to the vet right away. In the meantime, you may have to perform the Heimlich maneuver, which will often dislodge objects right away. (For instructions on performing the Heimlich, see "Choking" on page 28.)

WHAT YOUR VET WILL DO

As part of a general checkup, your vet will rub the outside of your pet's throat. If he has kennel cough or an infection of the pharynx, rubbing the throat will instantly cause gagging. Kennel cough is caused by a virus, so antibiotics aren't always needed. Other infections, however, can be treated with antibiotics, which will clear up the problem within a week or two.

If your vet suspects a tumor or another serious problem, she may recommend putting your pet under general anesthesia to perform a thorough throat exam. Besides looking for a tumor, she will check for things such as swollen tonsils, polyps, and foreign objects. It is not unheard of for pets to swallow something irritating, like a twig, that can cause gagging for weeks afterward. If there is something stuck deep in the throat or if your pet has polyps or tumors, he is probably going to need surgery to get them out.

See also Chapter 12: Coughing

SYMPTOM) GUM BLEEDING

Clues

- Your pet's gums are red or swollen.
- There are purple bruises or red spots on his gums.

In pets (as in people), bleeding gums usually mean that they have periodontal disease, and it is not a good sign. "When there is blood, there is cause for concern," says J. M. Tibbs, D.V.M., a veterinarian in private practice in District Heights, Maryland.

Periodontal disease occurs when bacteria in the mouth get beneath the gums, causing infection, swelling, and bleeding. If it is not treated quickly, it can weaken the teeth, causing them to loosen or fall out.

Minor injuries can also cause the gums to bleed. When dogs and cats chomp down on something hard or sharp, such as a stick, they may cut their gums. This type of bleeding usually stops within five minutes, says Dr. Tibbs.

Bleeding can also be a sign of internal problems. Cats with chlamydia, a bacterial infection that originates in their upper respiratory tract, will often have swollen and bloody gums, says Patricia Shema, V.M.D., a veterinarian in private practice in Glenn Dale, Maryland.

Feline leukemia, kidney disease, and cancer can also cause the gums to bleed. So can an immune system disorder called thrombocytopenia, which damages platelets, the cell-like structures in the blood that aid in clotting. "I've seen a lot of immune system problems in smaller dog breeds like cocker spaniels and poodles," says Dr. Tibbs.

WHAT YOU CAN DO

When a bleeding gum is caused by a cut, you can usually stop it by pressing with your finger or a towel for a few minutes, says Dr. Tibbs. You can put pressure directly on the cut or simply press on the outside of your pet's mouth, which pushes the lip against the cut. To help cuts heal faster, take away a dog's chew toys for a day or two. You may also want to feed your pet wet food since dry food can scrape the cut and start it bleeding again, he adds.

Red and swollen gums almost always mean that your pet has periodontal disease, which requires a veterinarian's care. There are things that you can do at home as well. "Brushing your pet's teeth is best, but some pets won't cooperate," says Dr. Shema.

An alternative is to dab the gums with a cotton swab dunked in 3 percent hydrogen peroxide or an oral rinse containing chlorhexidine, which

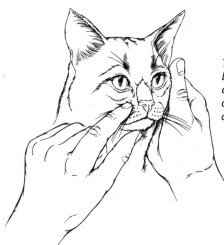

The easiest way to stop a cut gum from bleeding is to apply gentle pressure to the outside of the mouth. This will press the inside of the lip against the cut, helping it clot more quickly.

you can get from your vet, says Grant Nisson, D.V.M., a veterinarian in private practice in West River, Maryland.

For dogs, an easy way to keep the gums healthy is to give them a type of chew toy called CET Chews. Available from vets, these toys are coated with an antiplaque enzyme that helps keep the gums healthy. "They can help a lot," says Dr. Shema. If your dog already has bad teeth, however, the chews won't reverse the problem, she adds.

Look for purple bruises or red spots in your pet's mouth, Dr. Tibbs adds. These are signs of an immune system problem or poisoning, which can cause quite a bit of bleeding under the skin. It is an emergency because the bleeding may not stop on its own.

WHAT YOUR VET WILL DO

Most mouth problems are easy to spot, and your vet probably won't have to spend more than a minute or two saying, "Open wide." But if there isn't a cut and the gums aren't infected, your vet will need to do additional tests to figure out what the problem is.

For periodontal disease, you will probably be advised to have your pet's teeth professionally cleaned. The procedure is done under general anesthesia. It removes all the plaque that has built up over the years. When it is all done, your pet will have much healthier teeth and gums—and a whiter smile, too.

See also Chapter 11: Bad Breath

SYMPTOM) GUM PALENESS

Clues

- Your pet is tired and weak.
- She has been taking estrogen supplements or other medications.
- She is scratching a lot, or you see flea dirt on her bedding.

Dermatologists place a high value on paleness because the less sun you get, the lower your risk for skin cancer. Veterinarians, however, have always preferred the color pink—at least when they are looking at your pet's gums. When the gums change from bubblegum pink to pale, oxygen is probably in short supply, and there is an internal problem that needs to be taken care of.

Pale gums usually mean that a pet doesn't have enough red blood cells, a condition called anemia. Anemia is serious because red blood cells carry oxygen throughout the body. When there aren't enough of them, oxygen levels fall, and pets get weak and tired, says Knox Inman, D.V.M., a veterinarian in private practice in West River, Maryland.

Parasites are one of the most common causes of anemia. Dogs and cats produce just enough red blood cells to stay healthy. When fleas, hookworms, or other blood-sucking parasites are drinking their fill, there may not be enough blood to go around. "I see a lot of pets that are badly anemic because of fleas," says Donald W. Zantop, D.V.M., a veterinarian in private practice in Fallston, Maryland.

Pale gums may be a sign of internal bleeding, resulting from ulcers or even cancer, says Dr. Zantop. Internal bleeding that goes on long enough can also cause anemia.

The light-colored gums can also be caused by a serious condition called autoimmune hemolytic anemia, in which the immune system mistakenly destroys red blood cells, says Dr. Inman. This type of anemia may be hereditary, with cocker spaniels, Shetland sheepdogs, collies, English springer spaniels, Old English sheepdogs, Irish setters, and poodles having the highest risk. Cats can get it, too, but much less often than dogs.

Finally, anemia may be a side effect of medications. Drugs such as estrogen, chloramphenicol (an antibiotic), and phenylbutazone (taken for pain) may inhibit the blood marrow from producing red blood cells, says Dr. Inman. Dogs that are taking aspirin for pain will sometimes develop ulcers and internal bleeding.

Pale gums don't always mean that your pet has anemia. After a serious accident, for example, blood pressure can fall to dangerously low levels because the heart is so busy pumping blood to vital organs that it neglects more-distant regions like the gums, toes, or the tips of the ears. This drop in blood pressure and the resulting pale gums mean that a pet is going into shock and needs emergency care, says Dr. Zantop.

WHAT YOU CAN DO

Giving pets a balanced diet will help them recover from many forms of anemia, says Craig N. Carter, D.V.M., Ph.D., head of epidemiology at the Texas Veterinary Medical Diagnostic Laboratory at Texas A&M University in College Station. Your vet may recommend putting your pet on a prescription diet that is high in minerals, protein, and vitamins. Don't give pets iron supplements without your veterinarian's advice because they can be toxic.

Even though anemia can be dangerous, it is usually not that difficult to restore the red blood cells to healthful levels. Pets that are plagued by fleas, for example, will often recover within three to four days once you get rid of the little pests. Since anemia can make pets very weak, however, it is a good idea to avoid flea dips, powders, or other strong medications, says Dr. Zantop. Instead, give them a bath once or twice a week with a regular pet shampoo. Between baths, use a flea comb to remove fleas that weren't washed off in the bath. This will get rid of most of the fleas, allowing the red blood cells to recover. Once your pet is feeling strong again, it is fine to use over-the-counter products to keep the fleas from coming back.

WHAT YOUR VET WILL DO

Most conditions that cause anemia can be detected with simple blood tests. If nothing turns up on the blood tests, however, your vet will begin looking for more-serious problems such as cancer. In addition, he may need to take a sample of bone marrow, a painful procedure that is done under general anesthesia.

Shock is perhaps the most serious cause of pale gums, and your vet will have to move very quickly to restore the flow of blood. He will give intravenous fluid and steroids to quickly build up your pet's blood pressure. Once your pet is getting enough blood, your vet will have time to figure out why the pressure was so low in the first place. When the problem is corrected, your pet's oxygen levels will quickly rise, and the gums will shift back to a healthy pink.

SYMPTOM) MOUTH LUMPS

The next time your pet yawns, take a peek in his mouth. Everything should be pink (maybe with some dark-colored splotches) and smooth. If you see a lump that wasn't there before, call your vet right away because some lumps can be dangerous.

The least serious type of lump—and possibly the ugliest—is caused by a virus. Similar to warts, these lumps usually appear on a dog's (but not a cat's) lips. They look horrible and can give you a scare but tend to go away in a month or so, says J. M. Tibbs, D.V.M., a veterinarian in private practice in District Heights, Maryland.

Another condition that is unique to the canine club is hyperplastic gingiva, in which large lumps suddenly form on the gums. It is not dangerous, although the lumps will need to be removed if they keep growing and get too big.

Dogs will sometimes develop a hard, purplish lump surrounding a tooth. Called epuli, these lumps occur when the underlying bone gets a little knobby and pushes the gum outward, says Grant Nisson, D.V.M., a veterinarian in private practice in West River, Maryland. As with lumpy gums, epuli are only a problem when they get big enough to interfere with chewing. They can grow quickly, however, so vets usually recommend removing them before they have a chance to cause problems.

A more serious type of lump, which can affect dogs and cats, is caused by an abscess, an infection deep within the gum or elsewhere in the mouth. Abscesses hurt, so your pet will probably be pawing at his mouth. He may have bad breath as well, says Dr. Tibbs. Infections from abscesses can enter the bloodstream, so they need to be treated promptly, he adds.

Cats with gum disease will occasionally develop small bumps on their gums. Two serious conditions, feline leukemia and feline AIDS can also cause bumpy gums, says Mark Riehl, D.V.M., a veterinarian in private practice in Bristol, Tennessee.

The most serious cause of mouth lumps—and one of the most common, especially in cats—is cancer, says Dr. Nisson. Other signs of mouth cancer include sores or little black spots in the mouth that weren't there before.

WHAT YOU CAN DO

Any lump in the mouth is potentially serious, and there is nothing you can do at home to treat them. What you can do is catch them early by giving your pet a mouth exam once a month, says Patricia Ashley, D.V.M., a veterinary resident in dermatology at the University of Tennessee College of Veterinary Medicine in Knoxville. If you see *anything* that wasn't there before, call your vet, she advises.

WHAT YOUR VET WILL DO

Most dogs and cats don't object too strenuously to a thorough mouth exam, although some will be given a sedative if they won't hold still. Your vet can often make a diagnosis after taking a quick look, although she may need to do blood tests to check for infections or feline leukemia. When cancer is a possibility, your vet will snip off a small piece of the lump and send it a laboratory for testing.

Cancers in the mouth tend to be serious, and surgery is almost always needed. In fact, surgery is the best option for most kinds of mouth lumps, even those that aren't cancerous.

MOUTH PAWING

Clues

- Your pet has been catching insects or toads.
- The pawing only occurs at mealtimes.
- He has just been vaccinated.

Unlike cats, who delight in using their front paws to wipe their whiskers clean, dogs don't willingly turn their feet into washcloths—they prefer to keep them pads-down on the ground. So when your dog is suddenly pawing at his mouth or when your cat's pawing seems more frantic than finicky, you can be pretty sure that there is a problem.

Pets that have bitten something that they shouldn't, like the business end of a bee, will try to paw away the pain, says Michele Sharkey, D.V.M., a veterinarian in private practice in West River, Maryland. Pawing during the dinner hour, on the other hand, usually points to sore or loose teeth.

Bitter tastes can also make your pet swipe at his face. For example, Florida, Hawaii, and some states in the Midwest are home to a species of toad that wears a coat of poisonous mucus. When a curious canine takes a lick or bite, the shockingly nasty taste will cause him to paw his mouth and drool, says Mark E. Hitt, D.V.M., a veterinarian in private practice in Annapolis, Maryland. Some antibiotics and other medications also have a very bitter taste, as do a number of houseplants and household cleaners.

Dogs and cats that get bits of bone or other objects stuck in their mouths or between their teeth will often paw to get them out, says Dr. Hitt. Even something as small as a grass seed can set their paws in motion.

It doesn't happen often, but some cats may experience a severe allergic reaction called anaphylaxis. Anaphylaxis can make it very hard for them to breathe, and they will often react by grabbing and clawing at their faces. Anything can potentially cause an allergic reaction, including vaccinations. If your pet has just received his shots and starts pawing his mouth, call your vet immediately. "It's definitely an emergency," says Dr. Sharkey.

WHAT YOU CAN DO

When you notice your pet pawing at his mouth, take a look. There may be a bone or stick jammed inside. If you can remove the object, there is no more problem, says Dr. Hitt. Of course, pets that are pawing their mouths won't appreciate having your fingers in there. Be careful that you don't get bitten while trying to explore.

If you suspect that your pet has been doing some noxious nibbling, it is important to rinse out his mouth. A turkey baster filled with water is ideal, says Dr. Hitt, although a garden hose with low pressure will also work well. Point the muzzle down and aim the water toward the back of the mouth,

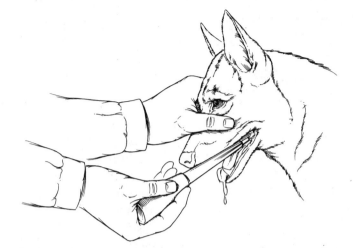

Dogs and cats aren't always careful about what they eat, and sometimes they will get into harmful substances that irritate their mouths. To flush away the danger, open your pet's mouth by holding the top of the muzzle and gently pressing against the upper lips. While holding the muzzle at a downward angle, squirt in water from a turkey baster or a hose. Aim the baster toward the back of the mouth to prevent harmful substances from being swallowed.

which will help prevent harmful substances from being swallowed.

Any substance that is strong enough to burn your pet's mouth could be a life-threatening poison. Call your vet immediately. (For more information on dealing with poisons, see "Purging the Poison" on page 33.) Swallowing or even licking any poison is always an emergency.

Allergic reactions to vaccines are rare, but it pays to watch for them, says Dr. Sharkey. The reactions usually take about 20 minutes to show up. If your pet just received a shot at the vet's office, don't be in too much of a hurry to pay your bill and head for home, she advises. Linger long enough to see if the vaccine will cause some aftereffects.

WHAT YOUR VET WILL DO

Your vet will begin the examination in the same way you did, by looking in your pet's mouth. Dogs and cats aren't willing to say "ahh" on command, so your vet may give him a sedative first. Most objects are fairly easy to remove. If something sharp is stuck in the mouth or gum, however, your vet will probably use a local anesthetic before taking it out.

Pets that are pawing because of dental problems often get better just by having their teeth cleaned, although loose or damaged teeth may need to be removed. Dental procedures usually aren't difficult, but they are uncomfortable. Your pet will put under general anesthesia beforehand.

Anaphylactic reactions are serious, but they are usually easy to treat. In most cases, a single injection of epinephrine will stop the problem immediately, although your pet may need intravenous fluids to counteract shock.

SYMPTOM) # MOUTH SWELLING

Clues

- There is a hard lump under your pet's eye.
- There is a bad smell in her mouth.
- Your cat's chin is swollen.
- Your puppy has swelling on the sides of her neck.

The Chinese shar-pei has thick, swollen lips and gums, which show judges refer to as mouth meat—they are a big plus in competitions. What is considered normal (and beautiful) in a shar-pei is a problem, however, in other dog breeds and in cats.

A swollen mouth is often caused by munching on bees or wasps, says Charles McLeod, D.V.M., a veterinary pathologist at Antech Diagnostics in Carney, Maryland. Unless your pet has serious allergies—and most dogs and cats don't—this type of swelling will go away within a day. More serious are injuries caused by snakes or scorpions. Their strong venom can result in severe swelling that should always be seen by a vet, he adds.

Swelling can also be caused by infections. A pet with an abscessed tooth, for example, may get swollen gums or a hard lump under the eye, says Michele Sharkey, D.V.M., a veterinarian in private practice in West River, Maryland. Infections in the mouth are potentially dangerous because the bacteria can easily spread to other parts of the body. Other signs of mouth infection include foul-smelling breath and warmth at the swollen area.

A type of swelling unique to puppies is "puppy strangles," in which lymph nodes in the neck swell to two or three times their normal size. Vets suspect that this condition is caused by an overactive immune system that reacts to "normal" bacteria in the mouth. Puppy strangles cause the entire head to swell, possibly making it hard to breath.

Cats have their own sets of problems. Vets don't know why, but some cats will develop a condition called chin edema, in which the chin swells to twice its normal size. It appears to be most common in cats with allergies or acne, says Dr. McLeod. Chin edema looks ugly, but it usually isn't serious, and your cat probably won't be overly bothered by it.

If your cat's mouth, face, and feet are all swollen, she may have gotten into a bottle of acetaminophen, says Dr. Sharkey. This common over-the-counter medication is mild for humans, but deadly for cats. (It is dangerous for dogs as well.) Other symptoms of acetaminophen poisoning include difficulty breathing and bluish gums. This is always an emergency that should be treated by a vet immediately, says Dr. Sharkey.

Tumors in the mouth are another cause of swelling. Because of the risk of cancer, it is essential to call your vet if any swelling doesn't go away within a few days.

WHAT YOU CAN DO

As long as your pet isn't having trouble breathing and seems okay otherwise, insect stings aren't likely to be serious, says Dr. McLeod. Giving your pet an antihistamine will reduce the swelling very quickly, Dr. Sharkey adds.

For dogs, vets recommend giving Benadryl—one milligram for every pound of dog, three times a day, says Karen L. Campbell, D.V.M., associate professor of dermatology and small animal internal medicine at the University of Illinois College of Veterinary Medicine at Urbana–Champaign. For cats, vets recommend Chlor-Trimeton, which contains an antihistamine called chlorpheniramine that is safer for cats. You can give half of a four-milligram tablet for every 10 pounds of cat, twice a day, she says. To be safe, check with your vet before giving antihistamines to pets.

If your cat is allergic to plastic, eating from a plastic bowl can make her chin swell, says Steven A. Melman, V.M.D., a veterinary dermatologist in private practice in Potomac, Maryland, and author of *Skin Diseases of Dogs and Cats*. He recommends using food and water bowls made of stainless steel, crockery, or glass. And since some cats love to lick plastic, it is smart to hide bread wrappers and grocery bags, he adds.

WHAT YOUR VET WILL DO

Your vet will probably be able to figure out what's causing the swelling just by looking in your pet's mouth, although he may need to take blood samples to check for acetaminophen poisoning.

In the rare cases when swelling doesn't go away fairly quickly, he may take a biopsy to check for cancer or other conditions.

Pets that have gotten into medications will need to stay at the hospital for several days and possibly get a blood transfusion, says Dr. McLeod. For snakebite, your pet may need intravenous fluids to flush out the poison and possibly an injection of antivenin to counteract the dangerous effects.

Swelling rarely is serious and will go away with simple treatment. A puppy with strangles, for example, may be given steroids to reduce swelling and antibiotics to fight infection. A cat with a swollen chin may be given a single injection of steroids, which will quickly get her face back to normal.

SYMPTOM) NOSE DISCHARGE

Clues

- Your pet's discharge is thick, bloody, whitish, or tinged with pink.
- There are bits of food or milk in the discharge.
- His discharge lasts more than a few days.

You won't see dogs and cats wiping their noses (they can't hold a tissue), but they get drippy just as often as people do and for some of the same reasons, like allergies, colds, and sinus problems. Most nasal discharges aren't serious, but some are, so you need to look at the discharge closely, says Grant Nisson, D.V.M., a veterinarian in private practice in West River, Maryland.

A discharge that is clear and watery is usually caused by colds or allergies and will go away fairly quickly. A thick, gooey discharge, on the other hand, occurs when something irritates the lining of the nose or sinuses and is more serious. It may be caused by a virus or, less often, by juices from the stomach that are backing up into the nose, says Mark E. Hitt, D.V.M., a veterinarian in private practice in Annapolis, Maryland.

A dog or cat will sometimes have a whitish nasal discharge, which is a sign of a serious bacterial or fungal infection. These can be caused by bad teeth, pneumonia, a tumor, or even a bit of debris that is stuck in the nose. This type of discharge should always be seen by a vet, says Dr. Hitt.

A discharge with a pink tinge means that your pet has broken some of the delicate blood vessels inside his nose. This bit of blood looks scary, but it only takes a few vigorous sneezes to damage the nasal lining, so it is usually no big deal. If you see pink for several days in a row, however, the inside of the nose may be severely irritated, and you will need to call your vet. This is especially true if the discharge is more red than pink, which means that there is a lot of bleeding.

You may notice that the discharge contains milk or bits of food. This usually means that there is a hole between your pet's nose and the roof of his mouth that is allowing food to go where it shouldn't. In newborn puppies or kittens, this may be caused by a defect known as a cleft palate. In older pets, an injury to the palate from taking a hard fall, for example, can cause a food-filled discharge.

WHAT YOU CAN DO

You usually don't have to worry about watery discharges. If they are happening often, however, your pet may have allergies and is probably feeling uncomfortable. In many cases, giving an antihistamine will clear up the drip within a day.

For dogs, vets often recommend Benadryl, an antihistamine that relieves allergy symptoms. The usual dose is one milligram for every pound of dog, three times a day, says Karen L. Campbell, D.V.M., associate professor of dermatology and small animal internal medicine at the University of Illinois College of Veterinary Medicine at Urbana–Champaign.

For cats, vets recommend Chlor-Trimeton, which contains an antihistamine called chlorpheniramine that is safer for cats than Benadryl. You can give half of a four-milligram tablet for every 10 pounds of cat, twice a day, she says. It is a good idea, however, to check with your vet before giving any type of human medications to pets.

In fact, you will want to call your vet about any discharge that isn't clear, Dr. Hitt adds. There is a good chance that your pet has an injury or infection that can't be treated at home.

WHAT YOUR VET WILL DO

Unless the inside of your pet's nose is obviously injured, your vet will probably need to take a blood sample to test for infection or other internal problems. She will probably recommend x-rays to check for tumors, abscessed teeth, or a sinus infection. Finally, she may do a nasal flush, in which water is squirted deep into the nose and then allowed to drain out. Your vet will then collect cells and other material that can be analyzed in a laboratory.

Most infections are easy to treat with antibiotics or other medications. Your vet may also squirt in a little steroid spray to reduce irritation and swelling.

| SYMPTOM | # NOSE DRYNESS |

Clues

- Your pet's nose looks dull and cracked.
- He has recently had a fever.
- He has a runny nose or has been spending time in the sun.

When you visit a dog or cat show, you are likely to hear someone mention the winner's unusually fine *leather*, the term for the skin on the nose. A healthy nose, like a fine leather glove, should be soft, shiny, and smooth. A dry nose, on the other hand, looks like a neglected saddle—dry and cracked.

Dogs and cats that are dehydrated because of kidney disease or fever, for example, will often have dry noses, says John Fioramonti, D.V.M., a veterinarian in private practice in Towson, Maryland. Paradoxically, a pet with a runny nose may also develop a dry nose because the dripping irritates the skin and robs it of internal moisture, he says.

If all of your pet's skin, including the skin on the nose, looks dry and thick, he could have a deficiency of zinc. Zinc is a mineral that is essential for skin health, says Charles McLeod, D.V.M., a veterinary pathologist at Antech Diagnostics in Carney, Maryland. Zinc deficiencies are especially common in some Siberian huskies and Alaskan malamutes because of an inherited condition that prevents the mineral from being absorbed. Pets that are given low-quality foods may also run low in this important nutrient, he adds.

Dogs and cats that spend a lot of time outdoors may get sunburned, which makes the nose look dry. The sun hurts in other ways as well. Some collies and shelties have an inherited disease in which the immune system reacts negatively to sunshine, causing nose damage.

Finally, some dogs and cats—especially those with light-skinned noses—may develop cancer, which can make the nose look dry.

WHAT YOU CAN DO

The easiest way to soothe a dry, chapped nose is to rub on a little moisturizer such as petroleum jelly or an ointment containing vitamins A and D (such as A&D ointment), available from your veterinarian or drugstore, says Dr. Fioramonti. Apply the moisturizer twice a day—more often if the nose still appears dry—and rub it in well.

When skin on the nose is thick and cracking, it is a little harder to get moisture deep inside. To help it penetrate, hold a warm, damp cloth on the nose for five minutes, followed by an application of moisturizer, says Patricia Ashley, D.V.M., a veterinary resident in dermatology at the University of Tennessee College of Veterinary Medicine in Knoxville. She recommends using a product called Kerasolv, an exfoliant that removes dead, calloused skin, and which is available from most veterinarians.

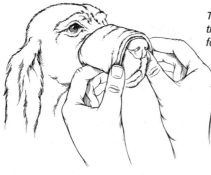

To soothe a dry, cracked nose, begin by softening the skin with a warm, damp cloth. Hold it in place for about five minutes.

When the skin is soft, apply a generous amount of moisturizer and rub it in well. Don't worry about being too neat. Your pet will quickly lick off the excess.

Once your pet gets sunburned, all you can do is apply a moisturizer and wait for the nose to heal. A better strategy is to protect your four-legged sun-worshipper by applying a very thin layer of sunscreen with a sun protection factor (SPF) of at least 30, suggests Dr. Fioramonti. Don't use a sunscreen containing PABA or zinc because some pets are sensitive to them, he adds.

WHAT YOUR VET WILL DO

Since a dry nose may be a sign of internal problems, you should call your vet if it doesn't return to normal fairly quickly, says Mark E. Hitt, D.V.M., a veterinarian in private practice in Annapolis, Maryland. Your vet will probably take a blood sample to check your pet's overall health. In addition, he may snip a small piece of tissue from the nose for a microscopic exam. Removing skin from the nose is painful, so the procedure may be done under general anesthesia.

If it turns out that your dog or cat has an internal problem, your vet is going to concentrate a lot more on the illness than on the nose itself. Pets with certain respiratory infections, for example, may be given antibiotics, which will relieve the infection and stop the nose from drip-drying. For a zinc deficiency, your vet may recommend giving your pet supplements as well as feeding her a high-quality, name-brand food, which will make it easier for her to absorb the zinc.

Kidney problems are more serious. Your pet may need to be hospitalized and receive intravenous fluids to restore his internal moisture. After that, you will be given instructions for keeping the illness under control.

SYMPTOM TONGUE SPOTS

Clues

- Your pet has a new spot or a spot that has changed its color.
- His tongue has raised bumps or white spots.
- Your pet has depressions in the tongue that look like sores.
- He is drooling or has trouble eating.

Dogs and cats have tongues that can do a hard lick of work or, if they need to, just a few tender laps. Those tongues are tough enough to do a number on hard bones, yet soft enough to gently lick a newborn clean. But whatever job they are doing, tongues have a typical color, and any change in the usual color of your pet's tongue may be a warning sign that something is wrong with your pet.

Most dogs and cats have tongues that are all pink. (Shar-peis and Chow Chows have black tongues, while mixed breeds sometimes have tongues with spots or speckles.) If you notice a black spot where there didn't used to be one, you should call your vet because it could be melanoma, a type of cancer, says Patricia Ashley, D.V.M., a veterinary resident in dermatology at the University of Tennessee College of Veterinary Medicine in Knoxville. Melanomas usually have an irregular border and appear to spread into the surrounding areas.

If your dog's tongue is naturally black, it won't be easy to detect dark spots, of course. But you can easily see flashes of pink, which are usually spots where the tongue is missing pigment. White spots on a dark tongue may occur if your pet has been licking irritating chemicals or even plastic, which may cause allergic reactions, says Steven A. Melman, V.M.D., a veterinary dermatologist in private practice in Potomac, Maryland, and author of *Skin Diseases of Dogs and Cats*. But in some cases, white marks signal immune system problems, he adds.

Usually, you don't need to worry about small, raised pink spots on your pet's tongue. These are probably just tastebuds that have been coated with milk or food, making themselves visible.

Apart from those pink spots, if your pet gets other types of lumps or bumps, he should be checked by a vet. Those marks could be tumors or a sign of infection, says Dr. Melman.

Pets will sometimes develop sores on the tongue called ulcers if they have been licking or chewing things like harsh chemicals or a plugged-in electrical cord. Ulcers on the tongue can be extremely painful, says Dr. Melman, and the pet will often drool or have trouble eating. Since ulcers may be caused by kidney disease, it is important to call your vet as soon as you notice them, he says.

What You Can Do

"When your pet takes a good, tongue-stretching yawn, peek at his tongue. You want to see what is normal for him," says Dr. Ashley. If you do that, you will see some spots that don't change; they are simply birthmarks. After you know what his tongue should look like, keep an eye out for ulcers or for spots that are new.

If your pet has been getting white spots on the tongue, you may want to swap his plastic dishes for dishes made of ceramic or metal. If he is just allergic to plastic, changing dishes will help prevent the white spots, Dr. Melman says. If the spots don't go away fairly quickly, you should ask your vet to take a look.

What Your Vet Will Do

Veterinarians spend a lot of time looking into open mouths, and a vet can let you know right away if the spots that you noticed are anything to worry about.

If your pet has ulcers or raised bumps, your vet will want to run blood tests to check for infection or kidney problems, says Dr. Melman. She may recommend snipping a tissue sample from one of the sores so that it can be examined in the laboratory. This is usually done under general anesthesia, and it is an easy procedure. Most pets bounce back so quickly that they won't even skip a meal.

If it turns out that your pet has an infection, you will probably need to give antibiotics for one to two weeks. Kidney disease requires lifelong therapy. In addition, your vet may give him large quantities of fluids to help remove toxins from the bloodstream.

If the problem is cancer, your vet will perform surgery to remove the spot, says Dr. Ashley. Many tumors won't cause your pet further problems, especially if they are caught early.

TOOTH DISCOLORATION

Clues

- One or more of your pet's teeth are brown, red, or black.
- Tooth discoloration is accompanied by bad breath.

When you consider that dogs and cats don't brush or floss their teeth, it is surprising that their teeth manage to stay as white as they do. But as pets get older, a lifetime accumulation of tartar—a bacteria-laden film that naturally forms on the teeth and hardens into rock-hard plaque—can stain their teeth an unhealthy brown.

"Brown tartar stains are a danger sign," says Carvel Tiekert, D.V.M., a veterinarian in private practice in Bel Air, Maryland, and executive director of the American Holistic Veterinary Medical Association. Brown stains on the teeth usually mean that large amounts of bacteria have already done their damage, increasing the risk of periodontal disease and causing bad breath as well.

When a tooth is red, on the other hand, you can bet that your pet has taken a solid knock by catching a hard object like a baseball, for example, or even biting a stone. Red means that there is bleeding deep inside the tooth, says Ira Luskin, D.V.M., a veterinary dentist in private practice in Baltimore. Without treatment, the injured tooth will eventually turn gray, meaning that the tissue has died, he explains.

A red tooth is bad, but a black tooth is even worse. "When you see a black tooth, you can bet it is not only dead but also badly infected," says Dr. Luskin.

Tooth discoloration isn't always a problem. Some dogs and cats will develop circles or streaks of dark brown on their teeth. These are usually caused by secondary dentin, a material that the tooth lays down to repair minor damage. In addition, puppies or kittens that were treated with the antibiotic tetracycline will sometimes have yellow or brown teeth when they are adults, says Dr. Tiekert.

WHAT YOU CAN DO

There is not a lot that you can do to whiten your pet's teeth at home. Since they are not appearing in toothpaste commercials anyway, it shouldn't be a problem. "Commercial tooth whiteners made for people don't help your pet," adds Dr. Luskin.

What you can do, however, is start brushing your pet's teeth every day—either with a toothbrush or a piece of gauze wrapped around your finger, say Dr. Luskin. Vets often recommend using pet toothpastes, although plain water also works well. Regular brushing will remove tartar from the teeth before it has a chance to harden into ugly and unhealthy stains.

You may want to pick up a black light at a lighting supply store and ask your pet to smile. Healthy teeth lit by a black light will be white with a purple tint, says Dr. Luskin. Teeth stained by tetracycline will turn orange, like they are glowing from within, and teeth coated with tartar will show orange right at the gum line.

WHAT YOUR VET WILL DO

Since discolored teeth often accompany periodontal disease, your vet will do a thorough mouth exam to make sure that the teeth are strong and that there aren't pockets of infection along the gums. He may recommend x-rays to check for tooth fractures or dead teeth. If a tooth has been damaged or has actually died, it may need a root canal or even to be taken out, says Dr. Luskin. If there is infection, your pet will need antibiotics as well, which will clear up the infection very quickly.

Cleaning and polishing won't remove deep stains, but they will make the teeth look brighter. In addition, cleaning the teeth removes accumulations of tartar and plaque, which will help prevent gum problems. The procedure can be somewhat uncomfortable, so it is usually done under general anesthetic, Dr. Luskin says.

See also Chapter 11: Bad Breath, Chewing Problems, Gum Bleeding

COMMON MOUTH, NOSE, AND TOOTH CONDITIONS

Broken teeth. Teeth are hard and durable, but they aren't indestructible. A fall from a tree or catching a baseball in mid-flight can crack or break a tooth. Puppies and kittens are especially vulnerable because they don't have their sturdy adult teeth. "Young teeth are a lot like eggs—they are nearly hollow inside," says Ira Luskin, D.V.M., a veterinary dentist in private practice in Baltimore.

An injured tooth hurts, but that is not the only problem. When a fracture is deep enough, the sensitive inner tissue of the tooth, called the pulp, gets exposed. Infection is almost sure to follow, says Dr. Luskin.

You have three choices when your pet has broken a tooth. If the break is small—perhaps a chip is missing and the pulp isn't exposed—you can ignore it, says Dr. Luskin. For more-serious breaks, your vet may recommend removing the tooth, which will prevent infection. A third option is for your vet to do a root canal, in which the pulp of the tooth is removed and the hole is filled with a strong material. This essentially cures the problem and allows your pet to chew and play normally, he says.

Fading nose. Some dogs and cats will occasionally lose pigment from their noses, causing this feature to turn white or red. In most cases, this isn't a health problem, but it looks unusual, to say the least. And for folks who show their pets, a fading nose can keep a pet out of competition until the normal black color returns—if, in fact, it ever does.

The most common cause of a fading nose is "snow nose," says Grant Nisson, D.V.M., a veterinarian in private practice in West River, Maryland. Vets aren't sure why, but many breeds of dogs will lose pigment from their noses during the cold months. (This rarely occurs in cats.) People once thought that snow nose was caused by bright sunlight reflecting off snow and bleaching the nose white—or by a combination of cold and trauma, since dogs often use their noses as miniature snow shovels. Vets have found, however, that even dogs living in warm, southern climates may get snow nose, so weather doesn't appear to be a factor.

There is no proven way to prevent snow nose, although some breeders swear that giving pets vitamin E and kelp will help restore the color. (Your vet can recommend safe amounts.) Vets sometimes advise getting rid of plastic food bowls and replacing them with metal or ceramic bowls since some pets may be allergic to plastic. Finally, your vet may suggest a thyroid test be done. There is no evidence to prove that it is true, but some vets believe that low thyroid levels can cause the nose to lose its color.

Snow nose isn't the only condition that can cause the nose to fade, although it is the only one in which the color eventually comes back. When a nose goes pale and stays that way, your pet may have vitiligo, a condition in which skin cells lose some of their melanin, or pigment. Pets with vitiligo may turn white on the paws, lips, and fur as well. Vitiligo appears to be a hereditary problem, affecting Doberman pinschers and Rottweilers more than other breeds. It will keep your pet out of the show ring but is otherwise harmless, says Dr. Nisson.

A more serious condition that can cause the nose to fade is Vogt-Koyanagi-Harada (VKH), or Harada's, syndrome, which occurs only in dogs. Vets suspect that it is caused by an immune system disorder that damages the eyes and the pigment in the skin. It can turn any part of your dog's body white, and without treatment, it can lead to blindness, says Dr. Nisson. Vets often prescribe steroids to pets with this condition, which help keep the immune system from going out of control.

Feline neck lesions. Despite the name, these painful sores don't occur on the neck but on the teeth near the gum line, an area that vets call the neck of the tooth. This is where the tooth's enamel meets the root underneath—and in cats (but not dogs), it is a prime spot for painful cavities.

Feline neck lesions are extremely common. Researchers have found that up to 67 percent of cats have at least one bad tooth, and some have more than one. It is hard to see feline neck lesions at home, although the gum surrounding the tooth may be red, swollen, and tender. If your cat is drooling, dropping food, chattering his teeth, or eating with his head tilted to one side, there is a good chance that he has one or more of these cavities.

There is no real cure for feline neck lesions, and vets usually recommend removing the entire tooth, says Dr. Nisson. What you shouldn't do is ignore the problem, he adds. Cats are stoic creatures, and it is hard to tell when they are hurting. Once the tooth is removed, you may be surprised to discover that your previously quiet cat suddenly starts acting like a kitten again.

Lip fold pyoderma. One of the charms of both Saint Bernards and cocker spaniels is their adorable floppy lips. But this visual asset can also be a liability if the lips get large enough to start forming little folds. Folds in the skin make natural traps for drool and bits of food. Over time, this can lead to a painful infection called lip fold pyoderma.

The infection is more than just uncomfortable. It can also give your pet horrific halitosis. "It is hard to believe that all that smell comes out of such a tiny crevice," says Dr. Nisson. Bad breath isn't always caused by this condition, of course. An easy test is to run a cotton swab around your pet's mouth and take a sniff. Then take a second swab and run it into a skin fold. If the second smell is overpowering, you will know exactly what the problem is.

The only way to quell the smell and prevent infection is to clean out the skin folds every day. Use a clean rag moistened with water or an antibacterial cleaner like benzoyl peroxide or an oral rinse containing chlorhexidine, says Dr. Nisson.

Despite daily cleaning, some pets will continue having problems. Your vet may recommend doing a simple nip-and-tuck plastic surgery to straighten the lip. Removing the food-trapping folds will prevent infections and make his breath a little sweeter.

Periodontal disease. Your pet's teeth are naturally self-cleaning. But even the cleanest teeth get coated with a thin film, called the pellicle, which is packed with bacteria. (Harder, longer-lasting versions of pellicle are known as plaque and tartar.) When bacteria migrate from this film and travel between the teeth and under the gums, they may cause an infection known as periodontal disease.

Periodontal disease isn't serious at first. But as time goes by, it gradually erodes the gums and sometimes the teeth. It can loosen the teeth, cause bad breath, and, in some cases, cause infections elsewhere in the body.

Researchers estimate that 60 to 80 percent of dogs and cats have periodontal disease by the age of five. It is an amazing statistic because this problem is entirely preventable. All you have to do is brush your pet's teeth. In one study, a group of beagles had one side of their mouths brushed daily, while the other side was left alone. Four years later, the brushed teeth were healthy and shining, while the "natural" side was in terrible shape.

Dr. Luskin recommends brushing your pet's teeth every day with a brush and pet toothpaste or just with plain water. Or you can rub the surfaces of the teeth with a bit of gauze. "It might not be possible to get a toothbrush into the tiny mouth of a fractious cat, says Patricia Shema, V.M.D., a veterinarian in private practice in Glenn Dale, Maryland.

When a pet's periodontal disease is well-advanced, your vet may recommend a professional cleaning. No sensible pet will sit still for all the scraping, rinsing, and polishing, so the procedure is usually done under general anesthesia. It typically takes about half an hour, says Dr. Shema.

Rodent ulcer. The term *rodent ulcer* has nothing to do with mice or rats, but everything to do with cats. Rodent ulcers are small sores that form on the outside of the upper lip beneath the nose. They start out as small red or brown bumps, but quickly turn into painful sores. They are called rodent ulcers because people once believed that cats got them after being bitten during their nocturnal hunts. Many cats today have never seen a rodent, let alone caught one. They still get rodent sores, however, so something else is clearly to blame. Vets suspect that they may be caused by allergies or some other kind of irritation of the upper lip.

Unlike most sores, rodent sores won't go away unless they are treated. In fact, they will only get worse, sometimes damaging large areas of the lip. But they can be very easy to get rid of. In most cases, injections of steroids given two weeks apart will make them disappear, says Dr. Nisson.

Respiratory System

Dogs and cats approach the world nose-first, breathing in thousands of intriguing scents every day. Along with the good, however, they also inhale the bad. With every breath they are exposed to bacteria, viruses, pollen, and other particles that can get into the airways, causing wheezing, sniffling, coughing, sneezing, and other respiratory symptoms.

In addition, the respiratory system can be disrupted by a variety of potentially serious conditions, from heartworms to asthma to overweight. Any underlying problem that puts strain on the heart or lungs can make it very difficult for pets to catch their breath.

Respiratory problems are scary because your pet needs large amounts of air simply to survive. Even slight reductions in airflow can make a dog or cat tired and weak. That is why it is so important to recognize respiratory problems as soon as possible and to take immediate action.

See Your Vet If:

- Your pet's voice has recently changed.
- Your pet is panting excessively.
- Your dog or cat is coughing, wheezing, sneezing, or gagging.
- Exercise makes him unusually tired or causes him to cough or wheeze.
- Your pet has recently begun snoring, wheezing, or panting at night.
- He is breathing rapidly or taking shallow breaths.
- His belly is heaving when he breathes.
- His nose is dry, crusty, or bleeding.
- There is a discharge from his mouth or nose for two days or longer.
- Your pet's tongue or gums are blue or pale.

COUGHING

Clues

- Your pet coughs after exercise.
- Coughing is accompanied by difficulty breathing or watery eyes.
- Her coughs are moist or last longer than a day or two.

Humans cough nearly every day, but you will rarely hear a dog or cat let loose with a good harumph. In fact, coughing in pets is usually a sign that something is wrong.

Dogs and cats tend to cough when they swallow something that they shouldn't have like hair or a piece of bone, says John Daugherty, D.V.M., a veterinarian in private practice in Poland, Ohio. They may also cough when they inhale something irritating, like cigarette smoke, dust, or pollen.

Pets often cough when they have an infection in the respiratory tract, says Dr. Daugherty. The sound of a cough gives a clue as to what the problem is. A moist cough, for example, is usually caused by a buildup of fluid and mucus in the throat or airways. A deep, wheezy cough or a sudden burst of coughing after exercise may be a sign of bronchitis. Dry coughing may simply mean that your pet has a scratchy throat—or, in dogs, a case of kennel cough, which is a viral infection.

"Probably 90 percent of the time, coughing in cats is caused by hair balls that they are trying to 'honk' up," says Alan Kirmayer, D.V.M., a veterinarian in private practice in Marysville, Pennsylvania. More seriously, cats cough when they have infections in the lungs or chest cavity, he says. If your cat is coughing and sneezing and has watery eyes, she probably has a viral infection.

Coughing that doesn't go away may be a sign of serious illness. Pets with heart disease, for example, will sometimes cough when fluids build up in the chest or airways. Asthma and parasites like heartworms can also cause coughing. In several toy breeds of dogs, such as Yorkshire terriers, coughing may be a sign that the trachea (the tube that carries oxygen from the mouth to the lungs) has collapsed, says Dr. Kirmayer.

WHAT YOU CAN DO

Not all coughs are cause for concern, says Dr. Daugherty. If your pet isn't coughing a lot, it may be that she simply got a muzzleful of dust or some other airborne irritant. If that's the case, the coughing will go away as soon as her system has a chance to clear itself.

If you smoke, plan on doing it outside since certain substances in cigarette smoke are heavier than air and will drift down to muzzle level. It is

also a good idea to keep your pet in another room when you are vacuuming or dusting the furniture.

If you suspect that your pet has a respiratory infection, you can give
her quick relief in the same way that you would take care of your own
cold, by filling the air with soothing moisture. "Steam from a warm
shower or a humidifier will help loosen up the phlegm," says Dr. Kirmayer.

If coughing seems to be making your pet miserable, your vet may recommend giving her an over-the-counter cough suppressant, says Annette
Carricato, V.M.D., a veterinarian in private practice in Harrisburg, Pennsylvania, and author of *Veterinary Notes for Dog Breeders*. There are many
different products on the market, however, and not all of them are safe
for dogs and cats. So it is important to talk to your vet before giving cough
suppressants to pets.

Since coughing in cats is often caused by hair balls, you can help prevent it simply by keeping your pet well-groomed. This will remove loose
hairs from her coat before she has a chance to lick (and swallow) them
herself. You can also get hair-ball remedies at pet supply stores or simply
put a little petroleum jelly on the roof of your cat's mouth. This will lubricate swallowed hairs so that they cause less irritation.

You shouldn't ignore coughing, Dr. Kirmayer warns. If the cough lasts
longer than a day or two, you should take your pet to the vet. This is particularly true if your pet has other symptoms such as fever, difficulty
breathing, or watery eyes.

WHAT YOUR VET WILL DO

Since long-term coughs may be a sign that something is seriously
wrong, your vet will probably give your pet a thorough examination. "I
take a good look in the mouth and throat to see if there are foreign objects, tumors, or inflammation, says Dr. Daugherty. "I look at the color of
the gums and tongue since poor oxygen levels in the blood, which may be
caused by an infection, can cause a bluish color."

Your vet may recommend x-rays to check for pneumonia or objects in
the windpipe. He will listen to your pet's heart and lungs to see if there is
a heart problem. And he may recommend blood tests to see if any parasites are present.

When coughs are caused by infections, your vet will probably recommend antibiotics or other medications, says Dr. Daugherty. In addition,
he may prescribe medications that will help clear clogged airways as well
as drugs to calm the cough.

SYMPTOM ⟩ # PANTING

Clues

- Your pet has gotten into toxic substances.
- He has been exercising vigorously.
- He is drooling, has deep red gums, or is very weak.
- Your pet's temperature is 104°F or higher.

You will never see your dog with sweat rings under his arms or your cat wiping his brow with a handkerchief. Dogs and cats don't sweat the way people do for the simple reason that they have hardly any sweat glands at all. (The few sweat glands that they do possess are on the pads of their feet.) One exception is the sphinx cat, which can sweat a surprising amount.

Unlike humans, who can shed jackets and sweaters when they start feeling warm, dogs and cats wear their fur coats all year-round. Having so few sweat glands makes them very sensitive to heat, but they do have another way of staying cool: They pant. Which is why, after a walk in the park or a fast game of chase-the-string, they will be puffing away with gusty, window-fogging breaths. (Cats are more discreet than dogs, and you won't see their tongues hanging out very often, but they also pant when they are feeling warm.)

"Panting is the main way that dogs and cats have of getting rid of body heat," said C. Dave Richards, D.V.M., a veterinarian in private practice in Valdosta, Georgia. "If they weren't able to pant, they would collapse from the heat."

Dogs and cats also pant when they are feeling nervous after a scolding, for example, or when they realize that they are going to the vet. In fact, fear is a common cause of panting.

If your pet is panting even when he is cool and relaxed, there is probably something wrong, says John Daugherty, D.V.M., a veterinarian in private practice in Poland, Ohio. A fever often causes panting. Anemia, a condition in which there aren't enough red blood cells to deliver adequate oxygen to the body, can cause pets to pant. So can problems with the thyroid gland, which may make your pet's metabolism run too fast, causing him to heat up too much. Poisoning is another cause of panting, Dr. Daugherty adds.

Perhaps the most serious thing to watch for is heatstroke, in which a pet's temperature can shoot above 104°F, causing very heavy panting and extreme exhaustion. Signs of heatstroke also include drooling, glassy eyes, deep red gums, and excessive weakness. Heatstroke may occur when a pet has been left in a parked car or if he has been exercising too vigorously in hot weather. This is an extremely serious condition that can cause brain damage or even death.

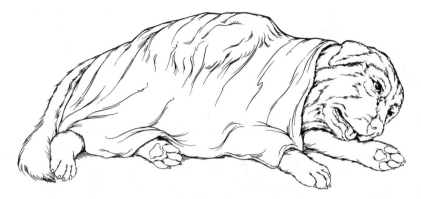

The only remedy for heatstroke is to cool your pet quickly. Wrap him in a layer of wet towels, followed by a plastic trash bag filled with ice. (An alternative is to place him in a bathtub filled with cool water.) Then get him to the vet right away.

What You Can Do

You usually don't have to worry about panting. Giving your dog or cat a drink of water and a cool place to rest—and a little extra attention if he is feeling tense—is really all you need to do, says Dr. Richards.

If you suspect that your pet has heatstroke, however, you need to act quickly. First, check your pet's temperature with a rectal thermometer. It should read somewhere between 100.5° and 102.5°F. If he is running hot—104°F or higher—you need to bring the temperature down *fast*, then you need to get him to the vet right away.

Dr. Richards recommends covering your pet with wet towels, then wrapping him with plastic trash bags filled with ice.

If you don't have a lot of ice, an alternative is to put your pet in a cool bath and hold a cool compress on his head, says Dr. Daugherty.

Take your pet's temperature every 5 to 10 minutes. Once it cools to 103°F, you can stop the treatments and let him rest until you can get him to a vet. "If your pet's temperature comes down too fast, it can cause hypothermia, which is an abnormally low body temperature," warns Linda T. Stern, D.V.M., a veterinarian in private practice in Mechanicsburg, Pennsylvania.

What Your Vet Will Do

Even though panting is usually normal, your vet will want to do a thorough exam to check for underlying problems like poisoning or an internal disease.

Don't be surprised when the vet takes a close look at the inside of your pet's mouth. The color of the gums can tell her whether or not your pet is getting enough blood and oxygen to various parts of his body. For a test, the vet will press against the gums to see if they quickly return to their normal pink hue. If they don't, your pet's circulation isn't working right, and heatstroke could be the cause. "I might give oxygen, which will help stabilize him," Dr. Daugherty adds.

Since pets with heatstroke are often dehydrated, your vet may give fluids intravenously. In addition, your pet may need medications in order to recover—anything from sedatives to stop seizures to steroids to prevent organ damage.

Most of the time, of course, the panting that had you worried will turn out to be entirely normal. But since there is no way to know for sure, it is best to be safe and get it checked. "Excessive panting can be very frightening," says Dr. Richards.

RAPID BREATHING

Clues

- Your pet is breathing rapidly and doesn't want to lie down.
- She seems to be in pain.
- Your pet has a fever.
- Her gums are blue or gray.

It is normal for dogs to pant when they have been running around and are feeling warm, and cats will, too, though usually less dramatically. But when your dog or cat is breathing fast and hard for no apparent reason, you need to figure out why.

Dogs normally breathe 12 to 20 times a minute; cats, 20 to 30 times. "Rapid breathing generally means one of two things: Your pet is in pain, or she isn't getting enough oxygen," says A. David Scheele, D.V.M., a veterinarian in private practice in Midland, Texas.

It is not always easy to tell when—or where—your pet is hurting, adds Robert L. Rooks, D.V.M., a veterinarian in private practice in Fountain Valley, California. Dogs and cats are much more stoic than people are. One reason that they cope with pain by taking rapid breaths rather than crying out may be that their ancestors attacked comrades that showed weakness. It is worth taking a few minutes to check your pet for injuries or other problems that might be causing pain.

- Look at your pet's eyes. If she is squinting or seems sensitive to light, she could have a scratched cornea or some other eye injury.
- Gently poke her abdomen. If she winces or pulls away, she could have an internal problem, something as innocent as constipation or as serious as an infection.
- Feel her legs and move them around a little. Conditions such as arthritis or hip dysplasia can be quite painful, and your pet could be having a flare-up.

If pain doesn't seem to be the problem, your pet could have a heart condition. Pets with congestive heart failure, for example, have trouble getting enough oxygen, so they will breathe more quickly. In addition, they may be reluctant to lie down. "Sitting upright helps them breathe a little easier, just as people with breathing problems will prop themselves up with pillows," says Ralph Barrett, D.V.M., a veterinarian in private practice in Carmichael, California.

One way to see if your pet is getting enough oxygen is to look at her gums. They are usually a healthy pink. If the gums seem slightly blue or gray, there may not be enough oxygen in the blood. (For pets with black gums, you can check for pink on the inside of a lower eyelid by gently pressing a finger below her eye and allowing the lower lid to droop a bit.)

Heart trouble isn't the only thing that can rob your pet of oxygen. Pneumonia or other respiratory tract infections can make it very hard for them to breathe. Pets with infections will usually seem quite sick, and they will often have a fever as well. (The normal temperature for dogs and cats is between 100.5° and 102.5°F.)

In cats, rapid breathing is sometimes caused by asthma. A cat that is having an asthma attack will breathe through her mouth, and she will probably be coughing and wheezing as well.

WHAT YOU CAN DO

Rapid breathing isn't a symptom that you can treat at home, especially if your pet isn't getting enough oxygen. Even when you are pretty sure that the problem is caused by pain, you will want to call your vet to make sure that there is nothing seriously wrong. On the way to the vet's office, it is a good idea to put your pet in front of the car's air-conditioning vent. This will make it easier for her to breathe.

WHAT YOUR VET WILL DO

Since rapid breathing is often caused by heart problems, your vet will probably want to take a chest x-ray. He may do an electrocardiogram as well. This is a test that provides a tracing of the heartbeat. It shows how well—or how poorly—the heart is working. In addition, he may give your pet oxygen to help her breathe.

"Be prepared to have your pet stay in the hospital until her condition improves," says Dr. Scheele. Many heart problems can be controlled with medications, including diuretics to remove excess water from the lungs.

If it turns out that your pet's heart and lungs are okay, your vet may take x-rays of the stomach and intestines. Rapid breathing is sometimes caused by a painful blockage in the intestinal tract. It can even be caused by gas, says Dr. Scheele. In some cases, all that she will need is an enema to clear things up.

Pneumonia and other respiratory infections can be very serious. They are usually treated with antibiotics. Since the drugs are typically given intravenously, however, your pet will still need to spend some time in the hospital.

Cats with asthma are given some of the same medications that people take, but in smaller doses. During an attack, the usual treatment is to use a steroid spray or mist, which reduces inflammation in the lungs. If your cat is having frequent attacks, your vet may recommend using medication on a daily basis to prevent them.

SHORTNESS OF BREATH

Clues

- Your pet is having trouble breathing even with mild exertion.
- He is getting overweight.
- He is short of breath, and it is mosquito season.

Before running a race or taking long hikes, humans will spend weeks or even months getting into shape. For dogs and cats, aerobic champs that they are, vigorous exercise just comes naturally. They can usually outrun (and outplay) us without even breathing hard. But if your pet is suddenly spending more time than usual catching his breath after exertion, you need to pay attention.

There are many physical problems that can cause pets to have shortness of breath. One of the most common—and the easiest to fix—is being overweight, says Richard L. Headley, D.V.M., a veterinarian in private practice in Mishawaka, Indiana. "We see many overweight pets develop significant respiratory problems due to added fat in their chests and stomachs," he says.

A more serious problem is heartworms. Transmitted by mosquitoes, heartworms are parasites that spend their lives in the heart or lungs, damaging tissue, blocking blood vessels, and making breathing difficult, says C. Dave Richards, D.V.M., a veterinarian in private practice in Valdosta, Georgia.

Asthma can also cause breathing difficulty. Dogs rarely get asthma, but it is very common in cats, says Lynne Boggs, D.V.M., a veterinarian in private practice in Austin, Texas. Pets with asthma may be short of breath after even mild exertion, like climbing the stairs. And during an asthma attack, they may have to struggle to breathe at all. Pets with heart disease will also have trouble breathing, she adds.

An obstruction in the windpipe can make it very difficult for a pet to catch his breath. Pets will occasionally swallow objects, such as a small ball, that can lodge in the trachea, blocking the flow of air, says Kenneth Drobatz, D.V.M., assistant professor of veterinary medicine and director of emergency service at the University of Pennsylvania School of Veterinary Medicine in Philadelphia. Obstructions are much more common in dogs than cats, simply because dogs are more likely to bite off more than they can chew. In addition, dogs and cats may develop tumors in the windpipe, which can also make breathing difficult.

Finally, dogs and cats sometimes get colds, flu, or other infections that cause large amounts of mucus or fluids to accumulate in the chest. "Fluid buildup in your pet's chest means that the lungs don't expand the way that they should," Dr. Drobatz explains. Injuries—falling from a tree, for example—can also cause fluids to accumulate in the chest. So can eating a poison, like rodent bait, he adds.

WHAT YOU CAN DO

Dogs normally breathe 12 to 20 times a minute. Cats breathe a little bit faster, 20 to 30 times a minute. If your pet is breathing significantly faster (or slower), you need to figure out what is going on.

Since overweight is a common cause of breathing difficulties, take a look at your pet's midsection. Better yet, feel his side: If you can't feel the ribs, he is probably too heavy and needs to shed a little weight. Once he slims down a bit, his breathing should come back to normal.

Daily exercise is important, but diet is absolutely essential for losing weight, says Dr. Headley. He recommends switching to a low-calorie, high-fiber food, which you can get from your vet or in pet supply stores. At the same time, avoid slipping leftovers from the dinner table into his food bowl since many human foods are high in fat and calories. If your pet hasn't lost any weight after a few weeks, you are going to need to feed him less.

Before starting any weight-loss plan, it is important to check with your vet. "You have to be careful about how much weight your pet loses and how quickly he loses it," says Dr. Headley. "You have to make sure that your pet is getting the proper nutrition while dieting."

Heartworms are extremely serious, so it is important to do everything that you can to prevent them. There are a number of medications—given either once a day or monthly—that will kill heartworms before they have a chance to mature and cause problems. It is also a good idea to avoid damp, swampy areas where mosquitoes thrive and where the risk for heartworms is high.

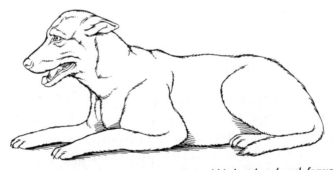

A dog that is having trouble breathing will often extend his head and neck forward, which makes it easier for air to get in. In addition, he may move his elbows away from his chest, giving the lungs more room to expand.

Pets with asthma always need to be under a veterinarian's care. If your cat is having an attack, however, you can help him breathe more easily by putting extra moisture in the air, either with a humidifier or by taking him into the bathroom and turning up the steam. The warm, moist air will help unclog his breathing tubes, explains Dr. Boggs.

Since asthma attacks are sometimes caused by dust, it is helpful to use dust-free litter, says Dr. Boggs. You should also use an unscented variety since the chemicals that give litter its scent may trigger attacks in some cats.

It is not always easy to tell if your pet has swallowed something that is blocking the flow of air. Even if you can see the object, it is not always safe—for your pet or for you—to remove it. "If your pet is having trouble breathing, don't open his mouth because the risk of a bite is high," advises Dr. Boggs. Instead, get him to the vet right away.

In fact, any breathing problem should be considered an emergency, Dr. Drobatz says. "If an owner calls and says that his pet is having trouble breathing, we don't mess around. "We tell them to come in right away." On the way to the office, put your pet in front of the car's air-conditioning vent. This will make it easier for him to breathe.

What Your Vet Will Do

The first thing that your vet will do is check to see if something is stuck in the windpipe. If the airways are clear, she may give your pet oxygen, which will replenish his natural supply and help him relax, says Dr. Boggs.

As part of a thorough checkup, your vet will listen to your pet's heart and lungs and take his temperature since fever is a sign of respiratory infections. She may take chest x-rays as well.

If your pet does have heartworms, he is going to need medication. This isn't as easy as it sounds since the drugs used to eradicate heartworms contain arsenic, which can have serious side effects. That is why prevention is so important, Dr. Richards says.

For asthma, your pet will probably need prednisone, a powerful anti-inflammatory drug that reduces swelling in the airways. In addition, your vet may give drugs such as albuterol (Salbutamol), which quickly dilate the airways, helping oxygen get through more quickly, says Dr. Boggs.

See also Chapter 12: Wheezing; Chapter 14: Weight Gain

SNEEZING

Clues

- Your pet is having nosebleeds.
- She is tired and listless and is running a fever.
- She is shaking her head or pawing her nose.

Dogs and cats have an exquisitely sensitive sense of smell, which is why their noses are at work nearly all the time sniffing strangers, identifying territory, or simply saying "Hi" to other pets.

Occasionally, of course, they sniff something that they shouldn't, and then erupt in a thunderous sneeze. "Sneezing is caused by anything that irritates the nasal passages or sinuses," says John Daugherty, D.V.M., a veterinarian in private practice in Poland, Ohio.

Pollen, smoke, and dust are common causes of sneezing, Dr. Daugherty says. Even a piece of grass can make their noses a little tickly. When your pet's sneeze is accompanied by head shaking or nose pawing, there is probably something in there that she wants to get out, and the next few sneezes will probably take care of it. Once it is out, the sneezing will probably stop right away.

As with humans, dogs and cats may sneeze when they have colds, flu, or other types of respiratory infections. In cats, frequent sneezing is often a sign of feline viral respiratory disease—cat flu, in other words. In dogs, all-day sneezing that is accompanied by a runny nose is usually a sign of canine viral infection.

"Most of the time, you are dealing with upper respiratory infections with cats," says Alan Kirmayer, D.V.M., a veterinarian in private practice in Marysville, Pennsylvania. "Foreign bodies in the nose aren't too common in cats because their noses are so small."

In rare cases, polyps and other growths can cause dogs and cats to sneeze. Even dental disease, which can spread infection to the sinuses, may be to blame, says Dr. Kirmayer.

While sneezing itself rarely causes problems, sometimes it goes on so long that the nasal passages get swollen and congested. Particularly vigorous sneezes can even result in nosebleeds.

WHAT YOU CAN DO

The occasional *achoo* is nothing to worry about. But if your pet has a respiratory infection, her nostrils may get clogged and gooey, which can make it hard for her to breathe.

It is a good idea to periodically wipe a runny nose with a paper towel moistened with a little warm water, says Dr. Kirmayer. In addition, dab-

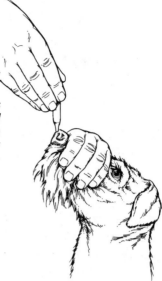

Vets sometimes recommend nasal decongestants for pets with allergies. To give the drops, hold the muzzle closed and tip the head back to a 45-degree angle. Hold the dropper just above the nostril and put in the necessary amount. Don't put the end of the dropper inside the nostril since that could damage the delicate tissues inside.

bing a little petroleum jelly on her nose will help prevent mucus from caking and blocking the airways, he adds. For a mild runny nose, place small dabs of the jelly below each nostril once or twice a day.

Veterinarians sometimes recommend giving nasal decongestants to pets with allergies in order to control sneezing. When the sneezing lasts for more than a day, however, and your pet seems tired and listless as well, you should play it safe and call your vet. "If she is running a fever, there is more going on than just sneezing," says Dr. Kirmayer. "We would have to be concerned that the cause is further down in her respiratory tract, and she might be developing pneumonia."

WHAT YOUR VET WILL DO

Since sneezing is often caused by infections, the veterinarian will check your pet's temperature and lungs to see if an infection has taken hold. He will also look at the inside of your pet's nose to see how serious the irritation is and to check for growths, says Dr. Daugherty.

Most of the time, the problem is simply an infection, which will go away within a week or two with the help of antibiotics, Dr. Daugherty says.

SYMPTOM) # SNORING

Clues

- Your pet gasps and wheezes even when he is awake.
- The snoring is worse during pollen season.
- Your pet is overweight.

It is hard enough sleeping with a spouse who snores. But lately your dog has been sawing logs, and even the cat lets loose with an occasional *szznx*. You can hardly sleep with all the noise.

Your pets' snoring may keep you awake, but it probably isn't bothering them at all, says David Tayman, D.V.M., a veterinarian in private practice in Columbia, Maryland. Snoring usually means that a slight obstruction—like postnasal drip or a loose bit of tissue in the throat—is rattling when your pet breathes. It may be noisy, but it is not a serious problem.

If your pet is snoring all the time, he could have allergies. In pets, as in people, being overweight can also cause some nighttime noise, adds Richard L. Headley, D.V.M., a veterinarian in private practice in Mishawaka, Indiana. "As the tissue in your pet's throat becomes thicker, he may start snoring."

Pugs and Pekingese are particularly prone to snoring because they have an elongated soft palate, the fleshy tissue at the rear of the mouth that separates the nose from the mouth. When they sleep, this tissue can hang down in the airways, causing them to snore, says Kenneth Drobatz, D.V.M., assistant professor of veterinary medicine and director of emergency service at the University of Pennsylvania School of Veterinary Medicine in Philadelphia.

Cats generally don't snore as much as dogs, although Persians sometimes have a problem because their nostrils are so small and the tissue vibrates when air goes out, says Annette Carricato, V.M.D., a veterinarian in private practice in Harrisburg, Pennsylvania, and author of *Veterinary Notes for Dog Breeders*.

Snoring can also be caused by polyps, growths that can form in the nose or throat. When your pet sleeps, muscles in the airways relax, causing the polyps to partially block the flow of air. This can result in a high-pitched snore, says Dr. Carricato.

WHAT YOU CAN DO

Since most pets occasionally snore and some do it all the time, you can get a little peace simply by having them sleep in another room, says Dr. Drobatz.

Giving your pet a different bed may also turn down the volume. Like people, dogs and cats have their favorite sleeping positions. When they sleep a little bit differently—in a long bed, for example, rather than a round one—their body positions change, and they will sometimes snore less. "Allowing him to sleep stretched out may reduce his breathing difficulty," says Dr. Carricato.

When snoring is caused by allergies, try to figure out what your pet is bothered by and then keep him away from it. For instance, if pollen is the problem, you may want to schedule your pet's outings for midday since pollen counts tend to be highest during the early morning and evening hours.

Since overweight is a common cause of snoring, it is worth checking to see if your pet is getting too portly. Run your hand across his ribs. If you can't feel them, he probably has too much padding and could stand to shed a little weight. For many pets, getting a little more exercise (vets usually recommend a minimum of 15 minutes, twice a day) and a little less food will be all it takes to keep them trim. Ask your vet if your pet would benefit from a weight-loss plan, says Dr. Headley.

Even though the occasional snore isn't anything to worry about, some pets gasp and wheeze all night long, or even during the day when they are relaxing. "Some pets may literally turn blue because they are not getting enough air," says Dr. Headley. When snoring seems unusually loud or goes on too long, it is a good idea to call your vet, he says.

WHAT YOUR VET WILL DO

Your vet will begin by taking a look inside your pet's nose and throat to see if polyps or other obstructions are causing the noise. She will probably take x-rays to check the sinuses as well.

Since snoring is often caused by allergies, your vet may recommend giving your pet antihistamines or other medications to reduce drainage and inflammation in the throat or airways.

When the snoring is severe and there is a chance that your pet isn't getting enough air, surgery may be the only solution. "If the cause is an elongated palate, we can sometimes cut that away and make their lives a little easier," says Dr. Drobatz.

SNORTING

Clues

- Your pet's snorting is seasonal or is accompanied by a runny nose.
- She is having other respiratory problems.

When humans have allergies or head colds, they sneeze. Dogs and cats, however, will sometimes let loose with a hearty snort—what veterinarians call a reverse sneeze. Sort of an *in-choo* instead of an *achoo.*

Snorting consists of a sudden series of noisy inhalations, which do pretty much the same thing that sneezes do. "It is an attempt to clear their nose or sinuses," says Edward A. Leonard, D.V.M., a veterinarian in private practice in Wayland, Massachusetts. Snorting usually lasts for a second or two, although it may continue for several minutes when there is a lot of mucus that your pet is trying to get rid of.

WHAT YOU CAN DO

The occasional snort is entirely normal, so you really don't have to worry about it. If your pet is snorting a lot, however, she may have allergies or an infection that is causing too much mucus to accumulate.

Perhaps the easiest way to relieve snort-causing congestion is to take your pet into the bathroom the next time you bathe or shower. "Breathing humid air eases the removal of secretions from your pet's airways," said Dr. Leonard.

Since snorting may be accompanied by a runny nose, it is a good idea to periodically wipe away mucus that can make it hard for her to breathe and which can lead to further snorting. Smearing a little petroleum jelly below your pet's nostrils will help her feel a little more comfortable, Dr. Leonard adds.

When snorting is caused by allergies, the only solution is to figure out what's provoking your pet's reaction and then keep her away from it. Since dogs and cats are often allergic to pollen, you may want to schedule your outings for midday since pollen counts tend to be highest during the early morning and evening hours. "Most pets will improve if the quality of the air that they are breathing also improves," says Dr. Leonard. Your vet may also recommend giving your pet antihistamines to ease the congestion.

Nose drops are another way to reduce nasal discharge and the accompanying snorting. "Saline nose drops work well," says Dr. Leonard. "Neo-Synephrine Mild Formula will sometimes help clear congestion as well." For dogs and cats, he recommends using one or two drops twice a day. This medication isn't safe, however, for older cats or cats with diabetes, heart trouble, or thyroid problems.

WHAT YOUR VET WILL DO

"When snorting goes on longer than a day or two or if it is accompanied by other respiratory problems, it should be evaluated by a veterinarian," says David S. Sobel, D.V.M., a veterinarian in private practice in Dover, New Hampshire.

To see what is causing the problem, your vet will do a thorough examination of your pet's airways: her nostrils, nasal passages, throat, and tonsils. He will also listen to her heart and lungs to make sure that her breathing and heartbeat are normal. Finally, your vet will feel around the windpipe to see how sensitive it is and to check for irregularities that may be causing the problem.

"If these things fail to reveal the cause of the problem, then I will take x-rays of the pet's chest and skull to look for possible obstructions, such as a tumor in the nasal passage," says Fred Goldenson, D.V.M., a veterinarian in private practice in Naperville, Illinois.

When allergies are to blame and decongestants or antihistamines don't seem to help, your vet may recommend a brief course of stronger medications such as steroids, which will reduce inflammation in the upper airways. He may also recommend that your pet undergo a series of injections that will desensitize her to whatever is making her snort. "But only about 50 percent of animals respond to the injections," Dr. Sobel adds.

Finally, since snorting may be caused by a bacterial infection in the upper respiratory tract, your vet may recommend that your pet take antibiotics, which will knock out the infection within a week or two.

WHEEZING

- Your pet's wheezing occurs in the spring or summer.
- She has been stung by an insect.
- She has lost her appetite.

Since air is so vital to life, nature made your pet's airways—the passages through which oxygen flows—exquisitely sensitive. The airways can expand and contract almost instantly, ensuring that the right amount of oxygen reaches the lungs. Sometimes, however, the airways narrow too much, forcing oxygen to push its way through. The result is a gasping, high-pitched wheeze.

"Wheezing in pets sounds just like a person having an asthma attack," explains Jeff Feinman, V.M.D., a holistic veterinarian in private practice in Weston, Connecticut.

Allergies are the most common cause of wheezing, says Dr. Feinman. With every breath, your pet inhales pollen, dust, or other particles that can potentially irritate the airways and cause allergic reactions. In addition, some pets are allergic to insect stings or the chemicals used in household cleaners. Even chemicals in new carpets may trigger wheezing in some pets.

There are a variety of upper airway conditions that can result in wheezing. Asthma is one of the most common, but it is much more of a problem for cats than for dogs, says Dr. Feinman. In addition, dogs and cats can get viral infections, such as colds or even pneumonia, which irritate the airways and cause mucus to accumulate. This makes it difficult for air to get through.

WHAT YOU CAN DO

An attack of wheezing usually stops as soon as your pet expels whatever it is that's tickling her airways. If the attack lasts 30 minutes or less, and your pet isn't wheezing on a regular basis, you probably don't have to worry about it, says William H. Craig, D.V.M., a veterinarian in private practice in San Antonio.

To make your pet more comfortable, however, you may want to pump some humidity into the air since this will be very soothing for the irritated airways, says Dr. Feinman. "If you don't have a humidifier, you can bring the pet into a steamy bathroom while you bathe or shower."

Allergies are trickier to control because it is often difficult to figure out what, exactly, your pet is allergic to. If the wheezing began recently, ask yourself what is new in your pet's environment, says Dr. Feinman. Are you cleaning the floors with a different cleaner? Did friends bring you a bouquet of pollen-filled flowers? Have you recently changed litter? Try to think of anything that occurred at the same time as the wheezing. Then, when you have a list of suspects, try eliminating them, one at time. If the wheezing goes away, you will have a pretty good idea what to avoid in the future.

You may find it helpful to keep your pet inside as much as possible during the spring and summer months. This is particularly important during the early morning and evening hours, when pollen counts tend to be highest.

"To help eliminate your pet's wheezing over the long haul, remove pollens and dust with a household air filter," says Lynne Boggs, D.V.M., a veterinarian in private practice in Austin, Texas.

For additional relief, you may need to give your pet an over-the-counter antihistamine. For dogs, vets usually recommend Benadryl—about one milligram for every pound of dog, three times a day, says Karen L. Campbell, D.V.M., associate professor of dermatology and small animal internal medicine at the University of Illinois College of Veterinary Medicine at Urbana–Champaign. For cats, Chlor-Trimeton is a better choice. The usual dose is half of a four-milligram tablet for every 10 pounds of cat, twice a day, she says. To be safe, however, check with your vet before giving human medications to pets.

Since wheezing can also be caused by aerosol sprays and smoke from fireplaces, cigarettes, and incense, you may want to keep your pet in an area where the air stays relatively clean, Dr. Boggs adds.

To help your cat breathe more easily, you may want to switch to a dust-free litter. At the very least, buy plain, unscented litter since the chemicals that give litter its scent may irritate the airways, causing wheezing and gasping, says Dr. Boggs.

Although wheezing itself usually isn't a problem, it may be a sign that something more serious is going on. To be safe, call your vet if the wheezing lasts a half-hour or longer, says Dr. Feinman. This is particularly true if your pet seems generally under the weather or hasn't been eating as well as usual.

WHAT YOUR VET WILL DO

Since wheezing is always a sign of respiratory problems, your vet will probably recommend giving your pet a chest x-ray to detect conditions such as asthma or pneumonia, says Dr. Feinman. X-rays can also detect tumors or other, more serious conditions that make breathing difficult.

To test for allergies, your vet may recommend that your pet spend several days in the hospital or clinic. If she gets better after staying in a sterile, stainless steel pen, there is a good chance that something at home is causing the wheezing. The next step, of course, is to figure out what that something is. "I ask pet owners to bring in carpet samples and other things to see if the pet reacts to them," says Larry A. Bernstein, V.M.D., a holistic veterinarian in private practice in North Miami Beach, Florida. "I had one couple bring in a cat with allergies. He was fine when the husband came to visit, but when the wife visited, the cat had an allergic reaction. We discovered her perfume was causing the cat to wheeze."

When allergies are severe, your vet may recommend that your pet undergo a desensitization procedure during which she would be given a series of shots to make her less sensitive to whatever it is that she's allergic to.

Since wheezing is caused by constricted, swollen airways, your vet may give anti-inflammatory medications, such as prednisone. He may also prescribe a bronchial dilator, an aerosol medication that will open blocked airways fast.

See also Chapter 12: Shortness of Breath

COMMON RESPIRATORY SYSTEM CONDITIONS

Asthma. Vets still are not sure what causes asthma, but it appears to be due to an allergic reaction to such things as pollen, litter-box dust, or even perfume that causes airways to get inflamed and swollen, reducing the flow of oxygen to the lungs. Dogs occasionally get asthma, but it is much more common in cats.

Asthma in cats is so common, in fact, that it is sometimes called feline allergic bronchitis, or simply, cat asthma. There are two forms of this condition. In cats with acute asthma, the attacks come on suddenly, causing loud wheezing. In addition, your cat may sit with his shoulders hunched—or lie down with his mouth open—straining to breathe.

"When your cat has an acute asthma attack, he needs emergency medical attention," says Lynne Boggs, D.V.M., a veterinarian in private practice in Austin, Texas.

The other form of cat asthma, called chronic asthma, is a lot less serious, at least in the short run, says Dr. Boggs. Your cat will breathe more rapidly and deeply than usual, but he won't be starved for air. The problem is that chronic asthma increases pressure inside the lungs, which can put pressure on the heart, causing additional problems.

There is no cure for asthma. If your pet has had one attack, he will probably have another. Veterinarians usually treat asthma with medications to open airways inside the lungs, along with anti-inflammatory drugs to reduce the swelling.

Bronchitis. Your pet's airways are lined with tiny, hairlike projections called cilia. Like little soldiers, cilia protect the lungs by trapping bacteria, viruses, and other irritants before they do harm. Sometimes, however, the cilia don't work as efficiently as they should, allowing harmful irritants to get inside. As a result, the bronchial tubes (tiny airways inside the lungs) may get inflamed and swollen, a condition called bronchitis.

Pets with bronchitis often have a dry, hacking cough, which may be accompanied by gagging. Bronchitis usually isn't serious, but it can make pets feel tired and run-down. It is important to encourage them to get plenty of rest. It is also helpful to turn on the humidifier because moisture in the air will help soothe irritated lungs.

Cat flu. A case of the flu will make your cat just as tired and miserable as it does you. Cat flu—which, as the name suggests, only affects cats—causes the nose and sinuses to get irritated and inflamed. Since the infection is extremely contagious, cats readily pass it back and forth by sneezing, sharing a food or water bowl, or even by swapping a loving lick or two.

"Cat flu most commonly occurs among cats kept in close confinement such as at breeders and shelters," says William H. Craig, D.V.M., a veterinarian in private practice in San Antonio. "It is the same principle as children at day care centers. One kid shows up with a runny nose, and before long, they all have it."

There isn't a cure for cat flu, so you have to let it run its course. (In most cases, it will start to clear up within a week or two.) In the meantime, you can expect your cat to do a lot of sneezing and to have a clear discharge from his eyes or nose.

If the discharge is cloudy or yellow, however, your cat may have developed a second, and more serious, bacterial infection. This means that he will need antibiotics, and you should take him to the vet.

Some cats are particularly susceptible to cat flu and will get it again and again. The repeated infections may permanently damage the linings of the nasal passages, causing a lifetime of sniffling, says Dr. Craig. "He may be healthy in all other respects and not have other symptoms. Persians, Siamese, and Himalayans seem to be more prone to this problem."

The best way to prevent cat flu is to make sure that your cat gets his annual vaccinations. "Vaccines are very important for preventing infection," says Dr. Craig. It is also helpful to make your home an inhospitable place for viruses to live. The cat-flu virus can live as long as 10 days outside your pet's body—in litter boxes, food bowls, and on blankets. Washing your cat's belongings every week will help wash away viruses before they cause infection. Washing your own hands several times a day will also help prevent the virus from spreading.

Hair balls. Cats love to be clean and will spend hours licking and rubbing their fur until it shines. With each lick, however, their coarse little tongues pick up loose fur, and the only place for it to go is down the hatch. The hairs tickle, which is why cats periodically give a good *harumph* and hack them up. "The vast majority of coughing in cats is due to hair," says Alan Kirmayer, D.V.M., a veterinarian in private practice in Marysville, Pennsylvania.

Not all hairs, unfortunately, are expelled by coughing. Many are simply swallowed. Eventually, they may form large, gooey clumps in the stomach. Some of the clumps pass out of the body in the stool. Others, too large to enter the intestine, get vomited back up—usually on your best carpet.

For cats, hair balls usually aren't a problem. But for owners who wake up in the middle of the night to noisy hacking or who clean up the resulting mess the next morning, they are a nuisance, to say the least. But they are not that hard to prevent. The easiest remedy is simply to groom your cat every day. This will remove loose hairs from his coat before he gets a chance to lick and swallow them.

In addition, there are ways to help hair balls pass through the digestive tract rather than being vomited back up. Pet supply stores sell a number of hair-ball remedies, which essentially lubricate the digestive tract so that the hairs pass out more easily. A less expensive strategy is to put about a quarter-teaspoon of petroleum jelly on your cat's front paws or on the roof of his mouth. When he licks the petroleum jelly, it will pass into his stomach, lubricating the hairs so that they move gently into the digestive tract. When your cat is coughing, apply the petroleum jelly once a day for about four days, says Craig N. Carter, D.V.M., Ph.D., head of epidemiology at the Texas Veterinary Medical Diagnostic Laboratory at Texas A&M University in College Station.

Hair balls generally come up fairly quickly when your cat starts hacking, says Dr. Kirmayer. If your cat is coughing and retching, but nothing is coming up, he could have a large hair ball stuck in his system. This can be serious, so it is important to call your vet right away.

Heartworms. You don't think of parasites as causing a respiratory problem, but that is one of the first symptoms of heartworms. These unpleasant worms, which live and grow inside the pulmonary arteries and the right side of your pet's heart, often cause shortness of breath, along with coughing, fatigue, and weight loss.

Heartworms begin their lives as larvae inside an infected mosquito. If your pet gets bitten, the larvae enter his bloodstream. Within six months, the larvae migrate to the heart, turning into spaghetti-like worms that can grow up to 12 inches long. Eventually, the worms may block the flow of blood. Since blood carries oxygen, reduced blood flow causes shortness of breath. Heartworms can also cause high blood pressure or heart failure.

There are drugs for treating heartworm. Unfortunately, the drugs may cause side effects that can be more dangerous than the worms themselves, says Kenneth Drobatz, D.V.M., assistant professor of veterinary medicine and director of emergency service at the University of Pennsylvania School of Veterinary Medicine in Philadelphia. That is why prevention is so important.

Heartworms are very easy to prevent with medications. Taken daily or monthly, depending on the kind you choose, the medications will kill heartworm larvae in your pet's bloodstream before they have a chance to mature and cause problems. Such preventive medications are generally recommended.

Heatstroke. Pets don't sweat the way people do, so they can easily overheat, particularly if they have been left in a parked car or in a yard without shade. When they get too hot, their internal temperatures rise to dangerous levels, possibly causing heatstroke, says C. Dave Richards, D.V.M., a veterinarian in private practice in Valdosta, Georgia.

In the early stages of heatstroke, your pet will be panting heavily. He may salivate a lot or even vomit. As his temperature rises above 104°F, he may begin staggering or even collapse entirely. His tongue and gums will probably turn a bright red.

Heatstroke can kill within hours, so it is essential to get to a veterinarian immediately, says Linda T. Stern, D.V.M., a veterinarian in private practice in Mechanicsburg, Pennsylvania. If, for some reason, you can't get him to a vet right away, you need to begin emergency first-aid. "It is critical to get the body temperature down," she says.

She recommends moving him to a cool place, then covering him with towels soaked in cool water. Or turn on the garden hose and let cool water run over his body for 10 to 15 minutes. When his temperature reaches 103°F, you can stop the treatments, she advises. Then get him to a vet as soon as you can.

Kennel cough. In the old days, dogs really did get kennel cough—a viral or bacterial infection of the upper airways—in kennels. Today, most kennels require dogs to be vaccinated before they check in, so the risk of getting kennel cough in a kennel is much lower than it used to be.

The germs that cause kennel cough are everywhere, however. And because they are contagious, kennel cough can readily be passed from dog to dog, says John Daugherty, D.V.M., a veterinarian in private practice in Poland, Ohio.

As the name suggests, the main symptom of kennel cough is a dry, hacking cough. This condition isn't particularly serious, Dr. Daugherty adds, and will usually clear up on its own in a week or two, particularly in grown, large dogs. Puppies and small dogs are more likely to have problems because they have smaller nasal passages than their larger kin.

The vaccinations against kennel cough aren't 100 percent effective simply because there are many germs that can cause this condition. Still, vaccines are helpful even when they don't prevent illness. "In most cases, they will prevent the infection from being severe," Dr. Daugherty explains.

When your dog is recuperating from kennel cough, don't put him on a leash because the airway inside his throat (the trachea) will be very tender. "Any pressure on the throat will cause him to cough," says Dr. Daugherty. If you are going for a walk, use a harness instead.

CHAPTER

13

Skin and Coat

Dogs and cats are well-protected from the elements by their thick fur coats, which repel water and trap heat next to the skin. But the skin underneath is surprisingly delicate. More than our own, their skin is vulnerable to a variety of itchy problems like infections, infestations, and allergic reactions. And the more pets scratch, the more the fur—quite literally—flies. Worse, they can scratch themselves raw, causing painful sores.

Most skin conditions are easy to diagnose and treat, but some are truly mysterious and unexpected. When dogs and cats get sick, such as with immune system disorders, their skins and coats often pay the price. Even vets can't always tell what is going on without doing extensive lab tests.

Fortunately, most skin problems aren't too serious and can be treated safely at home. In the following pages, you will find lots of information that will help cut through the confusion, along with practical tips for helping your pet look and feel better and heal more quickly.

See Your Vet If:

- Your pet is shedding or scratching more than usual.
- He has scales, bald patches, or a rash.
- He has severe dandruff or dry skin.
- His fur is greasy or smelly even after baths.
- Your pet has broken out in hives and is having trouble breathing.
- He has a bad sunburn.
- There has been a significant change in skin color, or the skin seems loose.
- There is a lump or swelling beneath his skin.
- Your pet has a sore on the skin that won't heal.
- The skin of the lips, abdomen, or rectal area is yellow.
- There are red or purple dots or splotches on his skin.

ACNE

Clues

- Your pet is rubbing her face on the floor or on other rough surfaces.
- Her chin is bumpy, itchy, and sore.
- She has started acting depressed and lethargic.

Dogs and cats don't get self-conscious about their pimples, but they can be as acne-prone as any bunch of human teenagers. And when pets get acne, they usually take it on the chin. That is where these eruptions appear, causing their chins to get bumpy, itchy, and sore.

Dogs usually get acne during their "teen-age" years, in part because changing hormone levels cause oil-producing glands in the skin to become overactive. This can clog their pores. In cats, acne usually occurs during their adult years.

No one really knows for sure why pets get acne. In dogs, there appears to be a genetic link since it tends to occur in short-coated breeds, such as Great Danes, Doberman pinschers, Rottweilers, and boxers, says Patricia Ashley, D.V.M., a veterinary resident in dermatology at the University of Tennessee College of Veterinary Medicine in Knoxville. Dogs can also get acne from allergies or from rubbing against objects that irritate the skin. In cats, acne may be triggered by allergies, ringworm, or even by problems with the immune system, she says.

Dogs usually get rid of it by the time they are about eight months old, and cats generally aren't bothered by it at all, according to Dr. Ashley. In some cases, however, the skin gets infected and swollen, and pets will rub their faces on the carpet or other rough surfaces to ease the irritation, says James Pelura III, D.V.M., a veterinarian in private practice in Davidsonville, Maryland. If the infection spreads, your pet may get a fever and feel sick as well.

WHAT YOU CAN DO

What is the best treatment? Often, hands-off is the best policy. Don't try to help by squeezing pimples, says Dr. Ashley, because you might damage the skin and cause the infection to spread.

If the acne seems to be painful, you may want to gently clean the area, to soften the oil plugging her pores. Dr. Ashley recommends washing the area with a shampoo containing benzoyl peroxide, chlorhexidine, povidone-iodine, or sulfur. These are available in some pet supply stores and from veterinarians. Repeat these treatments about once a week or as often as your vet suggests. Just be sure to rinse your pet thoroughly when you are done because medicated shampoos can irritate the skin, she warns.

A less messy way to loosen oily plugs is to use a compress, says Margie Scherk, D.V.M., a veterinarian in private practice in Vancouver, British Columbia. Use a thick towel soaked in warm water, and hold it on your pet's chin for five minutes at a time, twice a day. After using the compress, rub her chin gently with a dry towel.

Another way to make a compress is to stuff a sock with uncooked brown rice and sew it shut, Dr. Scherk suggests. Soak the compress in warm water and apply it. The rice holds moist heat longer than a towel.

When acne is inflamed or infected, you may want to apply a product that will help dry the skin. Domeboro Astringent Solution, available in drugstores and grocery stores, works well, says Dr. Ashley. Mix a packet of Domeboro in a pint of warm water, then soak a compress and apply it for five minutes. Start out using this three times a day until the chin gets drier, then use it only as needed.

You can also use medications. Your vet may recommend that you use an over-the-counter cleanser containing benzoyl peroxide (such as Fostex), or he may give you mupirocin (Bactoderm) ointment. Both of these medications help kill bacteria, says Mark W. Hanlon, V.M.D., a veterinarian in private practice in Slatington, Pennsylvania. (While mupirocin is available with a prescription from drugstores, it is much less expensive when you get it from your vet.)

Dogs and cats can't lick their chins easily, so the medication will stay on long enough to be effective. When using benzoyl peroxide, however, be sure to keep your pet off the Oriental rug because it can bleach the fabric.

WHAT YOUR VET WILL DO

If the acne doesn't start getting better within a week or two or if your pet also seems to be feeling sick, it is time to call your vet because there may be an underlying cause.

Your vet will look carefully at your pet's chin and mouth. He may recommend blood tests to check for serious internal problems such as feline leukemia or immune system disorders. If the chin itself requires a closer look, your vet will take a skin scraping and look at it under a microscope to check for bacterial infection, parasites, or yeast. He may also want to check for ringworm fungus, which tends to occur in long-haired cats. When checking for a fungal infection, your vet will cultivate cultures from hairs taken from the infected area. You will have to wait up to three weeks for results because these are slow-growing organisms, said Dr. Ashley.

Acne that keeps coming back could be caused by allergies, so your vet may recommend running allergy tests for your pet.

For severe acne, your vet will probably want to clip away the chin hair and wash the area thoroughly. Not surprisingly, most cats hate this, and your vet may recommend giving her a sedative and keeping her in the office for the afternoon. For dogs and cats, your vet may recommend giving oral antibiotics if there is a serious infection. He may also use an anti-inflammatory drug such as prednisone to relieve the swelling.

BLACK SPECKS IN FUR

Clues

- Your pet is scratching a lot.
- The specks are only on her face.

It is difficult to see black specks in dark-colored pets, but they can make dogs and cats with white coats look as though someone sprinkled them with black pepper. Don't yell at your toddler just yet: There is a good chance that something else is responsible for giving them that speckled look.

Black specks in the fur are often a sign of fleas, says Richard K. Anderson, D.V.M., a veterinary dermatologist at Angell Memorial Animal Hospital in Boston. Even when you can't see the fleas themselves, the black specks, which are their wastes, are a sure giveaway, he explains. If you look closely, you may also see eggs, which appear as very small whitish specks.

"When the black specks are on the chin and above the lip, especially on a cat, the problem is most likely some form of acne," says Dr. Anderson. Like people, cats have a large number of oil-producing sebaceous glands on their chins. The oils oxidize and turn black when they leave the glands, forming blackheads. Unlike flea dirt, the black material produced by sebaceous glands will feel slightly waxy. And, of course, it won't easily rub off on your finger when you touch it.

WHAT YOU CAN DO

If you have ever done battle with fleas, you know how hard it can be to rid your house and your pets of these obnoxious little pests. Apart from using flea shampoos, sprays, powders, or medications, it is essential to clean your house thoroughly to eliminate fleas and their eggs. "If your pet is infested, chances are her bed and your carpets are, too," says Dr. Anderson.

He recommends washing your pet's bedding often. While you are at it, you may want to check your pet for tapeworms since pets with fleas often have these intestinal parasites as well. To check for tapeworms, look at your pet's stool. If it contains little flat white segments that resemble uncooked rice, she probably has them. (For more information on stopping fleas, see Scratching on page 372.)

Acne usually isn't a health threat, but it can be uncomfortable. If your pet will hold still for it, it is a good idea to wash the area every day with a pet shampoo containing benzoyl peroxide. "You can also clean the area with cotton balls soaked in Listerine mouthwash," says Dr. Anderson. "It dissolves the wax and helps prevent infections."

WHAT YOUR VET WILL DO

Fleas can usually be treated with over-the-counter products, although your vet may recommend an oral medication like Program or a topical product such as Advantage, which help prevent fleas from reproducing, says Donna Angarano, D.V.M., professor of small animal surgery and medicine at Auburn University College of Veterinary Medicine in Auburn, Alabama.

See also Chapter 13: Acne

BLISTERS

Clues

- Your pet has blisters inside his mouth.
- Your pet is taking antibiotics or other medications.

If your cat jumps on top of a red-hot burner or your dog knocks a steaming cup of coffee from your hands, your pet may pay for his exuberance with a painful burn and blister.

But blisters aren't only caused by burns, says Donna Angarano, D.V.M., professor of small animal surgery and medicine at Auburn University College of Veterinary Medicine in Auburn, Alabama. Blisters can also be a reaction to other, less-obvious problems.

For example, some pets will develop blisters after taking antibiotics or getting a flea spray. "The blisters can occur within minutes of taking a medication or not until after a few days," says Dr. Angarano. In addition, pets with allergies, such as to pollen, may develop blisterlike bumps or hives.

It doesn't happen often, but blisters may be caused by immune system disorders such as lupus or pemphigus, in which the immune system attacks the skin, essentially causing sores from the inside out. These kinds of blisters may appear on the skin or inside the mouth, and they can be an unnerving sight, says Dr. Angarano. "Pets with autoimmune disorders such as lupus generally appear much sicker than pets with pollen allergies," she adds.

WHAT YOU CAN DO

Unlike humans, dogs and cats rarely burn themselves, so it is not always easy to figure out what is causing the blisters. It is worth taking a look around to see if there is anything new or different in your pet's life, such as a new food. Allergies don't cause blisters very often, but it is worth taking the time to explore that possibility. If you can figure out what your pet is sensitive to, it will be easy to prevent the blisters in the future.

In the meantime, you can help your pet feel better with a soothing soak. Adding colloidal oatmeal (like Aveeno) to the bathwater helps turn down the discomfort and itch, says Tiffany Tapp, D.V.M., a veterinarian in private practice in Garden Grove, California. Of course, most cats (and some dogs) won't hold still for baths. An alternative is to soak a washcloth in warm water mixed with Aveeno and hold it on the blisters for a few minutes.

WHAT YOUR VET WILL DO

Unless you know for sure what is causing the blisters, you should take your pet to the vet. Before you go, make a list of any medications that the pet is taking. If it turns out that he is having a drug reaction, swapping the medication for something else may clear up the problem within a few days. In addition, your vet may recommend giving your pet cortisone pills, which will "calm" the immune system until the blister-causing medication is out of his system, says Dr. Angarano.

Pets with long-term problems such as lupus will often need to take cortisone or other immune system suppressants for the rest of their lives, Dr. Angarano explains.

BOILS

Clues

- Boils are accompanied by bald patches in the fur.
- Your pet spends a lot of time outdoors.

It is hard to imagine, but your pet's skin (and yours, for that matter) is covered with bacteria. For the most part, these are "friendly" germs that don't cause any problems. But sometimes they slip into a hair follicle in the skin and begin multiplying. If they multiply fast enough, they can cause a painful, pus-filled boil (also called a furuncle). Dogs are more likely than cats to get boils because they are more prone to skin infections of all kinds, says Donna Angarano, D.V.M., professor of small animal surgery and medicine at Auburn University College of Veterinary Medicine in Auburn, Alabama.

Along with bacteria, dogs play host to a tiny parasite called demodex. This is a mite that normally lives peacefully inside the hair follicles. But when the immune system is weak because of stress, for example, or because of physical problems such as diabetes, the mites thrive, possibly causing boils or bald patches on the face, forelegs, and around the eyes, says E. Ann Lystrup, D.V.M., a veterinarian in private practice in Eau Claire, Wisconsin.

Pets that spend a lot of time outdoors will sometimes get boils between their toes. This usually occurs when something irritating—a grass seed, for example—sticks into the skin. When they try to lick away the annoyance, they will sometimes drive tiny hairs under the skin, causing deep infections, says Tiffany Tapp, D.V.M., a veterinarian in private practice in Garden Grove, California.

WHAT YOU CAN DO

Boils can be extremely tender. The only way to stop infection and ease the pain is to encourage them to drain. Dr. Tapp recommends applying a warm compress. Soak a washcloth in warm water and place it over the swollen area for about five minutes. Doing this every few hours will soften the tissue, making it more likely to open up and drain. Once this occurs, apply an antibiotic ointment several times a day, she advises. It is not a good idea to squeeze or lance boils, she adds, which can drive the infection deeper under the skin. If the boil does not get better within two days, it is probably time to call your vet.

You can treat most boils at home. Those that form between the toes, however, are more troublesome because whatever caused the irritation in the first place will often stay inside the skin, or worse, travel elsewhere in the body. Boils between the toes should always be treated by a vet, she advises.

If your dog gets boils often, you may want to bathe him once or twice a month with an antibacterial shampoo, suggests Dr. Angarano. These shampoos, available from your vet, will reduce the amount of infection-causing bacteria on the skin, she explains.

WHAT YOUR VET WILL DO

Boils are usually a sign of infection, and it is important to know what is causing it. Your vet will probably begin by taking a skin scraping to examine under the microscope. This may reveal such things as demodex mites, bacteria, or a yeast infection, says Dr. Tapp. Your vet may need to take a biopsy or surgical sample of skin to make an accurate diagnosis. This isn't very painful, although it can be done with a local anesthetic if your pet is uncomfortable. In addition, she may culture fluid from the boil to identify the type of infection.

Pets with demodex mites are often given oral antibiotics to fight infection. In addition, washing your pet with an antibacterial shampoo will help prevent future infections by preventing bacteria from getting established. Your vet may give him anti-mite dips, along with an oral anti-mite medication. The dips are usually given every two weeks for a month or two. "We perform skin scrapings just before each treatment and continue the treatments until two scrapings show the pet is clear of demodex," Dr. Angarano explains.

Even when mites aren't causing the boils, your pet may need antibiotics to stop the infection and possibly minor surgery if there are particles embedded in the skin that are festering. In addition, your vet may want to perform blood tests to check for internal problems such as diabetes or other hormonal problems, which can weaken immunity and allow boils to form.

COLOR CHANGES

Clues

- Your pet is licking or scratching the same spot.
- She has a slightly rancid odor.
- Your pet spends a lot of time in the sun.
- Her skin is slightly yellow.

Beneath their furry coats, dogs and cats come in a variety of hues. Some have pink skin. Others are gray, freckled, or black. As long as the color stays constant from year to year, there isn't a problem. Changes in skin color, on the other hand, mean that something is going on.

A yeast infection, for example, will cause the skin to get darker in places. Vets call this condition hyperpigmentation, says Richard K. Anderson, D.V.M., a veterinary dermatologist at Angell Memorial Animal Hospital in Boston. The yeast organism is most comfortable in warm, moist places, so you are most likely to see these dark patches on the neck, armpits, or groin. Pets with yeast infections often have a slightly rancid odor, and they may be itchy as well.

Changes in skin color can also be caused by simple friction. When pets lick or scratch the same area for a long time because of allergies, for example, pigment-producing cells in the skin get overactive making the area look darker.

Dark patches aren't always harmless, adds Thomas P. Lewis II, D.V.M., a veterinary dermatologist in private practice in Mesa, Arizona. They may be caused by a type of skin cancer called melanoma, which typically occurs on the feet or around the mouth. Other skin cancers may cause white or red crusty areas. "These often occur on the face, ear tips, or other areas that get a lot of sun," he says.

A number of the body's hormones, including those produced by the thyroid and pituitary glands, play a role in regulating melanin, the skin's natural pigment. Pets with a hormonal imbalance may produce too much melanin, causing the skin to get darker in places or even all over.

Dogs and cats that have spent too much time in the sun will occasionally get a little pink on their faces, the tips of their ears, or on their soft, hairless bellies. In addition, pets with lupus or other immune system problems will sometimes get a slight rash after even brief exposure to sunlight, says James Jeffers, V.M.D., a veterinary dermatologist in private practice in Gaithersburg, Maryland.

In pets as in people, jaundice—a condition caused by liver disease or sometimes internal bleeding—can turn the skin an unhealthy-looking yellow, says Vance Case, D.V.M., a veterinarian in private practice in Sunbury, Pennsylvania. At first, pets with jaundice will show a little yellow in the ears, on the gums, or in the whites the eyes. Over time, the color changes will appear elsewhere on the body and may darken to more of a pumpkin color. Jaundice is serious and always needs to be treated by a vet, says Dr. Case.

What You Can Do

Yeast is easy to beat by washing your pet with a medicated shampoo that contains povidine-iodine, available in pet supply stores or from your vet. Once she is yeast-free, bathing her once or twice a month will help prevent infections in the future. "Pay special attention to infection-prone areas such as the armpits and skin-fold areas," says Dr. Lewis. After bathing, dry these moisture-grabbing areas thoroughly to make them even less hospitable to germs.

Blackened or reddened skin caused by friction isn't easy to reverse simply because pets' licking and scratching habits can be hard to break. It is essential to figure out what originally caused the itching. Treating the underlying problem—both fleas and allergies are common offenders— will give the skin a chance to heal. In the meantime, keep the area clean to prevent infections, says Dr. Jeffers.

"Sunscreen is important for pets with autoimmune disorders since sun exposure can activate the immune response," says Dr. Jeffers. Areas that need the most protection are the ones that get the most sun: the face and other thinly haired areas. Also, be sure to cover the areas of the body where the rash is most likely to occur, he says.

What Your Vet Will Do

Since dogs and cats never take their coats off, they are protected to some extent from the sun's harsh rays. But every year, some pets get skin cancer due to sun exposure. That is why any new dark spot should be checked by your vet right away, says Dr. Lewis.

Most skin-color changes aren't that serious, of course. Even if you haven't been able to stop a yeast infection at home, your vet will have a solution. "Your vet may recommend a different bathing program, either more frequently or with a stronger, prescription shampoo," says Dr. Lewis.

Allergies sound like they would be easy to treat, and they are—if you can figure out what your pet is allergic to. Pets can be allergic to all sorts of things, from pollen in the air to mold in the living-room carpet. Your vet may need to take blood samples and do skin tests to figure out what is causing the problem and what things your pet needs to avoid in the future. In the meantime, he may recommend giving an antihistamine to stop your pet's itching. For dogs, vets often recommend Benadryl—one milligram for every pound of dog, three times a day, says Karen L.

Campbell, D.V.M., associate professor of dermatology and small animal internal medicine at the University of Illinois College of Veterinary Medicine at Urbana–Champaign. For cats, a better antihistamine is Chlor-Trimeton. Give half of a four-milligram tablet for every 10 pounds of cat, twice a day, she says. It is a good idea to check with your vet before giving antihistamines to pets.

Hormone or immune system problems can become quite serious without early treatment, but they can usually be controlled with medications (or, in some cases, with surgery). Pets with jaundice, on the other hand, usually need to be hospitalized in order to receive intravenous fluids, antibiotics, and special diets. When the jaundice is caused by a type of anemia that causes internal bleeding, pets often need a blood transfusion in order to recover.

SYMPTOM) # DANDRUFF

Dogs and cats don't wear blue blazers or black scarves, so dandruff doesn't show up as much as it does on people. But they get it just as often, usually for the same reason: Their skin is a little drier than it should be, and it is flaking off fast enough to become visible in their coats, says Peter S. Sakas, D.V.M., a veterinarian in private practice in Niles, Illinois.

Some pets have dry skin simply because that is how nature made them. Vets call this condition dry seborrhea. "The itching can drive your pet crazy," says Robert Rizzitano, D.V.M., a veterinarian in private practice in Los Angeles. Dry skin and dandruff are much more common in the winter, he adds, because indoor heat removes large amounts of moisture from the air. Frequent bathing can also lead to dry skin.

Dandruff itself isn't a problem, but the dry skin that causes it may be. Pets with dry skin get very itchy. Since dogs and cats don't know when to stop scratching, they may dig in so hard that they will scratch themselves raw, getting skin infections in the process. Allergies, parasites, or infections of any kind can also be a cause of flaky skin.

Dry skin and dandruff may be a sign that something is wrong in the diet. Dogs and cats need certain nutrients, especially fatty acids, to keep their skin healthy. Most pet foods contain plenty of fatty acids. But some dogs and cats either don't get enough fatty acids or they need more than the usual amounts. This can disturb the skin's normal balance, leading to dry skin and dandruff, Dr. Sakas says.

A tiny parasite known as walking dandruff can cause large white flakes to appear on the neck and back. It can cause fur loss as well. All pets can get walking dandruff, but it is most common in puppies.

It doesn't happen often, but dandruff may be a sign that the thyroid gland is underactive and producing too little hormone, a condition called hypothyroidism. Other symptoms of thyroid disease include weight gain, thinning fur, and a loss of energy.

WHAT YOU CAN DO

The easiest way to treat both dandruff and itching is to pay a little more attention to your pet's skin and coat. "Most pets need a bath monthly or less, but those with seborrhea should get a weekly bath with an antiseborrhea shampoo until the condition is under control," says Dr. Rizzitano. "Then use the shampoo every two to four weeks."

If your pet only has dry skin in the winter months, you can try bathing her with a conditioning shampoo and finish with a cream rinse and moisturizing spray, says Dr. Sakas.

Adding a little oil to your pet's food can also be helpful, Dr. Sakas adds. Corn, sunflower, and safflower oils all contain essential fatty acids. You can give cats up to a half-teaspoon of oil a day. Dogs need more, between one teaspoon (for dogs under 30 pounds) and one tablespoon (for dogs over 60 pounds) a day. Some dogs will get diarrhea after eating the extra oil, so it is a good idea to start with a smaller amount and gradually increase it over time. You can also get supplements that contain fatty acids from vets and pet supply stores.

In winter, plugging in a humidifier may help clear up dandruff. And in all seasons, frequent brushing will remove dandruff before it builds up to noticeable levels.

Walking dandruff jumps easily between pets—and from pets to people—so it is important to get rid of it quickly. Your vet will probably recommend using anti-mite shampoos or dips, which will usually do the trick.

WHAT YOUR VET WILL DO

Pets with dandruff often have other, potentially more serious problems, so it is a good idea to call your vet as soon as the flakes appear. Even though mild dandruff is often easy to treat at home, stubborn cases may require prescription-strength shampoos, creams, or supplements, says Dr. Sakas.

When dandruff is caused by an infection, your vet will prescribe antibiotics to get it under control. Mites can often be stopped with shampoos and dips, but some pets may need an injection of an anti-mite medication called ivermectin as well.

Thyroid problems are a bit trickier. Your pet may be given a blood test to measure the amount of thyroid hormone in the bloodstream. If it is running low, she may need medications to restore it to healthful levels. Thyroid supplements are safe, but they are not a temporary treatment. Most pets with underactive glands will need to take the medication for the rest of their lives.

See also Chapter 13: Scratching

DRY COAT

Clues

- There is dandruff on the furniture.
- You have been giving your pet a generic food.
- Your pet has recently been scratching or has runny eyes.

Has your pet's coat lost its luster? Does his hair feel like a Brillo pad? Are you finding dandruff on his favorite chair?

A dry coat says a lot about your pet's health. "Sometimes they are not getting enough of the right types of fatty acids to maintain a healthy coat," says Karen L. Campbell, D.V.M., associate professor of dermatology and small animal internal medicine at the University of Illinois College of Veterinary Medicine at Urbana–Champaign.

Even though commercial pet foods usually provide all the nutrients that your pet needs, some dogs and cats may have digestive problems, such as bowel or liver disease, that prevent fatty acids and other essential nutrients from being absorbed, says William H. Miller Jr., V.M.D., professor of dermatology in the department of clinical sciences at the College of Veterinary Medicine at Cornell University in Ithaca, New York.

In fact, any internal illness, from flu to diabetes, can cause a dry coat. In older dogs, hypothyroidism—a condition in which the thyroid gland doesn't produce enough hormone—may be to blame. Allergies can cause irritation of the skin, causing a dry coat. Or worms, fleas, and other parasites can cause your pet's coat to look dry and lifeless.

With some breeds, a dry coat comes naturally. Dogs such as cocker and springer spaniels are sometimes a little dry. This type of dryness usually appears before your pet is a year old and continues for the rest of his life.

Finally, don't overlook the obvious when trying to figure out what's taking the shine out of your pet's coat. Is your dog taking a dip in the chlorinated pool every chance that he gets? Does your cat enjoy sleeping next to the woodstove? Are you bathing your pet frequently, perhaps too often, or using a shampoo that is too harsh? "Anything that can damage human hair can do the same thing to a dog's or cat's hair," says Dr. Miller.

WHAT YOU CAN DO

If you have been giving your pet a low-cost generic food, you may want to try switching to a name-brand chow. Or if you are currently using a name-brand food, ask your vet if it is worth switching to a premium food, sold by vets and in pet supply stores. If it turns out that the food was the problem, you will start to see improvements in 8 to 12 weeks, says Dr. Miller.

Some vets recommend fatty-acid supplements to help nourish a dry coat. While those supplements can be helpful, they are generally not necessary as long as you are using a quality food and your pet is in good health, says Dr. Miller. "By the time you add the cost of supplements to the cost of cheaper foods, you will end up spending as much money as you would to upgrade to a better-quality food." If you are giving your pet a high-quality food and he is still having problems, ask your vet if supplements would be a wise choice.

Pets with dry skin caused by allergies, for example, will often have a dry coat as well. Bathing your pet and then using a moisturizer made specifically for pets will lubricate the skin, helping the hair regain its natural sheen.

- Use a shampoo that is made for pets since human shampoos are too harsh, says Melissa Verplank, a certified master groomer and director of Paragon School of Pet Grooming in Jenison, Michigan.
- Vets recommend looking for pet shampoos with the words *mild* or *hypoallergenic* on the labels. These are specially formulated for pets with dry skin, says Dr. Campbell.
- Shampoos for dogs and cats aren't interchangeable, Dr. Campbell adds. Shampoos that are designed for dogs may contain strong ingredients that can be dangerous for cats, so it is important to buy a shampoo that is dog- or cat-specific.
- When bathing your pet, keep the water on the cool side since warm water will tend to irritate dry skin.
- After shampooing, rinse your pet thoroughly. "You can't rinse too much," says Pam Lauritzen, a master pet stylist meritus, publisher of *PetStylist* magazine, and executive director of the International Society of Canine Cosmetologists in Garland, Texas.
- After bathing, apply a moisturizing rinse while the coat is still wet. In between baths, you can spritz on a little moisturizing spray. Moisturizers for pets usually contain lanolin, glycerine, or urea.
- Brush your pet after he is dry. In fact, you should brush him at least once a day since brushing helps distribute natural oils through the coat, keeping it soft and shiny.

Most dogs willingly take baths, but cats usually put up quite a fight. "If you have a kitty that is good enough to take a bath, go for it," says Dr. Miller. If not, you may want to spray on a little moisturizer and give him a quick brushing whenever he will hold still for it.

In summer, you can bathe your pet as often as once a week. During the cold (and dry) winter months, however, you will want to keep baths to a minimum. "When the humidity drops down below 40 percent, you can just suck water right out of the skin," says Dr. Miller.

WHAT YOUR VET WILL DO

Even though a dry coat is usually nothing more than a cosmetic problem, it can also be a mirror of your pet's overall health. So it is a good idea to have your vet check it out.

When you call for your appointment, ask your vet if you should take a stool sample so that she can test for worms or other parasites. In addition, be prepared to answer questions about your pet's daily habits—what he eats, how he spends his days, and what products, if any, you use to clean him.

Blood tests are often necessary to determine if there are internal problems such as a hormonal imbalance or bowel or liver disease. Blood tests will also reveal if there is a nutritional deficiency. Pets that are seriously low in fatty acids may require supplements for a short time until their fatty-acid levels are back up to normal. Fish-oil supplements, which are high in fatty acids, can be very helpful. "They seem to decrease inflammation on the skin," Dr. Campbell explains. Ask your vet what the right dosage is for your pet.

Finally, your vet may recommend that you use a specialty shampoo or moisturizer. Products that are available from your vet may be of higher quality than those sold in pet stores. Of course, they will probably be pricier as well.

FUR LOSS

Clues

- The skin has circular patches that are red and crusty.
- Your pet is always itchy.
- Her fur is brittle and coarse.

With the exception of a few hairless breeds, all dogs and cats have a smooth, even coat, no matter what their age. If your pet is developing bare spots or has a patchy, moth-eaten look, there is almost certainly something wrong—anything from parasites to infections, nutritional deficiencies to hormonal problems.

It is almost impossible to tell at home what is causing fur to fall out, but you can get a few clues from the appearance of the coat, says Karen L. Campbell, D.V.M., associate professor of dermatology and small animal internal medicine at the University of Illinois College of Veterinary Medicine at Urbana–Champaign.

Pets with circular patches of red or crusty skin, for example, often have ringworm, a type of fungus that is readily passed from pet to pet. Ringworm occurs throughout the country, but it is most common in places with hot, steamy weather. Cats are more likely than dogs to get ringworm, says Dr. Campbell. In addition, some cats may be asymptomatic carriers, meaning that they can spread the fungus without having symptoms themselves.

Fur loss in dogs is sometimes caused by demodex mites. These are tiny parasites that normally live peacefully in the hair follicles of dogs. But sometimes the mites multiply—and when they do, they can cause substantial hair loss, explains Dr. Campbell. The hair loss starts around the eyelids, mouth, and front legs, causing bare patches about an inch around. Eventually, the patches may enlarge, causing very large bare patches that often get infected.

When your pet is scratching hard enough to make the fur fly, you should always suspect fleas. Another itchy condition is seborrhea, in which oil glands in the skin get overactive, causing greasy, foul-smelling fur and bare patches that may resemble those caused by ringworm.

A thinning coat can be caused by a hormone imbalance. Too little thyroid hormone, for example, will cause hair to fall out all over your pet's body, and the hair that remains will be brittle and coarse. Too much estrogen can have the same effect, says Donna Angarano, D.V.M., professor of small animal surgery and medicine at Auburn University College of Veterinary Medicine in Auburn, Alabama.

"Nutritional deficiencies are rare these days, but they do occur and can cause hair loss or a dull, thin hair coat," says Craig N. Carter, D.V.M., Ph.D., head of epidemiology at Texas Veterinary Medical Diagnostic Laboratory at Texas A&M University in College Station. Pets that don't get enough protein or essential fatty acids may develop a dry, thin coat, he explains. "Nutritional deficiencies generally happen when people don't feed their pets commercial pet foods, most of which are formulated to meet your pet's nutritional needs, and instead rely on table scraps," he says. And if you are feeding your pet a generic food, you might want to upgrade her to a brand-name chow.

In addition, some Arctic breeds like Siberian huskies and Alaskan malamutes have a genetic tendency to absorb too little zinc. This can cause hair loss along with scaly, crusty patches on the skin.

What You Can Do

One way to find out if your pet has ringworm is to shine an ultraviolet light on her coat. These lights, available from plant and garden stores, will often cause the infected areas to glow green. The test isn't always effective, however, so the lack of a jolly green glow doesn't necessarily mean that your pet is ringworm-free. And other substances on your pet's fur, like medications or natural skin oils, may also glow.

To eliminate ringworm, put on a pair of gloves and clip around the infected area with blunt scissors or clippers. Be careful not to touch yourself or other pets with the gloves or the clipped hair because ringworm is highly contagious—to people as well as to pets, says Dr. Angarano. After the clip job, wash your pet's entire body with an antifungal shampoo. Let your pet air-dry so as not to rub the product off, she advises.

You don't need special equipment to recognize fleas, of course, but it

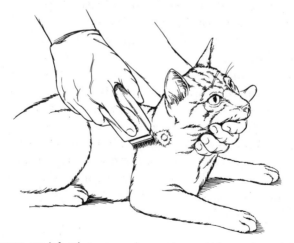

Your pet's ringworm can infect humans, so be sure to wear gloves when trimming fur from around the affected area. The fur clippings also contain contagious matter, so keep them away from bare skin or other pets. After clipping, wash your pet thoroughly with an antifungal shampoo and let her dry.

can take an army to get rid of them. Once your pet is infested, you might want to take a combination approach, using flea shampoos, powders, and possibly oral medications to get their numbers down.

Seborrhea is not always easy to control. "But you can keep it at a dull roar," says Dr. Angarano. When you first notice that your pet's coat is getting greasy, wash her once a week with an oil-dissolving shampoo, available in pet supply stores. This will keep her coat comfortable and help reduce the itching.

Finally, be sure to feed your pet a name-brand, quality food, says Dr. Carter. For most pets, this will provide all the nutrients that they need to keep the coat healthy. In some cases, your vet may recommend giving supplements as well. Severe illnesses will increase your pet's need for vitamins and minerals, so supplements may be prescribed along with the other drugs necessary to cure the primary problem. Those breeds that don't readily absorb zinc may be given zinc supplements to keep the coat healthy, he adds.

WHAT YOUR VET WILL DO

When your pet's fur doesn't improve within a few weeks with home treatments, you are going to need professional help. The first thing your vet will want to know is if the fur loss is caused by a skin problem or something else. He will probably begin by taking a skin scraping. Viewed under a microscope, this will reveal whether or not your pet has parasites.

Mite infestations can be very difficult to treat, and you are going to need your veterinarian's help. Your pet may be given an anti-parasitic dip at your vet's office every two weeks for at least six weeks. She may need injections of an anti-parasitic medicine as well.

Ringworm and seborrhea can usually be treated at home under the direction of a veterinarian. When baths and ointments don't help, however, your vet may recommend using an oral medication and possibly a steroid ointment to control itching and inflammation.

When fur loss isn't caused by skin problems, your vet will recommend a blood test to check for a hormone imbalance. He may recommend x-rays or ultrasound as well since some hormonal problems are caused by tumors in the reproductive organs or elsewhere in the body.

Most hormonal problems can be controlled with medications, although in some cases surgery—either to neuter your pet or to remove tumors—will be needed.

See also Chapter 13: Color Changes, Skin Crusts and Scabs

GREASY COAT

Clues

- Your pet is scratching a lot.
- His fur has a rancid odor.
- Your pet is drinking much more water than usual.

Your pet hasn't been in the bathroom lately, but you are beginning to suspect that he has been swiping the Brylcreem. His coat feels slick and greasy, and he is starting to smell like old french fries. What is making his coat so greasy?

Except when they have been playing in the dirt, dogs and cats usually have smooth, clean coats. But some pets, like humans, naturally have oily skin. If they are not bathed regularly, they get greasy coats. Some cocker and springer spaniels are particularly prone to getting this problem. In addition, pets with a condition called seborrhea can produce tremendous amounts of skin oil, which can result in sores and patches of missing fur as well as a greasy coat.

Dogs and cats will sometimes get greasy coats when they have fleas, mites, or even allergies, all of which can cause the skin's sebaceous glands to work overtime and secrete more oil than usual. Less often, a greasy coat can be a sign of internal problems such as diabetes or a hormonal imbalance.

"A lot of times, they will get almost a rancid type of an odor to them, which is unpleasant," says Karen L. Campbell, D.V.M., associate professor of dermatology and small animal internal medicine at the University of Illinois College of Veterinary Medicine at Urbana–Champaign. A greasy coat can be more than a cosmetic problem. It makes a comfortable breeding ground for bacteria and other organisms. As a result, pets with greasy coats are prone to skin infections, which can make their skin itchy and sore.

WHAT YOU CAN DO

Before you treat your pet's greasy coat, you need to find out if it is a natural problem or if your pet simply rolled in something oily. "If the coat is all matted and sticky, sometimes it is easier just to trim it back and start from the beginning," says Christine A. Rees, D.V.M., clinical assistant professor of dermatology in the department of small animal medicine and surgery at the Texas A&M University College of Veterinary Medicine in College Station.

If the hair grows back just as greasy as it was before, you have no alternative but to give your pet a bath. Bathing pets isn't anyone's idea of a good time, but it is really the only solution. Here are some guidelines to make it easier.

- Look for a medicated shampoo that is made specifically for oily-skinned pets, says Dr. Rees. These shampoos usually contain ingredients such as coal tar, salicylic acid, benzoyl peroxide, or sulfur, which are very effective at cutting through the oil and for removing built-up scales from the surface of the skin. Pet supply stores carry a variety of shampoos, among them, the medicated type. Don't use shampoos containing coal tar, phenol, or selenium sulfide on cats because they can be toxic.

- Depending how greasy your pet's coat is, he may need baths as often as every other day until the problem clears up. More often, once or twice a month will be enough, says Dr. Rees.

- Medicated shampoos are much stronger than regular cleansing shampoos, so you don't want to use them too often, Dr. Campbell says. Plus, the medications require at least 10 minutes of contact time to do their job. It is a good idea to rinse the skin and hair well to avoid irritation. The switch to a medicated shampoo may have to be permanent, unless you want the condition to come back.

- Applying a coat conditioner after shampooing will help restore moisture to the skin that the shampoo took out, Dr. Campbell adds. But check with your vet before using these products.

- Pet shampoos aren't interchangeable, says William H. Miller Jr., V.M.D., professor of dermatology in the department of clinical sciences at the College of Veterinary Medicine at Cornell University in Ithaca, New York. "If you use a tar-containing product on a cat, you are asking for trouble," he warns. Always read the label to be sure that the shampoo you are choosing is right for your pet.

- Shampoos containing tar can also be a problem for light-colored dogs because the tar may stain their fur. If you don't want your pet to re-

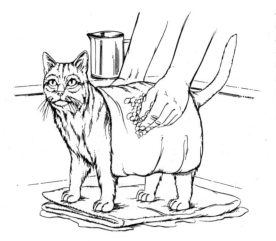

Bathing a cat is seldom trouble-free, but you can make it easier by putting a towel in the bottom of the sink so that he has something to dig his claws into. To keep a good grip yourself, you can wrap a wet dishtowel around his body and rub the shampoo right through the fabric.

semble a white shirt that accidentally went into the color wash, get a shampoo with other active ingredients, says Dr. Campbell.

In addition to regular baths, you may want to try giving your pet supplements containing fatty acids, such as those containing fish oil. "Sometimes the supplements can help calm down the hypersecreting oil glands," says Dr. Campbell. Call your vet to get supplement recommendations.

What Your Vet Will Do

Fleas are easy to spot at home, but other parasites, like mites, aren't. And allergies are notoriously difficult to diagnose. When your pet's coat keeps getting greasy or, in the case of seborrhea, your pet is still itchy and uncomfortable, even after regular shampooings, it is time to see your vet.

The doctor may want to take a skin sample to examine under a microscope. Pets with parasites can often be treated with over-the-counter medications. For more-serious problems like a skin infection, your vet will probably recommend using oral antibiotics.

If the problem doesn't seem to reside in the skin, your vet may draw some blood or get a urine sample to test for internal problems such as diabetes or hormonal imbalances. Your pet might need an allergy test as well. Once the underlying problem is taken care of, your pet's coat should quickly regain its normal shine and stop looking greasy.

HIVES

Clues

- Your pet is scratching, and there are bumps under her fur.
- Patches of fur appear slightly raised.

Dogs and cats tend to be itchier than humans, especially when these animals have allergies. The slightest contact with the wrong thing—anything from plants in the backyard to insect stings to certain foods—may cause them to break out in hives, itchy welts that resemble mosquito bites.

Hives aren't particularly serious and rarely last more than a few days. But they can be ferociously itchy. Some pets, dogs especially, have been known to scratch themselves raw in their vigorous attempts to make the itching go away.

Hives are easy to see in humans, but in pets they are all but invisible under the fur. "Run your hand through your pet's hair, and you will feel little welts if hives are present," says Robert Rizzitano, D.V.M., a veterinarian in private practice in Los Angeles. In addition, hives occasionally cause the fur overlying the area to appear slightly raised.

Hives aren't very common, so there is a good chance that you will never have to deal with them. But some pets get them all the time, and even vets may have a hard time figuring out what the allergen is. "Your pet may have encountered the now-troublesome substance her whole life without suffering an allergic reaction. And then one day she suddenly develops an allergy to it," says A. David Scheele, D.V.M., a veterinarian in private practice in Midland, Texas.

WHAT YOU CAN DO

There isn't a quick cure for hives, but you can relieve the itching until they go away. Over-the-counter antihistamines can be very effective. Vets often recommend giving antihistamines containing diphenhydramine (such as Benadryl) to dogs. The usual dose is one milligram for every pound of dog, three times a day, says Karen L. Campbell, D.V.M., associate professor of dermatology and small animal internal medicine at the University of Illinois College of Veterinary Medicine at Urbana–Champaign. For cats, vets recommend Chlor-Trimeton. You can give half of a four-milligram tablet for every 10 pounds of cat, twice a day, she says. Check with your vet to make sure that the dose is right for your pet.

Ointments to stop itching don't always work because dogs and cats tend to lick them off. If your pet will leave it alone, however, over-the-counter hydrocortisone ointment can be very helpful. It will quickly stop the inflammation and irritation that lead to itching. "Coating the hives with a baking-soda-and-water paste can also bring your pet relief," says Dr. Scheele. Cool baths with an oatmeal shampoo and cream rinse—or simply a five-minute soak in cool water to which you have added a little colloidal oatmeal (like Aveeno) are time-tested ways to ease itching. Many owners may feel, however, that these are a lot of work for a problem that will be gone in a day or two anyway.

The one time that you should definitely give your pet a bath, or a least a thorough washing, is when you suspect that the hives are caused by direct contact with an irritating substance—chemicals on the lawn, for example. Washing her thoroughly with a mild soap will remove any lingering substances before they have time to cause more itching.

Even though hives are nearly always harmless, sometimes they are only the beginning of a more serious allergic reaction. "If she shows any signs of breathing trouble, like coughing or breathing rapidly, or if she is having an allergic reaction that does not immediately respond to antihistamines, rush her to the vet immediately," Dr. Rizzitano says.

What Your Vet Will Do

One case of hives is annoying. Two or three cases—or more—may mean that your pet's immune system is overactive, and she may need medications to calm it down.

One way to quickly stop hives is to give intravenous corticosteroids. These are powerful drugs, so they are not used routinely. When hives are out of control, however, giving steroids will stop the immune system from working so vigorously, giving the skin a chance to heal. Once the outbreak is under control, your vet will need to do further tests, including allergy testing, to find out what the underlying problem is, Dr. Scheele explains.

See also Chapter 5: Chewing Skin, Coat, or Tail; Chapter 10: Foot Licking; Chapter 13: Scratching

LUMPS AND BUMPS

Clues

- Your pet has lumps that are hard and immobile.
- His lumps are red, warm, or filled with pus.
- Your pet recently had an injection.

It is natural for dogs to get a little gray around their muzzles and to put on an extra pound or two when they get older. They also tend to get a little lumpy in their senior years, as though their skin were filled with miniature water balloons.

When you don't know what is causing them, lumps and bumps can be scary and should be checked by a vet. But most lumps aren't cancer, says Richard K. Anderson, D.V.M., a veterinary dermatologist at Angell Memorial Animal Hospital in Boston. You may be feeling a harmless fatty tumor or a fluid-filled cyst, he says.

In dogs, small lumps on the surface of the skin are usually caused by infections, especially when they are warm, red, or tender. "If you look carefully, you may see that the infected bump started in a hair follicle," says Dr. Anderson. Infected hair follicles can be very sensitive, and your pet will probably wince when you touch him.

Dogs and cats that have recently had an injection will sometimes develop a small bump, which should slowly disappear, he adds. And they sometimes develop warts, which can look like small pieces of chewing gum stuck to the skin.

WHAT YOU CAN DO

There is no way to tell at home if a lump or bump is serious or not, which is why it is always a good idea to call your vet as soon as you notice any changes. Hard lumps or bumps that grow quickly may be cancer, and you need to get them checked quickly, Dr. Anderson says. You should also be suspicious of lumps that appear to be growing from a bone or from inside the breast or a nipple.

Lumps that feel soft and spongy and which glide freely under the skin are probably just lipomas, harmless accumulations of fat cells. Or they may be hair-follicle cysts, fluid-filled sacs that may go away on their own once they break open and drain.

Skin infections should be washed regularly, says Dr. Anderson. If there is redness and pus, he recommends applying a warm, moist compress several times a day for five minutes at a time. This will help drain the infection so that it heals more quickly. After applying the compress, dry the area well, then apply an over-the-counter triple-antibiotic ointment once or twice a day.

WHAT YOUR VET WILL DO

Even though most lumps aren't serious, you should ask your vet to take a look at any lump to make sure that it is not cancer, says Dr. Anderson. "Don't wait just because your pet doesn't seem to have much pain," he adds. "Most cancerous lumps don't hurt."

Since most lumps are near the surface of the skin, they are usually easy to remove—either by draining them, in the case of hair-follicle cysts or infections, or by removing them surgically. "When infected areas are especially large and painful, we may drain off the pus by lancing the area," adds Dr. Anderson, which will provide immediate relief. The area will heal within a few days.

See also Chapter 11: Mouth Lumps

SYMPTOM) NIPPLE REDNESS

Clues

- Your pet is scratching a lot.
- She has an infection.
- There are black specks in her fur.

All dogs and cats (males and females) have two rows of nipples running down their bellies, with five pairs in all. The nipples may be pale and almost invisible or red and slightly raised.

When the nipples are redder than usual or a rash is near them, your pet may have a skin problem. The nipples within reach of the back legs usually take the worst beating since dogs and cats scratch with their back paws. "Knowing what's normal for your pet is the key to detecting troublesome nipple inflammation," adds James Jeffers, V.M.D., a veterinary dermatologist in private practice in Gaithersburg, Maryland.

WHAT YOU CAN DO

The only way to stop your pet from scratching her belly is to figure out what's causing the itching in the first place. Allergies—especially flea allergies—are often to blame, says Dr. Jeffers. Even if you don't spot any fleas, look for little black specks in the fur, which are the wastes they leave behind.

In addition to treating your pet with a flea shampoo or other medications, you will want to vacuum the house thoroughly and wash her bedding to eliminate any fleas (and eggs) that may be in the wings. In the meantime, you can relieve itching by giving your pet antihistamines. For dogs, vets usually recommend Benadryl—one milligram for every pound of dog, three times a day, says Karen L. Campbell, D.V.M., associate professor of dermatology and small animal internal medicine at the University of Illinois College of Veterinary Medicine at Urbana–Champaign. For cats, vets recommend Chlor-Trimeton, which contains an antihistamine called chlorpheniramine that is safer for cats. You can give half of a four-milligram tablet for every 10 pounds of cat, twice a day, she says. Be sure to check with your vet before giving human medications to pets.

"If the itching is so severe that your pet has scratched enough to cause bleeding, take her to the vet," Dr. Jeffers says. The animal could have a bacterial infection that needs quick attention.

WHAT YOUR VET WILL DO

If your vet feels that the nipple inflammation is due to an allergy, he may treat the condition with antihistimines. But if the nipples are infected, he may culture some of the fluid to identify the underlying problem. In most cases, the vet will send you home with oral or topical antibiotics. In rare cases, an infection-damaged nipple will have to be surgically removed.

ODORS

Clues

- Your pet has a skin rash or open sores.
- He has deep wrinkles or skin folds.
- He has yellowish brown scales on his elbows or around the ears.
- Your dog spends a lot of time in the water.

When your pet is starting to smell as though he ran a marathon without deodorant—and he smells this way not just occasionally, but all the time—you can be pretty sure that there is a skin problem that needs attention.

"Some skin infections can brew undetected for a long time, especially in thicker-coated pets," says Donna Angarano, D.V.M., professor of small animal surgery and medicine at Auburn University College of Veterinary Medicine in Auburn, Alabama. A sour or rancid odor is often the first sign of a skin infection, she adds.

When your nose knows that something is wrong, part the fur and take a look at the skin. Infections will usually cause boils or pimples, scaly red rashes, or even open sores, says Dr. Angarano.

Pets with a lot of wrinkles and skin folds are especially prone to skin problems. "Skin wrinkles and folds are moist and warm, providing an ideal place for bacteria and yeast to grow," says Dr. Angarano. Pugs, sharpeis, and Pekingese often get infections in their facial folds, while bulldogs tend to get them in their tail folds. Pets that are overweight also develop skin wrinkles and tend to have a higher risk of infection, she says.

Yeast infections are common in retrievers, spaniels, and other dogs that love the water, says Dr. Angarano. A quick shake doesn't always do the drying trick, leaving warm, moist areas on your pet's body (especially in the ears) where yeast love to breed. Pets that have greasy coats, allergies, or weakened immune systems are also good candidates for yeast infections, says Dr. Angarano.

Another problem that can make your pet odoriferous is seborrhea, in which the skin's oil-producing glands are overactive. Pets with this condition typically have greasy, yellowish brown scales on their elbows, hocks (ankles), and the border around their ears.

An outdoor pet that has annoyed a skunk at close range will have a truly horrendous odor. You won't need any help knowing when your pet has been "skunked." The smell is so powerful and penetrating that it can be detected literally blocks away.

WHAT YOU CAN DO

Regular baths are the best way to clear up most odor problems. "Using a harsh detergent isn't good, but regular bathing with a gentle shampoo can be a real help, especially in dogs predisposed to skin infections," says Karen L. Campbell, D.V.M., associate professor of dermatology and small animal internal medicine at the University of Illinois College of Veterinary Medicine at Urbana–Champaign. A regular pet shampoo will often do the trick, although your vet may recommend a medicated shampoo instead.

Most pets, especially dogs, will benefit from monthly baths. Dogs that are especially wrinkly, however, may need to be washed as often as once a week. After bathing, take a few minutes to dry your pet thoroughly, especially inside his skin folds. Also, clip away the hair from these areas with blunt scissors, which helps cut down on bacterial growth caused by trapped skin secretions, says Dr. Campbell.

A weekly treatment with a solution made from equal parts white vinegar and water will often help prevent yeast infections, says Dr. Angarano. The vinegar lowers the pH on the skin, creating an acid environment that is inhospitable for yeast. Store the mixture in a spray bottle and spritz it on your pet's coat, especially where there are skin folds and wrinkles. Let the solution go to work without rinsing it off. Don't forget to dab inside the ears with a cotton ball dipped in the solution, says Dr. Angarano. But don't use a cotton swab, which can damage the eardrum if it slips too far inside the ear.

Pets with seborrhea also need weekly baths, preferably with an oil-dissolving shampoo that will clean away the scales. Follow the instructions on the bottle, leaving the product on for the specified time, and then rinse well, says Dr. Campbell.

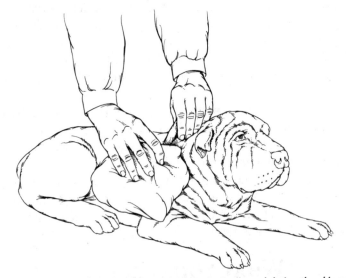

Cleaning out your dog's wrinkles and skin folds periodically and drying the skin well will help prevent bad odors from developing.

There are almost as many remedies for skunk-sprayed pets as there are skunks, says Marci Berman, a certified master groomer in Willoughby Hills, Ohio. "Forget the tomato juice and milk, which only create a bigger mess."

Pets usually get skunked when they stick their faces where they didn't belong. So the first thing to do, suggests Berman, is to rinse your pet's eyes with saline solution or water. Then scrub your pet with a mixture made with equal parts dish-washing detergent (like Dawn or Palmolive), 3 percent hydrogen peroxide, and baking soda, taking care to avoid eyes. (But continue rinsing the eyes with saline solution or water to flush away any lingering traces of skunk spray.) When you are done, rinse him thoroughly with a mixture made with equal parts red-wine vinegar and water. Don't be surprised when your pet takes on a pinkish tinge after this treatment. Red-wine vinegar will stain the fur slightly, but his usual color will come back fairly quickly. Let the vinegar dry on his coat to absorb the odor. You can rinse it off in 6 to 12 hours, or let it wear off naturally, says Berman.

Skunk spray is very hard to get rid of, Berman adds. The smell gets even worse when it rains since water reactivates the odor. She recommends mixing the vinegar-water solution and keeping it handy in a spray bottle for about six months. This makes it easy to give your pet a deodorizing spritz whenever he starts smelling lively again.

WHAT YOUR VET WILL DO

Skin infections can be simple to diagnose, although your vet may need to take skin scrapings or do a blood test to find out exactly what is causing them. Your pet may not need anything stronger than a medicated shampoo, although oral antibiotics may be necessary if the infection is severe, says Dr. Angarano. For pets with seborrhea, which are often itchy as well as smelly, your vet may prescribe a medicated shampoo, which will reduce itching and inflammation.

Pets that are unusually wrinkly and are getting frequent skin infections may need a little plastic surgery to remove excess skin. The procedure will reduce or eliminate the skin folds, making it more difficult for infections to get started.

PRESSURE SORES

Clues

- Your pet's elbows look sore or swollen.
- He is having trouble moving.

Most pets are easy sleepers and are happy to lie down whenever and wherever the urge strikes. When they decide to ease their tired bones, they will sometimes drop down and "hit the bricks," puting tremendous pressure on the skin over bony areas like on the elbows. This can lead to painful, fluid-filled pressure sores called hygromas, says John Brooks, D.V.M., a veterinarian in private practice in Fork, Maryland.

You are most likely to see this type of pressure sore on big dogs like Great Danes or mastiffs because they are usually not very graceful when they lie down; they often just drop the last few inches. Their elbows can hit the ground with as much force as a 10-pound can falling from a countertop, and their skin pays the price.

Even when they don't get pressure sores, large dogs often develop calloused skin in areas where they exert a lot of pressure—on the elbows or even over the breastbone. "Calluses are so common that they are almost normal in big dogs," says John Fioramonti, D.V.M. a veterinarian in private practice in Towson, Maryland. As long as the calluses don't turn into actual sores (and in most cases, they won't), you don't need to worry about them, he says.

Another type of pressure sore—one that is a lot more serious—is a bedsore. Also called decubital ulcers, these sores usually occur in elderly or ill pets who can't move around very much. Because they spend a lot of time in the same position, they lose circulation in parts of the skin, causing the cells to die. Bedsores are usually deep, infected, and painful and can be very hard to cure.

WHAT YOU CAN DO

There isn't a home cure for pressure sores, but there are ways to help them heal more quickly. Pets with hygromas, for example, will often get better if they are given a soft place to sleep, says Elvira L. Hall, D.V.M., a veterinarian in private practice in Odenton, Maryland. Vets often recommend using thick foam mattresses that resemble egg crates. Available in hospital supply stores and some pet catalogs, the mattresses provide good support with less pressure than flat mattresses.

Bedsores are a much more serious problem. The key to helping them heal is to keep blood flowing to areas where the sores are forming—and this means helping your pet move around a little more often, says Dr. Fioramonti. Pets with bedsores should be turned from one side to the other about every two hours. For small, minor sores, turning them once a night is probably enough.

WHAT YOUR VET WILL DO

Fluid-filled pressure sores that result from thumping down on the floor are tough to cure, says Dr. Hall. After putting your pet under general anesthesia, your vet will drain fluid from the sore, then insert a sterile rubber tube to prevent the fluid from accumulating again. If this doesn't work, your vet will probably recommend surgery to remove the fluid as well as the thick, unhealthy skin that surrounds the sore. Once the area has been cleaned up, it will heal fairly quickly.

Bedsores are even more of a problem because they tend to be badly infected. Your vet will need to clean the sores thoroughly, give topical and oral antibiotics, and possibly refer your pet to a hospital for around-the-clock care, which will include whirlpool baths and frequent turning to keep pressure off the sores.

Because bedsores usually occur in pets that are too ill to move, your vet will want to know what the underlying problem is. Expect her to take a blood sample and a variety of tests to look for internal problems such as infections or kidney failure. She will also recommend x-rays to check for arthritis, and possibly ultrasound tests to check for such things as cancer or heart failure.

SCRATCHING

Clues

- You see black specks in your pet's fur or on his belly.
- He is licking or biting his feet.
- There are bare batches in the fur or crusty sores on the skin.

When your pet's hind leg is whirling like a windmill, and the *thump, thump, thump* of his elbow is shaking the walls, you know there is a whole lot of scratching going on.

But sometimes the itch doesn't go away. So he keeps on scratching. In some cases, he will scratch so long and so hard that he will wear away the fur, making the skin red and sore.

It is not always easy to figure out why your dog or cat is scratching. It may be something as simple as a flea bite or as complex as a food allergy. In fact, allergies of one kind or another are among the most common reasons that pets scratch.

Many are allergic to fleas—a condition vets call flea-allergy dermatitis. When fleas bite, they inject a little saliva under the skin. This can induce a flood of histamine, a chemical that causes itching, runny, eyes, and other allergy symptoms. It doesn't take a lot of bites to set off this reaction. In pets with flea allergies, a single bite can trigger a week's worth of scratching.

Flea allergies usually flare in late spring and summer, when fleas are at their worst. But once your pet starts scratching, he will often get itchier and itchier, even when the fleas themselves are gone. "This can start as a seasonal thing and then become yearlong itching," says Carla L. Weinberg, D.V.M., a veterinarian in private practice in Davis, California. "The itching is usually concentrated in the back half of the animal, mainly around the rump near the base of the tail."

Food allergies also feed the itch. "Ingredients that can cause food allergies include beef, pork, and milk as well as some vegetable products," says Dr. Weinberg. Vets aren't sure why, but even pets that have been eating the same food for years may suddenly develop an allergy to one of the ingredients, she says.

In addition, some pets have hay fever and start scratching when they are exposed to pollen or even house dust, says Richard L. Headley, D.V.M., a veterinarian in private practice in Mishawaka, Indiana. A severe form of hay fever, called atopy, may occur in pets—usually dogs—that are sensitive to pollens or other airborne particles. Atopy is a very itchy condition, causing pets to scratch at their faces and armpits and to lick and bite their feet, says Dr. Weinberg.

The main problem with allergies—and the attendant scratching—is that pets can rub their skin raw, setting the stage for more-serious skin infections. All pets can get skin infections, but they are especially common in golden retrievers, German shepherds, Labrador retrievers, collies, and Saint Bernards.

Another common cause of scratching is skin mites. There are several kinds of mites, including ear mites, which live in the ears, and sarcoptic mites, which can cause itching anywhere on the skin. Dogs usually get sarcoptic mites, also known as scabies. These mites are highly contagious and readily passed from dog to dog. Cats don't get skin mites very often, but they are prone to ear mites, which can make their ears intensely itchy, says Dr. Weinberg. Pets with mites will often have other symptoms, like reddened, crusty areas of skin and possibly patches of baldness. Dogs with mites are itchiest on the chest, abdomen, legs, and the edges of the ears. In cats, the head and ears suffer the most.

WHAT YOU CAN DO

Fleas are always the first thing to suspect when your pet starts scratching. To tell if that is the problem, begin by looking at your pet's bare belly since fleas will be easier to spot there than elsewhere in the coat.

Fleas are very hard to get rid of for the simple reason that they are incredibly prolific. A few fleas can produce hundreds of thousands of offspring within a few months. What's more, for every flea that you see on your pet, there may be hundreds more in the yard, on the carpets, and in your pet's bedding. To get rid of fleas, you have to hit them everywhere they live. Here are some strategies that vets recommend.

• Bathe your pet with a medicated flea shampoo. That will send many fleas right down the drain. Products that are safe for dogs may be dangerous for cats, so be sure to read the label carefully. If your pet doesn't

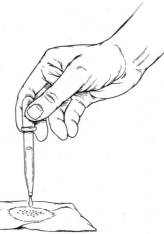

It is not always easy to tell if your pet has fleas. Here is a simple test. Look through his coat to see if there are any black specks. If there are, collect a few, put them on a piece of white paper, and moisten them with a little water. Fleas drink blood, and their wastes will turn red when they get wet.

cooperate, you can take him to the groomer for the bath. It is a good idea to wash your pet's bedding as well.

- Pull a flea comb through your pet's coat once a day. In between strokes, dip the comb in a bowl of soapy water to drown the fleas. This will remove many of the critters that are causing the scratching, says Dr. Weinberg.
- Use over-the-counter flea sprays and powders. Vets often recommend products that contain D-limonene or pyrethrins, which are effective and less toxic than some other chemicals. Flea collars will help as well.
- "Bomb" your house with a product containing a flea-larvae growth regulator such as Precor, following the directions on the label.
- Talk to your vet about long-lasting flea-control medications. Oral medications like Program, for example, contain a medication that prevents flea eggs from hatching. Other products, such as Advantage and Frontline, are applied to your pet's skin and will kill adult fleas for a month or more.

In the short run, the only way to stop your pet's scratching is to halt the itching. A lukewarm bath can be very soothing, especially if you use an oatmeal shampoo or add a little colloidal oatmeal (like Aveeno) to the water, says David A. Gordon, D.V.M., a veterinarian in private practice in Lake Forest, California. Cats, of course, hate getting wet even more than they hate itching. One way to keep them calm for a bath is to put something in the tub that they can grip, like a plastic milk crate or a rubber mat.

To relieve the discomfort of sores caused by scratching, apply some aloe vera several times a day, says Dr. Gordon. You can buy aloe vera creams or gels, but the juice from the plant is usually more effective and possibly safer, he adds.

If you suspect that your pet has ear mites—a telltale sign is an accumulation of dark-colored debris in the ears—you will need to clean the ears thoroughly and apply a mite-killing medication, available at pet supply stores, following the directions on the label.

WHAT YOUR VET WILL DO

If you treat your pet for fleas and the scratching continues, your vet will probably recommend an allergy test—shaving off a little fur and injecting some common allergens under the skin. The skin reaction tells your vet what your pet is allergic to and what he will need to avoid in the future.

One problem is that many common allergens, like pollen, are nearly impossible to avoid. Your vet may recommend over-the-counter antihistamines like Benadryl or Chlor-Trimeton, which will help relieve the itching. Ask your vet which antihistamine is most likely to be effective and how much of it you will need to give.

Food allergies are among the toughest allergies to diagnose. To identify food allergies, your vet will help you put your pet on an elimination diet, says Dr. Headley. You start with a new food having none of the ingredients in his usual chow. Within a few weeks, your pet may stop scratching. Then your vet will begin introducing various kinds of protein, one at a time, to see if the scratching flares up again. When it does, you will know what ingredient you will need to avoid in the future, he explains.

Pets with scabies usually need a series of insecticidal dips. In some cases, your vet may use oral medications to fight the mites from the inside out, says Donna Angarano, D.V.M., professor of small animal surgery and medicine at Auburn University College of Veterinary Medicine in Auburn, Alabama.

Skin sores that are caused by scratching will often need to be treated to speed healing. In some cases, your vet will apply a cortisone spray to reduce inflammation. For infections, your pet may need antibiotics as well, says Leslie Sinclair, D.V.M., director of Companion Animal Care for the Humane Society of the United States in Washington, D.C. Though antibiotics are often given orally, your vet may recommend using an antibacterial ointment or shampoo instead.

See also Chapter 7: Scratching and Shaking; Chapter 13: Black Specks in Fur

| SYMPTOM | # SHEDDING |

Clues

- Your pet is shedding heavily all year.
- Clumps of fur are appearing on the floor or furniture.
- She has dry, flaky skin.

The carpet looks like it came from a barber shop, and your silk skirt is starting to resemble mohair. From the looks of things, your pets are having one heck of a "bad hair day."

Dogs and cats shed hair all the time. But the rate and volume of shedding increases significantly in the warm months, when temperatures rise and they get more sunlight, says Ann Hohenhaus, D.V.M., a veterinarian in private practice in New York City. All cats shed, and there is not much difference among breeds. Dogs vary more. Those originally bred for cool climates, like huskies and collies, are notorious shedders, and female dogs that have just had a litter will also shed heavily.

Since pets always shed, it is not easy to tell from looking at the furniture if they are shedding more than usual. Here is a simple test: pull gently on your pet's hair. You should get some hair, but just a few strands—not big tufts. "In an excessive shed, a large number of hairs can be removed," says Richard L. Headley, D.V.M., a veterinarian in private practice in Mishawaka, Indiana.

Heavy shedding may be caused by hormonal problems such as hypothyroidism (in which the thyroid gland produces too little hormone) or Cushing's disease (in which the pituitary gland triggers the release of too much cortisol). Chow Chows and Pomeranians are particularly prone to hormonal problems.

WHAT YOU CAN DO

Most shedding means that your pet is doing what nature intended—taking off her coat when the seasons change. To keep things a little bit cleaner, you need to brush her often. Once a day is best, although you can get by with once or twice a week, says Dr. Headley.

You will need a good brush. Many vets recommend using a slicker brush, which has bent wire bristles. The bristles help trap hair so that it doesn't drift from your pet to the carpet.

Since pets shed more in warm weather, you can help reduce shedding by creating a more wintry state. "Try to keep the temperature cooler and keep the lights off longer," Dr. Headley suggests.

Another way to reduce shedding is to make sure that you are giving your pet a high-quality commercial food, says Dr. Headley. This will make the coat look healthier as well. You may also want to add fatty-acid sup-

GROOMING TOOLS

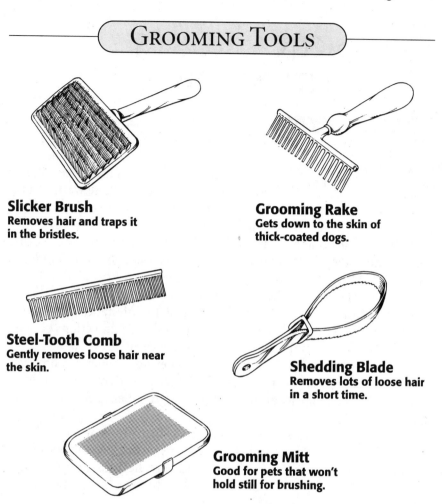

Slicker Brush
Removes hair and traps it
in the bristles.

Grooming Rake
Gets down to the skin of
thick-coated dogs.

Steel-Tooth Comb
Gently removes loose hair near
the skin.

Shedding Blade
Removes lots of loose hair
in a short time.

Grooming Mitt
Good for pets that won't
hold still for brushing.

plements to your pet's diet. These supplements are available from vets, pet supply stores, and health food stores. Fatty acids are good for the coat and can help cut down on shedding. Ask your vet which supplements (and doses) he recommends.

WHAT YOUR VET WILL DO

Virtually any illness can cause an increase in shedding, but hormonal problems are always a likely offender, says Dr. Headley. Your vet will need to run blood tests to check if your pet has the proper balance of the various hormones.

Untreated, hormonal problems can be extremely serious. While medications can help control the imbalances, your pet will probably need to take the drugs for the rest of her life.

Skin Crusts and Scabs

Clues

- Your pet is scratching a lot.
- There are white flakes or round bare patches in her coat.

Pets get cuts and scrapes just as often as people do, and their skin responds in the same way: by forming scabs to seal the wound. But sometimes you will see scabs or a bit of crust even where there wasn't an injury—at least, not one that you could see— and that makes it difficult to figure out why.

In dogs, scabs that appear on the belly or chest and spread to other parts of the body are often caused by a bacterial infection, says Randall S. Dugal, D.V.M., a veterinarian in private practice in Royal Palm Beach, Florida. Dogs tend to get these infections when something else has weakened their immune systems—anything from a flea infestation to a thyroid problem, or even cancer, he says. Fleas can also lead to infections because dogs will often scratch themselves raw to get at the itch.

Cats rarely get bacterial skin infections. They do get allergies, however, which can cause crusty bumps to appear on their heads or necks or down their backs. "The majority of the time, it is a sign of flea allergies," says Dr. Dugal.

In both dogs and cats, fungal infections such as ringworm can also be the culprit, says Dr. Dugal. You can suspect ringworm when you see one or two isolated patches that are round and bare, he adds. Some cats can be asymptomatic carriers, which means that they can spread the fungus without showing any signs of having it.

Mites are harder to recognize, with one exception: A kind of mite known as walking dandruff will cause bare patches and large white flakes on the neck and back. All pets can get walking dandruff, but it is most common in puppies.

What You Can Do

The easiest way to soothe crusty, irritated skin is to soak a washcloth in a mixture of cool water and colloidal oatmeal (like Aveeno) and apply it to the area for a few minutes. Once the crusts and scabs soften, they will often come right off.

Another approach is to apply a dab of over-the-counter hydrocortisone ointment. "That will help stop the itching and allow the area to heal," says Thomas P. Lewis II, D.V.M., a veterinary dermatologist in private practice in Mesa, Arizona. If your pet will put up with it, it is a good idea to bathe crusty areas with cool water and an antibacterial shampoo. This will wash away germs and help the skin heal more quickly.

Some parasites and fungal infections can be treated at home with medicated shampoos and ointments. When you are treating your pet for ringworm, however, remember that it is highly contagious. You may have to treat all your pets to stop it from making the rounds again. Ringworm isn't only contagious from pet to pet but also from pet to human. "Keep children away from pets with ringworm since their immune systems are less able to resist it," says Dr. Dugal.

WHAT YOUR VET WILL DO

Some parasites can be killed with over-the-counter medications, but others need something stronger. This may involve giving your pet oral medications and bringing her to the vet's office several times a month for a powerful anti-parasitic dip. Parasites can be tenacious, so you will need patience to get rid of them all.

If your vet suspects that the problem is internal, he may recommend a blood test or skin biopsy. Your pet may be tested for allergies as well. Once your vet figures out what is causing the scabs or crusting, he will recommend a complete treatment plan. If it turns out that your pet is allergic, she may need a series of allergy shots. For bacterial infections, of course, she is probably going to need antibiotics—either given orally or applied to the skin. Your pet will also need to be treated for the underlying problem that is allowing her skin to act up.

See also Chapter 13: Fur Loss, Scratching

SYMPTOM) **SORES**

Clues

- Your dog is constantly licking his paws or flanks.
- He has sores on the tips of the ears or other lightly furred areas.

Skin is tough and durable, but it isn't damage-proof. Almost any minor injury—from cuts and scrapes to scratching too hard at a flea bite—can cause a sore. Sores look ugly and are often painful, but they usually heal within in a few days. A sore that doesn't heal means that something more serious is going on.

A particularly troublesome type of sore is called a lick granuloma. Most common in middle-aged or older large-breed dogs like Labrador retrievers, lick granulomas occur when a dog constantly licks the same spot—usually on the paws, wrists, or ankles, says James Jeffers, V.M.D., a veterinary dermatologist in private practice Gaithersburg, Maryland. The constant moisture and friction can cause a deep, painful sore. And the more the sore hurts, the more the dog licks. It can take months for lick granulomas to finally heal. Even then, the fur doesn't always grow back, he says.

Vets aren't sure what causes dogs to become obsessed with licking. Boredom and anxiety may play a role. Dogs will also lick to relieve long-term discomfort such as that caused by allergies or arthritis, says Dr. Jeffers. Even when the pain is gone, they may keep licking out of habit, he adds.

Skin infections can also cause sores, especially in dogs, says Donna Angarano, D.V.M., professor of small animal surgery and medicine at Auburn University College of Veterinary Medicine in Auburn, Alabama. "Dogs have trouble keeping normal skin bacteria under control," she explains. Pets with weakened immune systems will often develop sores because normal bacteria populations on the skin are able to reproduce out of control, she adds.

Sores can also be caused by ringworm (a fungal infection), skin mites, allergies, or hormonal problems like low thyroid levels. Sores that won't heal are particularly worrisome because they may be a sign of cancer. Cancerous sores often appear on the face or ears—areas that get the most sun—and are common in white cats.

WHAT YOU CAN DO

It is difficult to treat lick granulomas because dogs won't leave the areas alone. The most important thing is to prevent further licking, which can cause infection. To stop your dog from worrying the wound, it is a good idea to fit him with an Elizabethan collar. These cone-shaped collars, available in pet supply stores, will prevent him from licking and will give the sores a chance to heal, says Dr. Angarano. The collars come in different sizes, so be sure to get the size that is right for your pet.

Another way to stop your dog from licking a sore is to use a bandage, says Dr. Jeffers. An elastic bandage wrapped loosely over the sore area works well, as does a sock with the toe cut out. You can fasten the bandage with white first-aid tape or masking tape wrapped in a spiral, with the last "turn" taped directly on your pet's leg, says Dr. Jeffers. Change the dressing when it gets dirty. Once the sore has healed, you can remove the bandage.

Pets with mites or other parasites need to be dipped or washed with a medicated shampoo every couple of weeks for six weeks or so. (Pets with ringworm usually need four or more baths a month.) The shampoos and dips aren't interchangeable, Dr. Angarano adds. Before you start spending money, ask your vet which active ingredient you will need to get your pet's parasites under control.

Baths do more than eliminate parasites, adds Tiffany Tapp, D.V.M., a veterinarian in private practice in Garden Grove, California. They also make the skin less itchy and can help sores heal, especially if you are using a medicated shampoo. Adding a little colloidal oatmeal (like Aveeno) to the water will make the baths even more soothing, she says. Be sure to rinse your pet thoroughly after a bath. Otherwise, the irritation will get even worse.

Finally, it is a good idea to clip the fur surrounding moist sores with blunt-nosed scissors. This allows more air to circulate, which will help the sores heal more quickly.

WHAT YOUR VET WILL DO

One way that your vet can tell what is causing sores is to remove a little bit of skin and examine it under a microscope. In addition, she may recommend sending a bit of tissue to a laboratory to check for cancer. She will also take blood to check for internal problems such as lupus. Your vet might recommend allergy tests as well.

Even though skin mites and other parasites can often be treated at home, any infestation that is serious enough to cause sores probably needs to be treated by your vet, who will use powerful medicated dips, says Dr. Angarano. Pets with parasites will often need to be dipped several times, she adds. Your pet may need oral medications as well.

See also Chapter 10: Foot Licking; Chapter 13: Fur Loss, Scratching

COMMON SKIN AND COAT CONDITIONS

Allergies. You can spot people with allergies because they are the ones blowing their noses and wiping their eyes. Pets with allergies, on the other hand, get very itchy. And the worse the allergy is, the more furiously they scratch.

Dogs and cats can develop allergies to just about anything, including pollen or ingredients in their food. Allergies can cause serious discomfort, and some pets will scratch themselves raw. It is worth taking a little time to figure out what is putting your pet's hind leg in perpetual motion.

One way to tell what kind of allergies your pet has is to watch *where* he scratches. Allergies to pollen usually cause itching around the armpits, paws, or head, says Randall S. Dugal, D.V.M., a veterinarian in private practice in Royal Palm Beach, Florida. Flea allergies usually cause itching on the back near the tail, he adds. And food allergies can cause itching almost anywhere on the body.

Once you know what is causing the itching, you will have to find ways to help your pet avoid it. In the meantime, vets often recommend giving an antihistamine, which will help relieve itching and other allergy symptoms. For dogs, Benadryl can be very helpful. The usual dose is one milligram for every pound of dog, three times a day, says Karen L. Campbell, D.V.M., associate professor of dermatology and small animal internal medicine at the University of Illinois College of Veterinary Medicine at Urbana–Champaign. For cats, vets recommend Chlor-Trimeton, which contains an antihistamine called chlorpheniramine that is safer for cats. You can give half of a four-milligram tablet for every 10 pounds of cat, twice a day, she says. To be safe, check with your vet before giving human medications to pets.

Autoimmune conditions. The immune system is constantly battling foreign invaders like bacteria and viruses, and usually it does a good job fending them off. But in pets with autoimmune conditions such as lupus, the immune system loses its aim. Rather than only attacking germs, it also goes after the body's healthy tissues. In dogs and cats, it is often the skin that gets in the line of fire, resulting in painful sores or blisters that seemingly come out of nowhere.

Autoimmune conditions may affect the whole body and can be difficult to treat. Vets often recommend applying hydrocortisone or other anti-inflammatory ointments to soothe the skin. You can also give your pet periodic soaks in a soothing mix of cool water and colloidal oatmeal (like Aveeno), says Dr. Campbell. In the long run, however, pets with autoimmune problems generally need more powerful treatments, such as oral medications that suppress the immune system and keep the attacks under control.

Fleas. Some pets get fleas and never seem to mind. But many dogs and cats are actually allergic to fleas—even one bite can make them intensely itchy.

Fleas have always been tough to get rid of. In the past, the only effective treatment was to use a combination of sprays, powders, shampoos, collars, and other products. But in recent years researchers have developed new flea products—such as the oral medication Program or a topical medication like Advantage—that are much more effective than their predecessors. It is worth using these new products, and not only because of the itching. Fleas are the main carriers of tapeworms. Pets with fleas are constantly licking or biting their coats. When they swallow an infected flea, they will get infected with tapeworms as well.

Hair-follicle cysts. Every hair on your pet's hide grows out of a tiny structure in the skin called a hair follicle. Sometimes these follicles get plugged with microscopic bits of skin or hair. This causes them to swell like little balloons, forming lumps beneath the skin. These lumps, called hair-follicle cysts, can be as small as the point of a pen or as large as the end of a crayon.

Finding a lump is always scary, but hair-follicle cysts aren't cancer. They aren't usually painful, and they don't cause long-term problems. And these cysts may go away on their own once they break open and drain. Don't try to get rid of them by squeezing because that can cause an infection beneath the skin, says Richard K. Anderson, D.V.M., a veterinary dermatologist at the Angell Memorial Animal Hospital in Boston.

Hormone imbalance. Hormones are extraordinarily powerful chemicals. Even tiny amounts can have powerful effects, which is why veterinarians use sophisticated tests to make sure that the body is producing the proper amounts. But you can also spot some hormonal problems at home. For example, when the thyroid gland fails to produce enough of the hormone thyroxin, your pet may lose hair or develop dry, flaky skin.

Another hormonal problem, called Cushing's disease, occurs when the adrenal gland produces too much cortisol. This can cause symptoms ranging from excessive thirst and frequent urination to a distended belly. In addition, pets with Cushing's disease tend to get sick a lot because it weakens the immune system.

It doesn't happen often, but pets that produce too much estrogen may lose fur along their flanks and belly, and their remaining fur may feel greasy. High estrogen levels are sometimes caused by ovarian cysts in cats and testicular tumors in male dogs or cats. Conversely, spayed females will occasionally produce too little estrogen. This also causes the fur to get thinner. In addition, the underlying skin may get thin and fragile.

There are different treatments for hormone imbalances, depending on the hormone and on whether your pet is producing too much or too little. Pets with low amounts of thyroid hormone usually need to take supplements for the rest of their lives. Cushing's disease is often treated with drugs that cause the adrenal gland to produce less cortisol. Pets with high estrogen levels, on the other hand, often need surgery because this condition is usually caused by tumors. Once the tumor is removed, estrogen levels should return to normal. Pets that produce too little estrogen, on the other hand, are better left untreated because estrogen supplements can cause dangerous side effects, says Donna Angarano, D.V.M., professor of small animal surgery and medicine at Auburn University College of Veterinary Medicine in Auburn, Alabama.

Mites. Mites are microscopic parasites that live on your pet's skin. There are several kinds of mites, including demodex and sarcoptic (scabies) mites. Demodex mites are permanent residents in your dog's hair follicles. (They live on humans, too, in the eyebrow follicles.) Most of the time, they are not a problem. But when your dog gets sick or stressed, his immune system gets weaker, which allows demodex mites to get stronger.

Demodex mites don't cause much itching, and mild cases will usually go away on their own, says Dr. Angarano. But a bad case can cause bacteria to attack the skin resulting in painful, open sores. It can take a long time—using medicated shampoos, antibiotics, and other medications—to get demodex under control.

Sarcoptic mites, on the other hand, cause pets to scratch themselves silly. Crusty patches may appear around the ears, elbows, and legs. This condition, also known as scabies, is often tough to diagnose. But once your vet knows that it is the problem, it is usually easy to treat.

Dogs and cats with scabies usually need a series of insecticidal dips. In some cases, your vet may use oral medications to fight the mites from the inside out, says Dr. Angarano.

Ringworm. Ringworm is a fungus that can wreak havoc on your pet's skin and coat, especially in adolescent dogs and cats. It often causes fur to fall out in circular patches, and the skin underneath can get red and crusty. And because it is contagious, you will rarely have just one pet with ringworm—other pets in the family can catch it, too. So can the human members of the family, Dr. Angarano adds. That is why it is important to wear disposable gloves and to wash your hands often when treating pets with ringworm, she advises.

Despite its ugly appearance, ringworm isn't particularly uncomfortable, but it can take a long time to go away. Most pets will need anti-ringworm dips or shampoos, and possibly oral medications. "Be very careful to keep young children away from ringworm-infected pets because the infection can spread quite easily to them," Dr. Angarano warns.

Seborrhea. Some pets have oil glands that are perpetually overactive. They churn out far more oil than the skin needs, particularly on the elbows, ankles, and around the ears. This condition, called seborrhea, results in greasy scales. Bacteria and yeast flourish on these scales, which is why pets with seborrhea often have an unpleasant odor.

Seborrhea usually accompanies other, more-serious conditions, like hormonal imbalances or infestations with parasites, although some pets seem to get it for no clear reason.

Seborrhea isn't dangerous, but it can make your pet very itchy and increase his risk for skin infections. "Bathing your pet every week with an oil-dissolving shampoo can be a big help when you are treating seborrhea," says Dr. Angarano.

Skin cancer. Dogs and cats don't spend their days on beach towels ordering margaritas and working on their tans. But many pets love the sun, and it is just as dangerous for them as it is for people. Too much sun exposure can dramatically raise the risk for skin cancer, especially on lightly furred areas—around the mouth, for example, or on the tips of the ears.

In people, cancerous skin changes are easy to see. In pets, however, fur often masks the problem until it is well-advanced and much more dangerous. Vets recommend periodically giving your four-legged sun-worshipper a careful once-over, parting the fur and looking for areas that are darker than the surrounding skin or for sores that never seem to heal. "Any change in color should be checked by a vet right away," says Thomas P. Lewis II, D.V.M., a veterinary dermatologist in private practice in Mesa, Arizona.

Skin infections. Skin infections usually aren't serious, but they can make dogs and cats itchy and sore. Dogs get skin infections much more often than cats, and some breeds, like bulldogs and shar-peis, get them the most because their wrinkly skin traps moisture and infection-causing bacteria.

You can prevent or reduce some skin infections by periodically bathing your pet with a medicated shampoo, says Dr. Angarano. Different ingredients are used for different types of infections, so be sure to ask your vet which product is best for your pet.

Whole Body

In the best mystery novels, the clue that solves the crime isn't all that obvious. It is usually a little thing: a bit of mud on the carpet, a weather report, a scrap of paper in a drawer. It is only later in the novel, when the clue gets the attention it deserves, that the entire mystery falls into place.

Whole-body symptoms are often like that. Signs that are seemingly trivial, such as lethargy, stiffness, or a little weight gain, may turn out to be profoundly important. In fact, even seemingly minor symptoms like fatigue may be early signs of serious illnesses.

Pets can't tell you when something is wrong. They can't explain that they are losing weight because their teeth hurt or that they are shaking because of a viral infection. It is up to you to play Sherlock Holmes by noticing any change in your pet's health or behavior and asking yourself what could be causing it.

This chapter covers some of the whole-body symptoms that you are most likely to see, along with some important clues for solving the case.

See Your Vet If:

- Your pet has been hit by a car or has taken a bad fall, even if she seems fine afterward.
- She is acting confused and disoriented.
- The joints are swollen or tender.
- Her sleep patterns have suddenly changed.
- She is fainting or having seizures.
- Your pet has gotten wobbly or clumsy.
- She is stiff or sore for no apparent reason.
- Her abdomen is bloated or feels tight.
- Your pet is pregnant and overdue or has passed a dead kitten or puppy.
- Her feet are cold or swollen.
- Her skin, gums, or mucous membranes are turning yellow.
- Your pet is reluctant to move or can't stand up.
- She is shivering or shaking even when it isn't cold.

CLUMSINESS

Clues

- **The clumsiness came on very suddenly.**
- **Your pet wobbles when he walks.**
- **He is dazed and disoriented.**

No one has ever mistaken your puppy for Fred Astaire. His feet are too big for his body, and his enthusiasm is greater than his common sense. He runs, gains speed, then *kerplunk*—does a belly flop right on the carpet.

It is natural for puppies to be clumsy. They are experiencing very rapid bone growth and haven't quite learned to coordinate their various parts, says John Saidla, D.V.M., director of continuing education at the College of Veterinary Medicine at Cornell University in Ithaca, New York. Breeds mature at different rates, but puppies between the ages of five and nine months are usually the most uncoordinated. "Teenage humans are clumsy, and teenage dogs are clumsy," he says.

As dogs age, however, they develop good muscular control. The same goes for cats: Kittens are pretty good on their feet, and they get even more graceful as they get older. So if your pet is suddenly showing signs of clumsiness, there is probably something wrong.

In cats, a loss of coordination could be caused by a mineral imbalance. In older cats particularly, the kidneys may remove too much potassium from the body. Since potassium (along with sodium) are critical for muscular control, an imbalance could cause the hindquarters to sag, making him clumsy and unsteady, says Dr. Saidla.

Hip dysplasia is a common cause of clumsiness in dogs and an occasional one in cats. This is an inherited condition in which the hipbones don't fit together the way that they should, and the hips wobble. Pets with hip dysplasia may have difficulty getting up, and their walk is often ungainly. Large breeds of dogs like German shepherds and golden retrievers are particularly prone to hip dysplasia. Among cats, Persians are most at risk, Dr. Saidla says.

Perhaps the most serious cause of clumsiness is poisoning. Pets that have gotten into antifreeze or other harmful chemicals will often appear clumsy, disoriented, and dazed because of damage to the nervous system, says Sheldon A. Steinberg, V.M.D., professor of neurology at the University of Pennsylvania School of Veterinary Medicine in Philadelphia.

WHAT YOU CAN DO

If your pet has hip dysplasia, there are many things that you can do to reduce the discomfort and, just as important, keep it from getting worse.

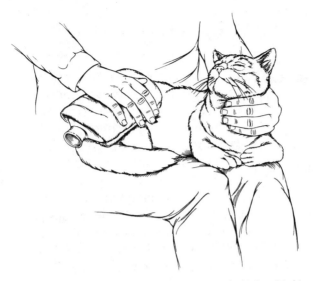

Heat can work wonders for your pet's aches and pains. When his hips are acting up, hold a hot-water bottle (filled with warm, not hot water) over the area for 10 minutes or so until he is feeling better.

Regular exercise—and, for pets that are overweight, slimming down—are very helpful for dogs and cats with hip dysplasia. Even if your pet isn't able to charge around the way he used to, taking regular walks will help lubricate the joint and strengthen the muscles that hold it together. This will reduce pain as well as prevent wear and tear on the joints, says Dr. Saidla. In addition, giving an occasional massage to your pet and applying heat—from warm-water bottles, for example—can be very soothing for pets with hip pain.

The one good thing about hip dysplasia is that it usually comes on slowly, and vets are alert to the warning signs, so there is plenty of time to take action. When clumsiness comes on very suddenly, however, there is a good chance that your pet has gotten into something dangerous, and you should get him to the vet immediately, says Dr. Steinberg.

What Your Vet Will Do

If your older cat has suddenly become clumsy, your vet will probably recommend blood tests to check for mineral imbalances or kidney problems, says Dr. Saidla. If he is low in potassium, supplements may be all that he will need to move gracefully again and, more important, to keep the kidneys in good shape.

Your vet will watch your pet walk around and observe how tight or sloppy the hip joints are. If the problem seems to be hip dysplasia, the vet will probably take x-rays to see how serious it is.

For young dogs that are showing signs of hip dysplasia, vets sometimes recommend reducing the amount of protein in their diets. This will help the bones grow more slowly and with better fit. For an older dog, your vet may recommend medications as well as a careful exercise program. Over-the-counter medications may be helpful, although some dogs will need more-powerful drugs to relieve pain and reduce swelling, says Dr. Saidla. In severe cases, pets may need surgery to repair or rebuild the damaged joint.

Poisoning is always an emergency, but there is a good chance for recovery if you get your pet to the vet right away, says Dennis O'Brien, D.V.M., Ph.D., a neurologist in the department of veterinary medicine and surgery at the University of Missouri College of Veterinary Medicine in Columbia. Before calling the vet, take a minute to figure out what your pet may have gotten into. This will make it easier for your vet to begin treatment as soon as you get to the office.

Don't try to make your pet vomit before calling your vet, Dr. Saidla adds. Make the phone call first. Your vet will know if vomiting is the best thing to do—or if you should try to get your pet to the office a little bit quicker. (For information on when to induce vomiting, see "Purging the Poison" on page 33.)

For poisons such as antifreeze, vomiting will eliminate some of the danger, and that is what your vet may recommend. To make your pet vomit, give about one teaspoon of 3 percent hydrogen peroxide for every 10 pounds of pet. (You can squirt it down his throat using a turkey baster.) He will probably vomit within a few minutes, says Steve Hansen, D.V.M., vice president of the American Society for the Prevention of Cruelty to Animals' National Animal Poison Control Center in Urbana, Illinois.

See also Chapter 10: Difficulty Getting Up; Chapter 14: Joint Swelling, Stiffness

CONFUSION

- Your pet seems disoriented and lost, even in familiar places.
- You have been using household cleaners or other chemicals.

Maybe he seems lost as he wanders from room to room. Or perhaps he can't find his food or water, or he has forgotten all his house training, or he seems nervous when you leave him alone. Confusion can be very frightening, both for you and for your pet.

When confusion lasts for more than a day or two, there could be a neurological problem, says Charles Lowrie, D.V.M., associate professor of neurology and neural surgery at the Veterinary Teaching Hospital at Michigan State University College of Veterinary Medicine in East Lansing. In older pets, it may be a sign of senility, a condition in which brain functions gradually diminish. A brain tumor can also result in mental confusion, he says.

Anything that puts pressure on the brain, like a tumor or an infection, can cause pets to become disoriented, says John Saidla, D.V.M., director of continuing education at the College of Veterinary Medicine at Cornell University in Ithaca, New York. Canine distemper, a viral infection, can sometimes cause confusion. So can hypoglycemia or diabetes, conditions in which not enough sugar reaches the brain, he says.

Temporary confusion may be nothing more than a reaction to an upsetting change such as when you are preparing to take a trip or when out-of-town guests have come to stay, says Dr. Lowrie. All pets can experience this type of confusion, but it is much more common in dogs than in cats.

Dogs and cats have thinner skulls than people do, and even minor injuries that can occur from falling off a ledge, for instance, can bruise the brain, causing confusion, says Dr. Saidla.

Finally, pets may experience confusion if they get into something that they shouldn't, like antifreeze or household cleaners. In fact, some pets get wobbly and confused merely from being around chemicals—in a room sprayed with pesticides or even in a new motor home that was sprayed with Scotchgard. Bites from a snake, spider, or scorpion can cause confusion, too. Any type of poisoning is extremely serious and should be treated by a veterinarian immediately.

WHAT YOU CAN DO

Mental confusion is a serious symptom and should always be a signal to take your pet to the vet. Even if your pet is elderly, don't assume that the problem is old age. Old dogs and cats shouldn't be confused by their surroundings, says Dr. Saidla. If they are, there is something wrong.

Of course, if the diagnosis *is* senility, you can't do much. Just keep your pet comfortable, safe, and reassured. Confused pets are often frightened pets, and giving them extra attention will help them stay calm and relaxed, says Dr. Lowrie.

Rearranging the furniture can heighten your pet's confusion, Dr. Saidla adds. Try to keep his surroundings the same. Knowing where everything is—including his food and water bowls—will help him feel more secure.

When your dog or cat goes outside, keep him on a leash, even if he used to play unsupervised, Dr. Lowrie adds.

Keeping your dog's vaccinations up-to-date is the only way to prevent canine distemper. Your vet will give the shots, but it is up to you to get your pet to the vet when the injections are due. It is worth doing because there isn't a cure for this viral illness. A few minutes of prevention now will help ensure that he stays sharp and alert later on.

WHAT YOUR VET WILL DO

Confusion can be caused by a variety of illnesses. In addition to a general physical exam, your vet may include a neurological exam to check the nervous system, brain, and spinal cord. She will probably take blood to check blood sugar levels and to see if there are harmful chemicals in the bloodstream. Your vet may recommend other, more-advanced tests, such as the MRI (magnetic resonance imaging) brain scan, which can detect small tumors or inflammation in the brain.

If there is a brain tumor, your vet may need to take a biopsy to determine if the tumor is harmful or not, and whether additional treatments like surgery, radiation, or chemotherapy will be needed.

If it turns out that your pet has low blood sugar, there are a number of medications, including insulin, that will help restore the blood sugar to healthy levels. In addition, your vet may recommend putting your pet on a special diet and exercise plan, which also will help keep blood sugar in balance.

For head injuries, your pet will probably need x-rays to find out where (and how serious) the problem is. Your vet may recommend that your pet stay in the office for a day or two, just in case there is a skull fracture or blood clot. In rare cases, surgery may be needed to repair damage to the brain or skull, says Dr. Saidla.

There are many different treatments for poisoning, including activated charcoal, which absorbs poisons inside the stomach, as well as medications that cause vomiting.

See also Chapter 14: Clumsiness

FAINTING

Clues

- Your pet's tongue or gums have a blue tint.
- She has been exposed to insecticides or other chemicals.

People faint for all kinds of reasons: the sight of blood, for example, or getting a glimpse of a favorite movie star. Unlike tender-hearted humans, however, dogs and cats don't simply swoon. If they pass out, there is something physically wrong with them, says John Saidla, D.V.M., director of continuing education at the College of Veterinary Medicine at Cornell University in Ithaca, New York.

Fainting usually occurs when blood flow to the brain temporarily slows or stops. This may be caused by a condition called heart block, in which the heart's electrical signals are suddenly interrupted. Dogs are more likely than cats to experience heart block, and schnauzers, which have an unusually narrow aorta (a major blood vessel leading from the heart), are particularly susceptible, says Dr. Saidla.

While heart problems are the main cause of fainting, there are a number of other conditions that can cause dogs and cats to lose consciousness. Pets with epilepsy, for example, may pass out when they have seizures, says Dr. Saidla. This is more than just fainting, however, since seizures are usually accompanied by other symptoms such as kicking, shaking, or urinating, he explains.

A pet may lose consciousness if she bangs her head or gets something in her windpipe that is blocking the flow of air, says Ronald Stone, D.V.M., a veterinarian and clinical assistant professor of surgery at the University of Miami School of Medicine in Florida. If you have recently painted your house or sprayed for pests, the concentrated fumes could cause fainting. Fumes that are strong enough to cause fainting are potentially strong enough to damage the lungs, so you need to see your vet right away, he adds.

Finally, pets with a neurological disorder called narcolepsy may suddenly fall over and fall asleep without warning. "One of our students has a narcoleptic dog, and if you clap your hands or startle that dog, he's going to pass out," says Dr. Saidla. Narcolepsy usually isn't dangerous, although a pet may fall asleep in a dangerous place, like on a stairway or in the street, he says.

WHAT YOU CAN DO

Even though fainting itself usually isn't a problem, the conditions that cause it often are, so it is critical to call your vet immediately. In the meantime, there are things that you can do to help your vet figure out what's wrong, says Dr. Stone.

Take a look inside your pet's mouth. If the tongue or gums are blue, she probably wasn't getting enough oxygen. This is an excellent test, but only if you are careful with your fingers. "An unconscious cat or dog can still clamp her jaw down hard," says Dr. Stone. If you can't see inside your pet's mouth, check the whites of the eyes, the inside of the eyelids, the vagina of a female, or the penile sheath of a male. If they are blue, a lack of oxygen is probably to blame.

If your pet has been diagnosed with narcolepsy, about the only thing you can do is to make sure that your pet is always in a safe place so that she won't get hurt if she suddenly falls asleep. If you have a swimming pool, for example, keep your pet away from it when you are not nearby. It is also a good idea to keep her away from stairs, balconies, and other high or uneven places since a pet can take a bad tumble if an attack comes at the wrong time, says Dr. Saidla.

Pets that have fainted because something is stuck in the windpipe can often be revived if you perform the Heimlich maneuver, a procedure in which you press on their sides and create enough internal pressure to "blow" the object out. (For information on doing the Heimlich maneuver, see "Choking" on page 28.)

What Your Vet Will Do

If your pet is still unconscious when you reach the office, your vet will begin by making sure that she is getting enough air. He will also ask a lot of questions: Did your pet run into anything? If it is a cat, did she fall from a tree? How often has she fainted before? Has she been tired, short of breath, or generally under the weather recently?

Since seizures can cause pets to lose consciousness, your vet may recommend tests to see if epilepsy is to blame, says Dr. Saidla. He will also check your pet's respiratory and circulatory systems to make sure that she is getting enough blood to the brain.

If it turns out that your pet has heart problems, she may need medications to help the heart beat more efficiently. For heart block, an implanted pacemaker can be very effective, adds Dr. Saidla. While some vets do the procedure themselves, heart surgery is usually done by a veterinarian who specializes in cardiology.

See also Chapter 14: Seizures

HEARTBEAT IRREGULARITY

Clues

- Your pet has fainted or seems fatigued.
- Her heartbeat seems more irregular than usual.

The heart does an astonishing amount of work. It can beat about 145,000 times a day in dogs and more than 170,000 times in cats. With every beat it pushes blood, oxygen, and nutrients throughout the body. If you happen to notice a pause or skip in your pet's heartbeat, you need to pay closer attention since even small changes in its predictable pace can have dangerous consequences.

There are probably a hundred reasons for uneven heartbeats, and not all of them are serious. Some dogs, for example, have a perfectly harmless condition called sinus arrhythmia, in which the heart periodically beats a little faster than usual, then slows down. Pets with this condition are basically healthy since the heart manages to keep blood flowing even when the beat is uneven, says William D. Tyrell, D.V.M., a veterinarian in private practice in Annapolis, Maryland.

Other kinds of heartbeat irregularities are more serious. For example, pets with a condition called sick sinus syndrome will sometimes have long pauses between beats or periods when their hearts speed up. The heart's poor rhythm means that blood has trouble getting to the brain and other organs, which can cause a pet to faint. Sick sinus syndrome usually occurs in pets with severe heart disease, and schnauzers, boxers, cocker spaniels, dachshunds, and pugs seem to be especially vulnerable to developing it.

Sometimes what feels like an uneven heartbeat is really a sign of fluid around the heart, says Paul D. Pion, D.V.M., a veterinary cardiologist in Davis, California, and founder of the Veterinary Information Network, an online service for veterinarians. Fluid around the heart is often caused by infections or tumors, and it allows the heart to swing like a pendulum with each beat. This can make the beat feel uneven even when it is perfectly regular, he explains.

WHAT YOU CAN DO

You can't treat your pet's heart problems at home any more than you could treat your own. What you can do, however, is periodically check her heartbeat to make sure that it is regular. When you know what is normal for your pet, it will be easy to tell if something changes, and you will know that it is time to call your vet, says Dr. Tyrell.

The easiest way to check the heart is to feel the left side of your pet's chest just behind her elbow, says Dr. Pion. You can also measure the strength of the pulse by feeling the inside of her thigh near the top of the leg.

WHAT YOUR VET WILL DO

It won't take your vet more than a minute or two to know if your pet's heartbeat is truly uneven. He may even be able to make a diagnosis after listening for a minute or two with a stethoscope. But it is usually not that simple. Your pet will probably need an electrocardiogram (ECG), a painless test that draws a picture of what is happening inside your pet's heart before, during, and after each beat.

Your pet will probably need a chest x-ray as well, says Dr. Tyrell. If the heart looks huge and round, there is probably fluid trapped in the sac (called the pericardium) that surrounds it. If the heart looks misshapen, your pet could be developing heart failure.

The best tool for diagnosing heart problems is called an echocardiogram. Done with ultrasound, it allows your vet to see the heart while it is actually beating. Most vets don't have the necessary equipment, however, so you will probably have to see a specialist, says Dr. Tyrell.

Since there are many causes of heart problems, there isn't a one-size-fits-all treatment plan. Pets with sick sinus syndrome, for example, often need to have a pacemaker implanted, which will help the heart beat regularly. Other heart problems can be treated with medications such as digoxin (Cardoxin), which makes the heart beat more strongly, or with diuretics to remove excess fluids from the body.

INSOMNIA

Clues

- Your pet is urinating more than usual.
- Your schedule is unusually hectic.
- There is a guest or someone new in the household.

For some reason, every night when you are ready to fall asleep, your dog wakes up. He doesn't just lie there either; he starts squirming around. He scratches his chin. Gives a good shake. Paces around the room, his nails clicking on the floor. Between the clicking, the jingling of his collar, and the occasional plaintive whine, it quickly becomes obvious that he is not the only one who is going to spend a sleepless night.

"A lot of owners end up in my office because their dogs are keeping them up at night," says Jane Shaw, D.V.M., an instructor in the department of anatomy at the College of Veterinary Medicine at Cornell University in Ithaca, New York. Cats also spend wakeful nights, but because they are naturally nocturnal, this isn't considered a problem.

For dogs (as with humans), temporary bouts of insomnia often occur when there is something upsetting in their lives, says James Dalley, D.V.M., associate professor of small animal clinical sciences at Michigan State University College of Veterinary Medicine in East Lansing. Dogs are very attuned to their human owners. If you have been fighting with your spouse or if there is someone new sleeping in the house, your dog may get nervous and restless, he says.

Another common reason dogs have sleepless nights is that they simply aren't getting enough exercise. If you have been too busy lately to be walking or playing with your dog, he could have so much pent-up energy that he is simply not tired enough to sleep. In addition, older pets tend to be more wakeful than when they were younger.

Some dogs are very sensitive to changes in the weather, Dr. Dalley adds. "Some make good weather forecasters. They will start pacing and acting nervous long before the skies get cloudy." Dogs also tend to be bothered by heat and will often be a little restless when the temperatures climb.

Both dogs and cats can have trouble sleeping when they are feeling uncomfortable. Pets with fleas or allergies, for example, may spend time scratching instead of sleeping. Conditions such as arthritis or hip dysplasia, which can make it difficult for pets to get comfortable, will often cause sleepless nights. So will internal problems such as diabetes or kidney disease: Pets that need to urinate frequently won't be able to sleep well, Dr. Shaw explains. In fact, almost any physical problem can result in sleepless nights.

WHAT YOU CAN DO

Insomnia is rarely serious and usually goes away on its own within a few days. In the meantime, you may want to move your pet out of the bedroom and into a cozy place of his own. This won't necessarily improve his sleep, but it might improve yours.

It is also helpful not to close your pet in at night. If he is restless in one place, he will appreciate the freedom to wander off to find a spot that is more comfortable, says Dr. Shaw. Dogs are naturally adaptable. In the summer, for example, they will often curl up on a bare floor, where it is a little bit cooler. In winter, they will appreciate a dog bed or a thick folded blanket, where they can curl up and stay warm. Both dogs and cats may sleep in several places in a night, so don't be surprised when you hear them moving around a bit.

If your pet is generally healthy, one of the best cures for insomnia is to get his paws moving during the day, says Dr. Shaw. Walking him or simply throwing a ball for 15 to 20 minutes, twice a day, will help tucker him out so that he will sleep more soundly at night.

It is also worth taking a few minutes to give him an at-home checkup, especially if he is whining or crying at night. Pets that normally sleep well but are suddenly restless may have physical problems, like fleas or painful rashes, that are making them uncomfortable, says Dr. Dalley. Or they may have to urinate more often than usual. Once you take care of the problem, they will usually start sleeping well again.

Dogs with mild aches and pains will often feel better if you give them a little bit of aspirin, says Dr. Shaw. (These medications are dangerous for cats and should never be used without a veterinarian's supervision.) Vets usually recommend 10 milligrams of coated aspirin (like Ascriptin) per pound of pooch, once or twice a day. Don't use plain aspirin because it can upset a pet's stomach. To be safe, check with your vet before giving aspirin or other human medications to pets.

If your pet needs to go outside much more often than usual or if he seems unusually stiff and sore, you will want to call your vet. There are a number of potentially serious problems—including diabetes and hip dysplasia—that can cause these symptoms, and you will want to get him checked out as soon as possible.

Things can get a bit tricky when your dog seems to be reacting to the emotions or activities in the household. You can't change your entire life simply because your dog can't sleep. What you can do, however, is give him extra love and attention, especially if there is a new person in the house, and the change is making him insecure. The more secure and accepted your dog feels, the more likely he is to sleep the night through, says Dr. Dalley.

WHAT YOUR VET WILL DO

If your pet's hind leg is in perpetual motion at night, there is a good chance that allergies are keeping him awake. Your vet may recommend giving him a skin test to find out what, if anything, he is allergic to. Skin tests give results very quickly and provide a good starting point for eliminating allergies.

Allergies aren't always easy to treat. Pets with food allergies, for example, need to be given an entirely new diet with none of the ingredients in their usual chow. Pets that are allergic to pollen or other airborne particles may be given antihistamines to ease the itching. You will also want to find ways to avoid the pollen by keeping the windows closed and using the air conditioner instead, for example. In severe cases, your vet may recommend giving your pet a series of shots that will make him less sensitive to whatever is bothering him.

If your pet isn't sleeping and is also urinating a lot, your vet will want to give him a thorough checkup, along with blood and urine tests. Conditions such as a kidney infection usually aren't difficult to treat, but they can be serious if they aren't stopped early. Once your pet has been given the appropriate medications, he should return to his normal sleep schedule very quickly. If you have been using over-the-counter pain pills without success, your vet may recommend using stronger, prescription drugs. Sleeping pills, however, are rarely used, says Dr. Dalley.

See also Chapter 9: Urinating Frequently; Chapter 13: Scratching

JOINT SWELLING

Clues

- Your pet's joints are red and tender.
- You have found ticks on your pet.
- Your cat has stiffness in the same joints on opposite sides of her body.

Every joint in your pet's body, from her elbows to her hips, has a number of moving parts. When something goes wrong with one or more of those parts, the body sends in blood and other fluids to control the damage. This is what causes joints to swell, says Jane Shaw, D.V.M., an instructor in the department of anatomy at the College of Veterinary Medicine at Cornell University in Ithaca, New York.

Any injury—from falling out of a tree to getting caught under the garage door—can cause swollen joints. Due to their adventurous natures, cats are somewhat more prone to these sorts of injuries than dogs, says James R. Richards, D.V.M., director of the Cornell Feline Health Center, also at the College of Veterinary Medicine at Cornell University.

Infections are a common cause of swollen joints, Dr. Richards adds. Sometimes the infection is local—that is, it is limited to one particular joint. This usually occurs when there has been an injury from a spat with another pet, for example, or from getting jabbed by something sharp.

Infections can also spread throughout the body, causing swelling in a number of different joints. For instance, pets with Lyme disease (a bacterial infection transmitted by ticks) often have trouble walking because many of their joints may be swollen and painful at the same time, says Dr. Shaw.

In older pets, swollen joints may be caused by arthritis. One kind of arthritis, called osteoarthritis or degenerative joint disease, is simply a result of years of wear and tear. This type of arthritis usually occurs in dogs, though older cats may get it, too. A more serious form of arthritis, called rheumatoid arthritis, occurs when the immune system periodically attacks tissue inside the joints, causing painful swelling.

A type of arthritis unique to cats is called feline chronic progressive polyarthritis, in which the same joints are affected on both sides of the body. An immune system condition, called lupus, can also cause joints to swell, says Dr. Shaw.

Cancer is probably the most serious cause of joint swelling, says Dr. Richards. If it turns out to be cancer, quick attention can make all the difference.

WHAT YOU CAN DO

One way to tell what is causing a joint to swell is to feel it. When it feels warmer than the surrounding area and if there is a bit of redness beneath the fur, it is probably infected, says Dr. Shaw. In fact, since joint swelling is often caused by injuries or other serious problems, it is really not something that you can handle at home without a lot of help from your veterinarian.

While you can't deal with the infection yourself, try to keep your pet comfortable until you get to the vet or after you bring her home. To reduce the swelling caused by infection or injury, vets sometimes advise putting cold packs (or ice wrapped in a washcloth) on the swollen area several times a day for about 10 minutes each time. This reduces the flow of blood to the joint, which can bring the swelling down. If swelling is due to arthritis, warm wraps will keep your pet more comfortable, but they won't have much effect on the swelling.

Swollen joints are usually painful, so your pet isn't going to want a lot of exercise. It is a good idea, however, to get her moving at least a little bit, says Dr. Shaw. Exercise increases blood flow, which will help remove fluids from the swollen area while allowing fresh blood and nutrients to get in.

To keep your pet comfortable, make sure that she has a warm, comfortable place to sleep. It is helpful to put her food and water bowls—and for cats, the litter box—nearby, so that she won't have to walk too far, says Dr. Richards. "Just plain old tender loving care at home makes a huge difference regardless of the problem."

Your vet may recommend giving your pet over-the-counter medications as well. For dogs, aspirin can be very helpful for reducing swelling. Give 10 milligrams of coated aspirin for every pound of pooch, once or twice a day. (Avoid regular aspirin because it is hard on the stomach.) Aspirin can be dangerous for cats, however, so never use it without your veterinarian's supervision.

WHAT YOUR VET WILL DO

It is usually not difficult to tell when swelling is caused by an infection. Your vet may remove fluid from the joint and give the liquid a quick look. Normal joint fluid is clear, almost colorless. Fluid from an infected joint, however, may contain pus, blood, or drifting particles. It will also contain bacteria or fungi, which can be identified in a laboratory. Unless the cause of the swelling is obvious—like a puncture wound over a joint—your vet will probably take an x-ray as well.

When swelling is caused by an abscess, which is a painful infection that can form in tissue over a joint, your vet will drain out the pus and apply an antibiotic ointment or liquid, says Dr. Richards. When the infection is occurring inside the joint or throughout the body, as with Lyme disease, the only treatment is to give antibiotics. In most cases, your pet will start feeling better with a day or two after taking the medication, and the infection will be gone within one to two weeks.

If your pet has an infection of the joint bone, however, she will probably need surgery to clear away infected bone from the area, says Dr. Richards.

The treatments for injuries, of course, are as varied as the injuries themselves. Dogs or cats that have fractured bones are often required to wear casts or splints, says Dr. Richards. In addition, surgery may be needed to wire or pin damaged bones together.

To help your pet recover, your vet may recommend prescription medications to reduce swelling and ease the pain. In some cases, powerful drugs such as steroids may be injected. This is not only done to reduce inflammation, but also to prevent the immune system from working so vigorously, which can play a role in arthritis flare-ups, says Dr. Shaw. Steroids take effect almost immediately, she adds.

See also Chapter 14: Stiffness

SYMPTOM LETHARGY

Clues

- Your pet has fleas.
- He is having trouble walking or chewing.
- He is middle-aged or over-weight.

You expect your pet to be pooped when you have spent a few hours throwing balls or walking in the woods. But what if he seems exhausted and listless *before* he puts his paws in motion?

Lethargic pets almost certainly have a physical problem, says Sheldon A. Steinberg, V.M.D., professor of neurology at the University of Pennsylvania School of Veterinary Medicine in Philadelphia. Lethargy is easier to recognize in dogs than in cats, he adds, since cats are naturally less excitable. "My cat may or may not get up to greet me, but the dog will always be alert and awake," he says.

Pets with anemia, a condition in which red blood cells are either in short supply or they aren't carrying enough oxygen, will often be tired and lethargic. Anemia can be caused by an ulcer, poor diet, or, more often, by parasites like fleas or hookworms, which can remove large amounts of energy-giving blood.

Lethargy can also be caused by pain. Conditions such as arthritis, hip dysplasia, and even dental problems will often make pets tired and reluctant to move, says Ronald Stone, D.V.M., a veterinarian and clinical assistant professor of surgery at the University of Miami School of Medicine in Florida.

The thyroid gland has been called the body's gas pedal because it controls the rate of metabolism. Pets with underactive thyroid glands, or hypothyroidism, can get extremely lethargic, says Charles Lowrie, D.V.M., associate professor of neurology and neural surgery at the Veterinary Teaching Hospital at Michigan State University College of Veterinary Medicine in East Lansing. This condition usually occurs in middle-aged dogs, although cats can get it, too. Dog breeds most susceptible to hypothyroidism include Doberman pinschers, dachshunds, English bulldogs, golden retrievers, and springer and cocker spaniels.

Finally, pets that are overweight will sometimes have low energy, says Dr. Stone. In pets as in humans, overweight is usually a result of eating too much or not getting enough exercise.

WHAT YOU CAN DO

If your pet is overweight, helping him shed a few pounds and increasing the amount of exercise he gets each day may be all it takes to get his energy up to par, says C. A. Tony Buffington, D.V.M., Ph.D., professor of veterinary clinical sciences at the Ohio State University Veterinary Hospital in Columbus. Here are a few things that he recommends.

- Cut back the amount you feed him by about 25 percent. If he hasn't lost any weight in about two weeks, reduce the serving sizes a little more. Continue doing this until you can just feel the ribs through the coat, which will mean that he is at a healthy weight.
- To keep him comfortable on his new diet, feed him several small meals a day instead of one big one. This will help keep his stomach satisfied even while he is slimming down to a livelier size. If you are only able to feed him in the evening, it is a good idea to have a play session before, rather than after, eating. If you serve dinner first, he may consider your playtime afterward to be a reward for cleaning his plate.
- Vigorous daily activity is essential for any weight-loss plan. Dogs need at least two 20-minute workouts each day. It is best to schedule the workouts either an hour before or an hour after eating since vigorous exercise too close to meals can lead to bloat. (For more on bloat, see page 130.)
- Cats aren't always walkable, of course, but they do love to play. Spend time each day encouraging her to put her paws into motion by chasing a length of string or attacking a catnip-filled mouse. (For more tips on losing weight, see Weight Gain on page 422.)

Since dental problems can sap your pet's energy, it is worth taking a few minutes to keep his teeth and gums healthy, says Mark M. Smith, V.M.D., associate professor of surgery in the department of small animal clinical sciences at Virginia–Maryland Regional College of Veterinary Medicine in Blacksburg, Virginia. Brushing your pet's teeth every day will help remove plaque and bacteria that can lead to tooth decay, he says. Just be sure to use a toothpaste made for pets; human toothpastes may upset a pet's stomach.

WHAT YOUR VET WILL DO

Vets worry when energy levels take a downturn because there are so many physical problems that can cause this. Your vet will want to do a thorough checkup. She will examine your pet's joints for signs of arthritis or other problems. She will also order blood tests to look into the state of his internal health.

Anemia usually isn't difficult to treat. If your pet has parasites, for example, there are a number of medications that will get rid of them. (Be sure to take a stool sample when you go to the vet since many parasites are diagnosed by examining the stool.) Once your pet stops losing blood to the parasites, his energy levels should quickly rebound. In addition, your vet may recommend giving your pet iron and B vitamins, which will help his red blood cells get back to normal.

If your pet's teeth are in bad shape, he may need to have them professionally cleaned or repaired, says Dr. Smith. These procedures can be somewhat painful and usually involve general anesthesia, which requires an overnight stay. Once the anesthesia wears off and the pain diminishes, he should start feeling better fairly soon.

There are many options for pets with hip dysplasia, says Dr. Stone. Acupuncture can be very effective at controlling pain. Your vet will be able to recommend a qualified acupuncturist in your area. In addition, your vet may put your pet on a regular exercise program, which will strengthen muscles in the hips as well as help keep the joints lubricated.

When your pet's flagging energy is due to low thyroid levels, your vet will probably give thyroid supplements to replenish the body's natural supply. The medications have to be taken for life, but they are very effective, says Dr. Lowrie.

See also Chapter 4: Overeating; Chapter 14: Joint Swelling, Stiffness

POTBELLY

- The swelling appeared quickly or after eating.
- Your pet is 12 weeks or younger.

Dogs and cats love to eat, and sometimes they pay for their hearty appetites by getting noticeably rotund. Unlike humans, however, overweight pets don't get a potbelly—they get round all over. A dog or cat that is generally lean but is pooched-out in the middle almost certainly has a medical problem.

In puppies and kittens, a big belly is usually a sign of parasites, says Kristin Varner, D.V.M., a veterinarian in private practice in Severn, Maryland. Parasites such as roundworms live in the intestines, robbing your pet of essential protein. When protein levels fall, pets may begin secreting fluids into the abdomen, causing a potbelly.

A potbelly that comes on very suddenly in dogs—within an hour or two—is probably caused by bloat, a life-threatening condition in which the stomach fills with gas, says Thomas Schmidt, D.V.M., a veterinarian in private practice in Fort Washington, Maryland. Vets aren't sure what causes bloat. It usually occurs after large meals and is most common in big, deep-chested dogs like Labrador retrievers and Great Danes.

It is normal for dogs and cats to have small amounts of fluid in their abdomens, just enough to keep the organs moist. But pets with internal problems such as cancer or liver or heart disease will often retain fluids, causing their bellies to swell to several times their normal size, says Knox Inman, D.V.M., a veterinarian in private practice in West River, Maryland.

Pets with a hormonal problem called Cushing's disease, which can occur when the adrenal glands are overactive or as a side effect of medications such as prednisone, will often get a potbelly. Because this condition weakens the abdominal muscles, the stomach may droop toward the ground as well. Cushing's disease is fairly common in dogs, but it rarely occurs in cats.

One of the most obvious causes of a potbelly—one which many owners forget to consider—is pregnancy. From the time a pet starts to show until the time she delivers, her belly may double or even triple in size. So if you have an unspayed female and you suspect that she has had some unauthorized visitors lately, you may want to ask your vet whether the pet is expecting.

WHAT YOU CAN DO

Unless you are sure that your pet is pregnant—you may be able to feel the babies wiggling inside—a swollen middle is always serious and may be an emergency. It is essential to call your vet as soon as you notice it.

Since worms may cause swelling in puppies and kittens, it is worth taking a look at their stool and the fur around the anal area. Roundworms resemble long strands of spaghetti and are easy to see. Over-the-counter deworming products containing pyrantel pamoate are effective and safe as long as you follow the directions exactly.

The problem with treating worms yourself, adds Dr. Varner, is that pets with one kind of parasite often have other kinds as well. The medications you buy at the pet supply store won't kill all of them. Your best bet is to call your vet, she advises.

What Your Vet Will Do

Since a potbelly often indicates serious problems, your first visit to your vet may be a long one. He will start by listening to your pet's chest to see if there are signs of heart disease. Your vet will also feel her belly to see if the swelling is caused by fluid, gas, or tumors.

Pets that are bloating need to get rid of the pressure—fast. The usual treatment is to pass a tube down the throat into the stomach, which allows the gas to escape. One problem with bloat, however, is that it may cause the stomach to twist on itself, making it impossible to get the tube in. Your vet may have to take a shortcut by poking a needle through your pet's side directly into the stomach in order to draw the gas out that way. More often, pets with bloat will need surgery to let the air out and correct the problem.

Once the gas is out of the stomach, most pets with bloat will be just fine. Pets that get bloat once will often get it again, however, so you will have to keep an eye out for problems.

A belly filled with fluid is also serious, and the treatment is similar to that for bloat. Your vet will stick a needle through the skin and into the abdominal cavity to remove the fluid. The procedure looks painful, but it is actually no worse than getting a shot—and once the needle is inserted, it doesn't hurt at all. By analyzing the fluid, your vet can diagnose a variety of illnesses, including cancer and infections.

Because so many things can cause a potbelly, your veterinarian will have lots of treatments to choose from. Some, like giving deworming medications, are simple. Others, like those for treating heart disease, can be quite extensive. Depending on the diagnosis, you may be making more than one visit to your vet to correct the problem and to restore your pet to good health.

See also Chapter 6: Bloat

| SYMPTOM |

ROLLING ON THE GROUND

Clues

- There is a strong odor coming from your pet's ear.
- His rolling is preceded by several weeks of dizziness or clumsiness.
- Your pet tilts his head before falling over and rolling.

Cats and dogs love to lie on their backs and roll from side to side. They do it to scratch itchy spots and just because it is fun. But sometimes you may see pets lose their balance and fall and then roll about helplessly because they can't get back up again. This usually means there is a problem with their balance system, and that's no fun at all.

The most common cause of rolling is an inner-ear infection, says John Fioramonti, D.V.M., a veterinarian in private practice in Towson, Maryland. The inner ear is one of your pet's balance centers (the other one is in the brain), and an infection can make him dizzy. You may see him tilt his head, fall, and then roll on the ground as he tries to regain his sense of balance. Infections can be smelly, so a strong odor coming from the ear is one hint that this may be the problem.

Another cause of rolling is a condition called idiopathic vestibular disease, which affects the part of the nervous system (the vestibular system) that controls balance. Pets with this mysterious condition will feel fine one minute, then suddenly lose their balance, says Stephen A. Smith, D.V.M., a veterinarian in private practice in Pasadena, Maryland. It is fairly common in older cats, but it may occur in dogs and cats of all ages.

Vets used to think idiopathic vestibular disease was caused by eating blue-tailed lizards—until they discovered that most pets that get the condition have never seen the lizard, much less eaten one. They now suspect it is caused by a chemical imbalance in fluids in the inner ear, and it sometimes occurs in pets that have had heatstroke. The attacks look scary, but most pets feel fine within three to five days, says Dr. Fioramonti.

Other, more-serious problems that can affect balance include strokes, brain tumors, liver disease, diabetes, or even rabies. Tumors grow slowly, so pets will get increasingly clumsy and uncoordinated before they actually start to roll. With other conditions, however, the symptoms usually come on very quickly, Dr. Fioramonti explains.

WHAT YOU CAN DO

Pets that lose their balance and start rolling aren't going to regain their balance right away. They will be frightened and probably nauseated, and there is not much you can do to help or comfort them. Even though most conditions that cause rolling aren't life-threatening, some are. You will want to call your vet right away.

WHAT YOUR VET WILL DO

Because inner-ear infections are a common cause of dizziness and rolling, your veterinarian will probably start by doing an ear exam. "If your pet struggles, he may need to be sedated to let your vet get a good look," says Dr. Fioramonti.

Your vet will also perform a quick neurological test by moving your pet's head up and down and side to side while looking at his eyes. The idea isn't to make him dizzier, but to look for signs of nystagmus—rapid eye movements that signal problems with one of the body's balance centers. The way the eyes move can provide clues as to which balance center is out of kilter: the one in the ears or the brain. Since problems in the brain are much more serious than those in the ears, it is an important distinction, Dr. Fioramonti explains.

Your vet will usually be able to tell what's wrong with a simple exam. If nothing shows up right away, she may need to do blood tests to check for internal problems such as diabetes or widespread infection. The next step, if the rolling is still a mystery, will be to see a veterinary neurologist. Your pet may be given a spinal tap to check for infection as well as an MRI (magnetic resonance imaging) or a CAT scan, painless ways to check for tumors in or on the brain.

Most ear infections are easily treated with oral antibiotics or ear drops. In fact, your pet may be given antibiotics even if he appears to have idiopathic vestibular disease since the two problems may appear very similar. Vets will often play it safe and give antibiotics right away, Dr. Fioramonti says.

For conditions other than an ear infection, your pet will probably need to be hospitalized for a few days. He may need medications to control his nausea, and possibly sedatives to keep him calm. After that, of course, his treatment—anything from surgery to medications—will depend on what the underlying problem is.

See also Chapter 14: Walking in Circles

SEIZURES

Clues

- Your pet trembles and seems confused.
- You have a working dog, and it is the off-season.
- She has been in an accident.
- Your dog is nursing a litter of puppies.

You can't see the surge of electricity going through the brain. But when it causes a dog or cat to have a seizure, the symptoms can be shockingly apparent. In the grip of a seizure, pets may collapse, drool, or thrash their legs uncontrollably, says C. B. Chastain, D.V.M., professor of small animal medicine in the department of veterinary medicine and surgery at the University of Missouri College of Veterinary Medicine in Columbia.

Seizures aren't always dramatic and frightening, he adds. Sometimes they are quite subtle, causing nothing more than a little trembling and momentary confusion. It is possible for your pet to have a seizure right in front of you without you noticing that there is a problem. But whether the seizure itself is big or small, the underlying condition that is causing it is potentially serious.

Many things can cause a seizure, but the most common cause is epilepsy, which occurs more often in dogs than in cats, says Charles Lowrie, D.V.M., associate professor of neurology and neural surgery at the Veterinary Teaching Hospital at Michigan State University College of Veterinary Medicine in East Lansing. Pets that have had one epileptic seizure are likely to have others. In severe cases, they may have many seizures in a single day, he adds.

Other conditions that can cause seizures include brain tumors and encephalitis, an infection and inflammation of the brain. In puppies, a viral infection called canine distemper is a common cause of seizures, says Dennis O'Brien, D.V.M., Ph.D., a neurologist in the department of veterinary medicine and surgery at the University of Missouri College of Veterinary Medicine in Columbia.

Dogs that are normally very active, like hunting dogs, will sometimes develop low blood sugar, or hypoglycemia, during the off-season when they are getting less exercise. In some dogs, the drop in blood sugar may cause seizures, says Ronald Stone, D.V.M., a veterinarian and clinical assistant professor of surgery at the University of Miami School of Medicine in Florida.

Another possible cause of seizures is low calcium levels, which typically occur in female dogs that are nursing. Seizures can also be caused by injuries to the brain from a car accident, for example, or from taking a bad fall.

WHAT YOU CAN DO

Even though seizures may look terrifying, they are unlikely to cause serious harm as long as they don't last too long. In fact, pets that are having seizures are temporarily unconscious and aren't feeling any discomfort, says Dr. O'Brien. But if your pet is prone to seizures, it is important to take a few precautions to make sure that she doesn't get hurt.

If you have stairs, for example, putting a guardrail around the stairwell will prevent dangerous falls, says Dr. O'Brien. If you suspect a seizure is coming—pets with seizures often show certain signs like a vacant expression, a moment's confusion, or restless behavior—make sure that there is nothing nearby that could get broken or could fall on your pet. Once a seizure begins, all you can really do is back off and let it run its course.

Don't try to restrain your pet, Dr. O'Brien adds. Unlike humans, a pet having a seizure won't swallow her tongue, so there is no reason to put anything in her mouth. In fact, pets can bite extremely hard during a seizure, so you will want to keep your distance. Most seizures are over in one to five minutes, he says. That is when it is time to call your vet.

"It's important to try to stay calm when your pet is having a seizure," says Dr. Chastain. The more you can tell your vet about the seizure, the easier it will be to make a diagnosis. How long did the seizure last? Was your pet yelping, trembling, or making paddling motions with her legs? What was she doing before the seizure began?

It is not always possible to prevent seizures, but there are things that can help. Vaccinating your puppy, for example, will prevent canine distemper, which in turn will prevent those types of seizures, says Dr. Chastain.

If your dog is prone to blood sugar problems, your vet may recommend giving her a high-protein food several times a day. Dr. Stone usually recommends that puppies up to six months old be fed four times a day. Puppies six months to a year can be fed three times a day, and dogs up to 18 months can be fed twice a day. After that, once a day should do it, he says.

Commercial pet foods have plenty of calcium, so it is usually easy to get enough of this mineral. If your dog is nursing, however, your vet may recommend giving her Pet-Tabs or other pet vitamins to keep her calcium levels high.

WHAT YOUR VET WILL DO

Most seizures don't last more than a few minutes. If your pet is having a seizure when you take her to the vet, she will probably be given a sedative such as diazepam (Valium) to keep the muscle spasms under control.

After that, your vet will need to do a series of tests, including blood tests, spinal taps, and CAT (brain) scans, to see what is causing the seizure to occur.

Seizures caused by bacterial infections are serious problems but are relatively easy to treat. If your pet has encephalitis, for example, antibiotics will knock out the infection and the risk for seizures. Pets with low blood sugar may also need medications and sometimes surgery. In some cases, though, simply modifying their diet will correct the problem, says Dr. Stone.

If it turns out that your pet has epilepsy, she will probably need to take medications for the rest of her life. "Phenobarbital is far and away the best drug we have," says Dr. O'Brien. While medications may not eliminate the seizures completely, they will reduce the frequency and severity, allowing a pet to live a normal life.

Not all pets with seizures need medication, adds Dr. Stone. If the seizures are happening once a month or less and your pet is otherwise in good health, your vet may decide that it is better simply to let the occasional seizure happen than to treat it with drugs. As long as you keep an eye on her during seizures to make sure that she doesn't get hurt, she will probably be just fine.

SHAKING

Clues

- Your pet is taking antibiotics or other medications.
- She is shaking even when she is dry.

Dogs think it is great fun: First they jump into a stream or pond—preferably one that is somewhat smelly—and then they run up to you and let loose with a vigorous, water-spraying shake.

Shaking is a very efficient way to remove excess water from the fur. Sometimes, however, dogs will shake frequently even when they are dry. Usually this just means that they are a little uncomfortable because one of their legs fell asleep, for example, or because they are being buzzed by a fly or mosquito. They will also shake when they are feeling a little itchy.

But frequent shaking may be a side effect of medications, such as antibiotics or drugs to prevent heartworms, says Ronald Hodges, D.V.M., a veterinarian in private practice in Allentown, Pennsylvania. Shaking may also be a sign of poisoning or neurological or heart problems. These causes of shaking aren't very common in dogs and even less so in cats. Still, it is a symptom that may need your attention.

WHAT YOU CAN DO

Most of the time, you don't have to do anything about your pet's shaking, except to stand back if she happens to be wet at the time. When she is shaking for no apparent reason and she is doing it all the time, you really need to call your vet, says Dr. Hodges.

WHAT YOUR VET WILL DO

After checking for obvious problems, your vet will probably check your pet's heart. It doesn't happen often, but pets may develop electrical problems in the heart that cause erratic signals to travel through the body, causing shaking. If your pet does have an irregular heartbeat, medications will usually keep it under control, although some pets will need to have a pacemaker installed, says James R. Richards, D.V.M., director of the Cornell Feline Health Center at the College of Veterinary Medicine at Cornell University in Ithaca, New York.

Your vet will also look for neurological problems that could be causing seizures. And of course, if your pet is taking medications that are causing her to shake, changing drugs may be all that is needed.

See also Chapter 14: Seizures

SYMPTOM # Shivering or Trembling

Clues

- Your dog is nursing puppies.
- Your pet is elderly or getting weak.
- She occasionally seems disoriented or loses her balance.

Unless you live in Hawaii, your dog will spend some of her time in cold, frosty air. And she will react just as humans do, by shivering or trembling. This is the body's technique for warming itself up a bit, explains James Dalley, D.V.M., associate professor of small animal clinical sciences at Michigan State University College of Veterinary Medicine in East Lansing. Cats also get cold, but they are less likely than dogs to shiver.

It is not just the cold that puts muscles in motion. Pets also tremble when they are scared or nervous, says Dr. Dalley. Some dogs, in fact, are so tightly wound and have such high levels of nervous energy that they tremble nearly all the time. This kind of trembling is normal and doesn't cause any problems.

In older pets, shivering and trembling may be a sign of underlying problems like arthritis or weak muscles. It can also be a sign of neurological problems, says Jerry W. Northington, D.V.M., a veterinarian in private practice in Valley Forge, Pennsylvania.

A variety of illnesses, including lupus (an immune system problem), hypothyroidism (a condition resulting from underactive thyroid gland), and some kinds of anemia can also cause pets to shiver. Pets with fever will often shiver and tremble. In rare cases, so will pets that have low levels of calcium. This tends to occur in female dogs that are nursing puppies and losing calcium through the milk, says Dennis O'Brien, D.V.M., Ph.D., a neurologist in the department of veterinary medicine and surgery at the University of Missouri College of Veterinary Medicine in Columbia.

Finally, pets with epilepsy may have seizures that cause them to shiver and tremble, says Sheldon A. Steinberg, V.M.D., professor of neurology at the University of Pennsylvania School of Veterinary Medicine in Philadelphia. Seizures are usually accompanied by other symptoms as well, such as falling down, disorientation, or salivating heavily.

What You Can Do

During the cold months, it is important to recognize your pet's limits when the mercury drops. While some northern breeds of dogs like huskies and Samoyeds can withstand quite a bit of cold, other breeds get

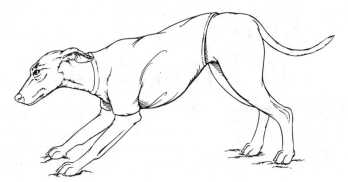

Dogs with short, thin coats don't enjoy being outside on blustery days. It is a good idea to add a layer of protection when cold weather hits. You can buy sweaters and other cold-weather wear at pet supply stores.

chilled in a hurry. And even the hardiest pets need protection from the wind and cold. If your pet is cold and trembling, don't leave her outside. Bring her in the house and give her a chance to warm up, says Dr. Dalley.

If your dog is naturally nervous and high-strung, there is nothing that you can do to stop the trembling. Just get used it to it, although a few soothing words and a gentle rub will calm her down somewhat, says Dr. Steinberg.

If your dog is trembling and nursing puppies, ask your vet if she needs to get more calcium in her diet, says Dr. Dalley. Otherwise, it is unlikely that a lack of calcium is causing the symptoms since most pets get enough in their diets. Brand-name pet foods contain plenty of calcium.

For either dogs or cats, you should see your vet if your pet is trembling a lot and for no apparent reason. This is especially true for cats since they rarely shiver or tremble unless they are sick, says Dr. Steinberg.

WHAT YOUR VET WILL DO

Most conditions that cause shivering, like arthritis or thyroid problems, are easy to diagnose. But your vet may also want to know if there is a neurological problem behind the trembling. Unfortunately, this often requires a number of tests, possibly including a spinal tap. Not all vets are well-versed in neurological problems, so don't be surprised if your vet recommends that you see a specialist.

When shivering and trembling are severe, your vet may give your pet muscle relaxants, says Dr. Dalley. More often, your vet will be less concerned about the shivering itself than what is causing it. Once the underlying problem has been treated, the shivering will usually go away fairly quickly.

See also Chapter 14: Seizures

STIFFNESS

Clues

- Your pet is having trouble getting up.
- The stiffness is affecting his jaw or other joints.
- The stiffness came on suddenly.
- Your pet is vomiting or has blood in his urine.

Dogs and cats are remarkably limber, which is why they are able to swerve around trees, run up and down hills, and bite at their own tails—almost at the same time. Even though they stiffen up a bit with the years, they usually maintain a grace and ease of movement that we can only envy.

That is why you should be alert if your formerly flexible friend is suddenly moving as stiffly as a mechanical toy. While stiffness often has minor causes, like pulling a muscle or simply sleeping on a cold floor, it can also mean that one or more joints is breaking down.

A common cause of stiffness in dogs is hip dysplasia, an inherited condition in which the hip joints don't fit together as tightly as they should, says Jane Shaw, D.V.M., an instructor in the department of anatomy at the College of Veterinary Medicine at Cornell University in Ithaca, New York. Hip dysplasia usually begins in the first six months of a dog's life, although the pain and stiffness usually don't appear until much later on. Dogs (especially large breeds) are much more likely to get hip dysplasia than cats, although Persians and Maine coon cats sometimes get it, too.

You can spot hip dysplasia in dogs because they may have trouble getting up, and they will have a distinctive sway when they walk. It is harder to recognize it in cats since they don't always have visible symptoms, says James R. Richards, D.V.M., director of the Cornell Feline Health Center also at the College of Veterinary Medicine at Cornell University.

Arthritis is another cause of stiffness that affects dogs more often than cats, says Dr. Richards. Arthritis typically appears in the hip joints, although it may affect the elbows, back, and neck as well.

In cats, stiffness is sometimes caused by an inflamed vertebrae. Both dogs and cats may have problems with the disks in their backs, which can make them slow and creaky. Anything that affects the nerves or spine—a bad fall, for example—can lead to stiffness, says Dr. Richards. In addition, internal problems such as infections or cancer can cause pain and stiffness.

A possible cause of stiffness is tetanus, a serious bacterial infection, which is also known as lockjaw. In pets with tetanus, the whole body, and particularly the jaw, may get stiff and very tender.

WHAT YOU CAN DO

Stiffness may be a sign of serious, underlying problems, so it is important to see your vet if it lasts longer than a day or two. In the meantime, you can do many simple things to help your pet feel a little bit better.

Since coldness and dampness invariably make stiff joints even stiffer, be sure to keep your pet warm, says Dr. Shaw. She recommends giving him a warm, well-padded place to sleep, such as a pile of blankets on a carpeted floor or his own pet bed placed in a warm area. If he spends a lot of time outdoors, you may want to shop for a heated bed, which will keep him comfortable even on the coldest days.

If your pet has a stiff neck, raise his food and water bowls to mouth level. That way he won't have to struggle to bend down to eat and drink.

For occasional stiffness, vets sometimes advise giving dogs coated aspirin. (These medications can be dangerous for cats, however, and should never be used without a veterinarian's supervision.) Vets usually recommend giving 10 milligrams for every pound of pooch, once or twice a day.

Since pets with stiff joints often have trouble on slippery floors or steep steps, it is a good idea to do a little remodeling. Put down throw rugs on wood or tile floors to make it easier for them to get around without slipping. If your house has steps leading to the yard, put down a simple carpeted ramp, which makes it easier for them to get in and out.

When your dog is hobbling around, you may be nervous about letting him run. Go ahead and put on your walking shoes and get out the leash and the play toys. Exercise is good for all pets, including those with joint problems, says Dr. Shaw. "Dogs should be taken on walks every day."

It is important, of course, not to overdo it. If your pet hasn't been getting around much, start with a leisurely 15- to 20-minute walk or play session and gradually work up from there, says Dr. Shaw. Regular walking will help keep your pet's muscles loose and limber. Plus, it helps lubricate the joints so that they move more smoothly.

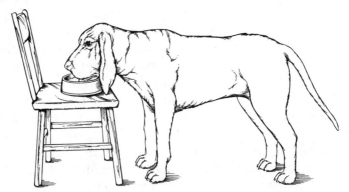

When your pet is having trouble lowering his head enough to eat, you can make life easier by putting his bowl on a short stool or chair.

Even though cats will do anything to avoid the water, most dogs enjoy getting wet, and swimming is a great exercise for easing stiffness. For one thing, it puts almost no stress on creaky joints. At the same time, it provides a vigorous workout that will keep them strong and loose.

Diet also plays a role in easing stiffness, says Dr. Richards. Keeping your pet trim—or, if he is heavy, helping him slim down—is one of the best ways to treat and prevent joint problems. Extra weight increases the wear and tear on their joints, he explains. What's more, heavy pets generally don't get a lot of exercise, which makes the stiffness even worse.

WHAT YOUR VET WILL DO

Since stiffness can be caused by so many different things, you will make your vet's job easier by writing down everything that you have noticed about your pet's problem. Did the stiffness come on very suddenly? If so, he may have been in an accident. Has he been vomiting? Is there blood in the urine? The more you can tell your vet, the quicker she will be able to find a solution, says Dr. Richards.

"A physical exam is probably the single most important thing that we can do," Dr. Richards adds. Besides giving your pet a thorough exam, your vet may perform a variety of tests, including urine analysis and x-rays, to see if something internally is wrong. She may take a blood sample to test for inflammation or infection. And if cancer is a possibility, your vet will probably need to perform a biopsy.

Medications can be very effective for easing stiffness. If over-the-counter drugs aren't helping, your vet may recommend something stronger. When stiffness is severe because of hip dysplasia, for example, surgery may be needed to repair or even replace the damaged joint, Dr. Shaw says.

One of the most exciting developments for relieving pain and stiffness in pets is acupuncture. This technique in which needles are inserted into specific parts of the skin causes the release of natural painkillers in the body, explains Andrea Looney, D.V.M., a veterinarian and certified acupuncturist in private practice in Springfield, Massachusetts.

Acupuncture works for dogs and cats, and the procedure is essentially painless. "Most dogs and cats suffering from chronic pain will fall asleep during the procedure," she says. "They get that comfortable."

Pets will usually be given one treatment a week at first. As they begin to improve, treatments are needed much less often, sometimes as little as once every three months, Dr. Looney says.

For cancer, unfortunately, there are no easy solutions. But the same treatments that work for humans, like chemotherapy and radiation, can be lifesavers for pets as well.

See also Chapter 10: Difficulty Getting Up

SYMPTOM # WALKING IN CIRCLES

Clues

- Your pet has been taking medications.
- She seems confused or disoriented.
- She is tilting her head or losing her balance.

Dogs and cats will often turn around once or twice before lying down, and they enjoy spinning around and chasing a tempting tail that is just out of reach. Circling is normal—most of the time. But there are also physical problems that can cause pets to aimlessly walk in circles or to stand in place and spin around.

In some pets, antibiotics such as gentamicin or metronidazole can damage the inner ear, disrupting their sense of balance and causing them to turn in circles, says Deena Tiches, D.V.M., a veterinary neurologist in private practice in Gaithersburg, Maryland. Even over-the-counter ear washes may be a problem. Products that contain antiseptics such as iodine or chlorhexidine can be quite dangerous if the eardrum happens to be damaged when you give them. Pets may react to these products by walking in circles. They could lose their hearing as well, she warns.

A more common cause of circling is an inner-ear infection. The inner ear is one of the body's balance centers, and an infection can cause pets to tilt their heads, fall over, or walk in circles, says Thomas Schmidt, D.V.M., a veterinarian in private practice in Fort Washington, Maryland.

Infections in the brain—caused by such things as distemper in dogs and feline infectious peritonitis (FIP) in cats—can result in the same problem, Dr. Tiches adds. "The sooner we can figure out what's causing the infection, the better the chance of finding a cure," she says.

An area of the brain called the cerebellum helps control walking and gives pets a sense of their surroundings. A tumor in this area can cause pets to be confused and walk in circles, says Karen Munana, D.V.M., associate professor of neurology at North Carolina State University College of Veterinary Medicine in Raleigh.

Brain tumors usually occur in pets eight years or older, Dr. Munana adds. Tumors that occur deep in the brain can be hard to treat. But one type, called a meningioma, grows in the membrane covering the brain and is often curable.

WHAT YOU CAN DO

Circling is always a serious warning sign, and you will want to call your vet as soon as it begins. If you can't see your vet right away, be sure to stop using ear medications or oral antibiotics in the meantime, Dr. Munana says. There is a good chance that the drugs are irritating the inner ear. Stopping them right away will help ensure that there isn't permanent damage. Your vet will recommend other, safer drugs to try.

Pets that are walking in circles are often dizzy and confused. To help your pet avoid simple dangers, like falling down a flight of stairs, keep her locked in a crate or a small room until you can see your vet, Dr. Schmidt advises.

What Your Vet Will Do

Anything that interferes with your pet's balance is going to look scary, and in fact, most of the conditions responsible for this symptom are quite serious. With fast diagnosis and treatment, however, you have the best chance to stop the circling and cure the underlying problem.

Your pet is going to need a thorough neurological exam, but the first part of it will be quite simple: Your vet will watch her walking in circles. The size and direction of the circles may tell your vet exactly what the problem is. He will also examine the eyes since they can provide valuable clues. Pets that move their eyes very rapidly, for example, probably have a problem with one of the body's balance centers, says Dr. Tiches. Brain tumors and some infections also cause eye changes, such as uneven pupils, that your vet can see during an exam.

Ear infections are the most common cause of circling, says Dr. Tiches. Giving antibiotics for a week or two will quickly clear things up, although it may take days or even weeks before your pet entirely regains her bearings and sense of balance.

Tumors are less common, of course, and they can be hard to detect. Your vet may refer you to a veterinary neurologist, who has the training and equipment to diagnose problems early on. Tests for tumors, infections, and other brain problems include the spinal tap, the MRI (magnetic resonance imaging), and the CAT scan.

Surgery is very effective for some types of tumors, says Dr. Munana. Even when a tumor can't be removed, drugs such as prednisone can cause it to shrink, eliminating the symptoms.

See also Chapter 14: Rolling on the Ground

WALKING WITH ARCHED BACK

Clues

- Your pet is vomiting or has a fever.
- There is blood in his urine.
- He has recently taken a hard fall.

Dogs and cats are much more flexible than humans and can bend their backs in some surprising ways. When they are walking, however, their spines are nearly flat—unless they are in pain. Then the back may arch upward like a camel's.

Dogs and cats with belly pain will instinctively pull up on the abdominal muscles to relieve it. Since the belly is attached to the back, raising one naturally raises the other, says Thomas Schmidt, D.V.M. a veterinarian in private practice in Fort Washington, Maryland.

Most bellyaches, especially in dogs, are caused by eating the wrong things, like yesterday's garbage or even stones from the yard, and the discomfort will go away fairly quickly. But belly pain and back arching can also be caused by painful internal problems like pancreatitis, peritonitis, or bloat, says Dr. Schmidt. Kidney or prostate gland infections, which may cause bloody urine as well as back arching, can also be responsible. If your pet is arching his back and is vomiting or has a fever, you need to call your vet immediately, he advises.

Arthritis of the spine or a ruptured spinal disk will often cause a pet to arch his back, adds Dr. Schmidt. Minor muscle strains and sprains can cause it, too.

WHAT YOU CAN DO

Since an arched back is often a red flag for serious problems, you should call your vet right away unless you are sure that it was caused by something minor—a bruise from taking a hard fall, for example, or a slight flare-up of arthritis.

The easiest way to relieve muscle and joint pain is to apply a warm compress to the sore spots, says Kristin Varner, D.V.M., a veterinarian in private practice in Severn, Maryland. She recommends applying a warm compress for about five minutes, three times a day. This will loosen up the muscles and help your pet move more comfortably.

For arthritis, a back rub can be very soothing, Dr. Varner adds. Encourage your pet to lie down, then use your fingers or palms to rub firm, gentle circles down the muscles on both sides of the spine. (Dogs and cats don't like having their fur ruffled, so start at the neck and work backward to the tail.) Doing this for several minutes, once or twice a day, will improve circulation to the back and help take the arch out of the spine, she says.

WHAT YOUR VET WILL DO

Most muscle aches and even problems with the spine can often be diagnosed with a little hands-on investigation. By moving your pet's legs and back in a variety of directions and seeing what hurts, your vet will get a pretty good idea of what the problem is. Since a ruptured spinal disk can cause nerve problems, she will also press on the hind feet to make sure that there is feeling there. Male dogs will usually get a digital rectal exam to check for prostate problems. Cats rarely get prostate infections, so they are spared this indignity.

If your vet can't find anything wrong during the physical part of the exam, she will probably take blood samples to check for infections and to see how well the kidneys and other organs are working. Your vet may recommend x-rays to check out the spine as well.

Spinal pain can usually be controlled (and sometimes eliminated) with anti-inflammatory medications. Dogs are often given aspirin. Cats can't take aspirin, so they are often given prednisone, a steroid that reduces inflammation.

Infections that are serious enough to cause back arching are sometimes difficult to treat. Pets will often need to take oral antibiotics for several weeks or even months. If your pet is truly sick, however, he may need to spend several days in the hospital to make sure that his organs are working properly and that the infection is under control.

WEIGHT GAIN

Clues

- Your pet is mooching or stealing food.
- You can't feel his ribs.
- He has a big belly but is otherwise thin.

If there is one pastime that dogs and cats love more than walks, more than a nap, and even more than chasing a ball, it is eating. And we, their owners, are all too happy to oblige, which is why there are lots of pudgy pets out there.

Being overweight can cause as many problems for pets as it does for people. Heavy dogs and cats are much more likely to develop diabetes, high blood pressure, and liver and joint problems than their thinner friends, says James R. Richards, D.V.M., director of the Cornell Feline Health Center at the College of Veterinary Medicine at Cornell University in Ithaca, New York.

The main cause of overweight, of course, is eating too much. It is hard to refuse when your dog stares longingly at his bowl or when your cat meows and rubs against your legs as you walk into the kitchen. Even people who are strict about mealtimes often provide a smorgasbord of snacks—a biscuit here, a tender piece of chicken there—all day long. Those extra calories start adding up, says Dr. Richards.

"Being overweight is probably the single most common nutritional disorder in cats," Dr. Richards adds. Not only are cat foods better tasting and higher in calories than they used to be, but cats, even more than dogs, spend most of their time indoors, so they don't get a lot of exercise.

Being overweight isn't necessarily a sign that your pet is spending too much time at the trough. If he has a potbelly but the rest of his body is thin, he could have a condition called abdominal distention, in which fluids leak into the abdomen, causing the belly to swell, says Jane Shaw, D.V.M., an instructor in the department of anatomy at the College of Veterinary Medicine at Cornell University.

Abdominal distention, which may be caused by a viral infection, can be quite serious, she adds. So if you suddenly notice a bulge where there didn't used to be one, you will want to get your pet to the vet right away.

WHAT YOU CAN DO

Since your pet doesn't jump on the bathroom scale each morning, it is not always easy to tell when he is gaining weight. One test you can do is to run your hands across his sides. If you can't feel his ribs, it is probably time to trim his tummy.

• Set regular mealtimes. Many people feed their pets buffet-style by leaving food in the bowl for them to pick at. While some pets show admirable restraint, others will insist on cleaning their plates—and then ask for more. Rather than making food available all the time, it is a good idea to establish regular mealtimes once or twice a day, says Dr. Richards. Give your pet his usual amount of food and allow about a half-hour for him to eat. If he doesn't eat it all, put away the leftovers until it is time for his next meal. He will eventually learn to eat when the dinner bell rings, and you will be able to control the amount of calories that he takes in.

• Check the quantities. Even when you are watching calories, you may be giving your pets too much food, says Dr. Shaw. When you pour out a

Fat or Thin

Dogs and cats don't step on bathroom scales first thing in the morning, so you won't always know their exact weight. But there is an easy way to tell when they need to slim down: Take a look at their figures.

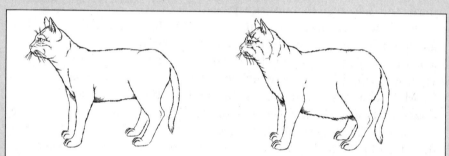

A fit cat will have a well-defined, slim figure, and you will be able to feel the ribs beneath the fur. If your cat's belly protrudes beneath the rib cage and you can't feel the ribs, he is probably overweight.

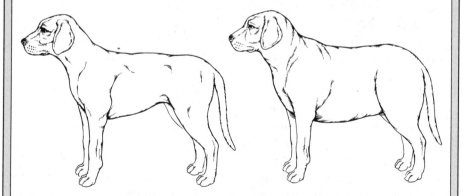

Your dog's ideal weight will depend on his breed, but all dogs should have a distinct waist behind the rib cage. If you can't feel your dog's ribs and he is looking a little thick around the waist, it is probably time to start planning a diet.

bowlful, for example, do you use a measuring cup or do you simply pour "about a cup"? Dr. Shaw recommends measuring the food *after* you have poured it out. You may be amazed at how much you are actually giving.

• Customize his diet. Every pet needs a different amount of food, Dr. Richards says. So even though the instructions on the bag provide a starting point, ask your vet how much you should be putting in the bowl.

• Scale back the servings. Try cutting back the amount you feed him by about 25 percent, says C. A. Tony Buffington, D.V.M., Ph.D., professor of veterinary clinical sciences at the Ohio State University Veterinary Hospital in Columbus. If he hasn't lost any weight in two weeks, reduce the amount a little more.

• Feed him more often. The problem with diets, as humans know all too well, is the constant feeling of hunger. To keep your pets feeling satisfied, Dr. Shaw recommends feeding them less food a little bit more often. Even though their total daily calories will be about the same, the more-frequent meals will help keep them comfortable.

• Read the labels. You may want to switch to a food that is higher in fiber and lower in calories than his usual chow, says Dr. Richards. When buying a new food, check the label to be sure that it is a better choice than his previous food. Or ask your vet which food will be best for your pet.

• Make changes gradually. The problem with switching foods is that dogs—and especially cats—tend to be creatures of habit. "There are some cats that will literally starve themselves before they accept a new food that they don't like," says Dr. Richards. Rather than switching foods all at once, he recommends making the transition slowly by mixing a little bit of the new food in with the old. Every day, add a little bit more of the new food, keeping the total amount the same. If you do this over a few weeks, your pets will probably never notice the difference.

• Stick to healthy snacks. Your pet won't lose weight if he is eating between meals. So cut back on between-meal snacks or at least switch to healthier snacks, like carrot sticks or popcorn cakes, says Dr. Shaw.

Don't be surprised when your pets don't take kindly to their new culinary routines. In fact, you can expect them to resort to surreptitious kitchen raids, digging through the trash, for example, or nabbing food off the counter. Some dogs even learn to open the refrigerator, says Dr. Shaw.

"In some cases, you can hardly live with an animal on a diet," she adds. It can become an almost daily test of wills. For the health of your pet, however, it is a test that you have to win. "Hang in there," Dr. Shaw says, "and after awhile your pet will adjust."

Cutting calories is an essential part of any weight-loss plan, but getting more exercise is also important. For dogs, it is usually easy to get more exercise since they love just about everything that gets them moving: going for walks, chasing balls, or running around the yard.

With cats, of course, going for walks is a bit trickier, especially if your cat isn't leash-trained and there are cars zipping about. But there are other ways to get your feline friend moving, says Dr. Richards. Take a few minutes each day to keep him entertained. Toss a toy mouse. Tease him with a piece of string. Roll a ball across the floor. Anything that gets him excited will get his legs moving and the pounds off. "I have a cat that fetches," he says. "She showed me that she could do it and that she likes it."

When you are helping your pet lose weight, be sure to do this gradually. Giving them too little food will make them hungry and possibly ill, says Dr. Shaw. This is particularly true for cats. They can get a serious liver problem called hepatic lipidosis when they lose too much weight too fast. In fact, cats can develop this condition in as little as a day or two if they don't get enough food.

A safe weight-loss limit is between ½ and 2 percent of his weight each week, says Dr. Buffington. If you have a 100-pound dog, for example, he can safely lose about 1 pound a week. For a 10-pound cat, losing 1 to 2 ounces a week is about right.

WHAT YOUR VET WILL DO

It really isn't necessary to see a vet if your pet is slightly overweight and you are helping him lose a pound or two. For heavier pets, however, vets recommend following a customized weight-loss plan to make sure that they are getting the necessary nutrients. This is particularly true for cats since they are very sensitive to changes in their weight.

Your vet will probably recommend that you come to the office once a month until your pet reaches his ideal weight, says Dr. Richards. This way you can be sure that he is staying healthy while losing weight at a safe pace. And of course, it is a lot easier to check his weight on your vet's large, comfortable scale than on the two-footed model at home. Most vets are happy to weigh pets between visits, he adds, so you can check his weight every few weeks to see how he is doing.

Since pets will sometimes gain weight because of underlying medical problems, your vet will probably do a thorough checkup and run some tests to make sure that nothing serious is happening inside. In rare cases, your vet may recommend a procedure called abdominocentesis, in which fluid is drawn from the abdomen and examined in the laboratory for signs of infection or other problems.

See also Chapter 14: Weight Loss

WEIGHT LOSS

Clues

- Your pet is extremely active and has a high energy level.
- There are worms in his stool.
- He is having trouble chewing.

Any symptom is cause for concern, but unexpected weight loss is a five-alarm warning. It can be caused by dozens of problems, and some of them are serious, says James R. Richards, D.V.M., director of the Cornell Feline Health Center at the College of Veterinary Medicine at Cornell University in Ithaca, New York.

At the very least, weight loss may be caused by a simple (and easy-to-fix) feeding problem. In families with more than one pet, for example, it is not uncommon for one of the more timid fellows not to get his share at mealtimes. In addition, cats are known to be choosy eaters. If you have recently changed foods, it is possible that your finicky feline isn't eating the way he should, which is causing him to lose weight, says Dr. Richards. Finally, some pets, such as those that participate in agility competitions, are extremely active, and their usual diet may not be meeting their needs.

Dogs and cats will occasionally stop eating when they are depressed or under stress, says Dr. Richards. A recent move, the death of another pet, or a change in the family's routine can cause pets to lose weight. This type of weight loss usually doesn't last long and isn't a serious health risk, he adds.

Weight loss often means that there is an internal problem, possibly diabetes or cancer, says Dr. Richards.

A variety of intestinal problems, including parasites, can also cause your pet to lose weight, says Jane Shaw, D.V.M., an instructor in the department of anatomy at the College of Veterinary Medicine at Cornell University.

In cats, weight loss is a common symptom of thyroid problems, says Dr. Richards. The thyroid gland helps regulate the body's metabolism. For pets with a condition called hyperthyroidism, the gland goes into overdrive, producing too much hormone and causing the body to burn more calories than it is taking in.

If your pet has been losing weight and he is also having trouble chewing, there is a good chance that he has dental problems, says Dr. Richards.

It could be, too, that your pet has fractured a tooth, which can make eating painful, says Mark M. Smith, V.M.D., associate professor of surgery in the department of small animal clinical sciences at Virginia–Maryland Regional College of Veterinary Medicine in Blacksburg, Virginia.

What You Can Do

Since many of the conditions that cause weight loss are potentially serious, it is important to catch them early. The problem, says Dr. Richards, is that it's not always easy to tell when your pet has started losing weight. This is particularly true of cats since they often don't show signs of illness until the problem is well-advanced.

It is a good idea to periodically check your pet's weight, he advises. One way to do this, of course, is to weigh him on the bathroom scale. An even simpler strategy is to pay attention to how he feels when you pet him. Your fingers will often notice changes—bonier ribs, for example, or a more prominent spine—that your eyes will miss.

If you suspect that your dog is losing weight because he is unusually active, you may want to start feeding him puppy food even if he is grown since puppy foods are higher in calories than adult foods, says Dr. Shaw. You may also want to feed your pets separately—at different times or in different rooms—to make sure that they all get their share. Elderly pets or those with kidney problems shouldn't be given puppy food, however.

Since cats don't always take kindly to changes in their diets, vets usually recommend feeding them the same food all the time. If you do make a change and your cat is turning up his whiskers at mealtimes, you may have to be a bit sneaky to get him eating again. Try mixing a little bit of the new food with a healthy serving of the old. After a few days, add a little bit more of the new food. If you do this gradually over a week or two, he will probably never notice that he is eating something new, says Dr. Richards.

Since diabetes is a common cause of weight loss in dogs and cats, it is important to keep it under control. (Many of the things that vets recommend for controlling diabetes will help prevent it as well.) Preventing young pets from getting fat will help them maintain healthy weights later on since lean pets are much less likely to get diabetes than their portlier peers. And a pet that already has diabetes will be less likely to develop complications if he doesn't get too fat. Vets also recommend that pets with diabetes eat several small meals a day instead of one big one. Feeding your pet a high-fiber food, which helps slow the absorption of sugars into the bloodstream, can also be very helpful.

To keep your pet's teeth and gums healthy and infection-free, it is important to brush them several times a week, every day is even better. "If we never brushed our teeth, we wouldn't have them very long, and it is the same situation with our pets," says Dr. Smith.

Most pets don't mind having their teeth brushed, especially if you get them used to it when they are young, says Dr. Smith. Some pets actually

The easiest way to brush your pet's teeth is to wrap a piece of gauze around your finger, smear on a little pet toothpaste, and rub the inner and outer surface of each tooth.

look forward to it because pet toothpastes come in tasty flavors, such as meat. Don't use human toothpastes in pets, however, because they contain ingredients that can upset their stomachs.

Another way to keep your pet's teeth and gums healthy is to feed him dry food. Because it is slightly abrasive, dry kibble actually scours the teeth every time he eats. The same is true of hard biscuits and, for pets that like the taste, baby carrots. Canned pet food, on the other hand, sticks to the teeth, making it easier for tooth-damaging bacteria to accumulate.

If your pet already has dental problems, of course, dry food may be too painful for him to eat. To get him back to a healthy weight, it is important to make his meals easier to chew. In this situation, canned food is a good choice, says Dr. Richards. Or you can simply add a bit of warm water to his kibble, which will make it softer and easier to chew.

WHAT YOUR VET WILL DO

Since weight loss can be caused by so many different things, your vet will do a thorough examination to see what the problem is. Your vet will probably want to test for intestinal parasites, so be sure to take along a fresh stool sample, Dr. Richards says.

Since diabetes is quite common, your vet will probably take a urine sample to see if it contains a lot of sugar—a telltale sign of this condition. If your pet does have diabetes, he will probably need daily shots of insulin, along with additional exercise and changes in his diet, to keep his blood sugar under control and his weight healthy, says John Saidla, D.V.M., director of continuing education at the College of Veterinary Medicine at Cornell University.

Your vet will show you how to give the injections, says Dr. Richards. Just be sure to give your pet a lot of love, and perhaps a small treat, after you give the shots. Eventually, your pet will learn that "shot time" is also fun time, and he will be less likely to struggle.

Thyroid problems can be serious, but they are generally easy to treat with oral medications, says Dr. Richards. Or your vet may recommend giving your pet an injection of radioactive iodine, which can help control—or even cure—the problem, he says. At the very worst, your vet may recommend surgery to remove part of the gland, which will reduce the amount of hormone it produces.

To keep your pet's teeth and gums healthy, vets sometimes recommend having the teeth professionally cleaned once a year. It is not a simple procedure, says Deborah S. Greco, D.V.M., Ph.D., associate professor of small animal medicine in the department of clinical sciences at Colorado State University College of Veterinary Medicine and Biomedical Sciences in Fort Collins. Your vet or an assistant will use an ultrasound scaler to chip away tartar on the teeth. Since the device can scratch the teeth, this is followed by a buffing to smooth the surfaces, she explains. The entire procedure usually takes about a half-hour.

As an experiment, Dr. Greco had the cleaning procedure done on *her* teeth. The procedure can be quite uncomfortable, she says, which is why pets are given anesthetic before having it done.

See also Chapter 14: Weight Gain

COMMON WHOLE-BODY CONDITIONS

Anemia. Your pets don't take the classic old blood-booster Geritol, but perhaps they should. Like humans, dogs and cats can get anemia, a condition in which the body's red blood cells either decline in number or aren't able to carry enough oxygen to tissues throughout the body.

There are many causes of anemia. One of the most common is blood loss due to intestinal parasites, for example, or internal bleeding caused by an ulcer. Pets with anemia get weak and tired because their bodies aren't getting enough oxygen, says James Dalley, D.V.M., associate professor of small animal clinical sciences at Michigan State University College of Veterinary Medicine in East Lansing. Pets with anemia often breathe rapidly as well, which is the body's attempt to deliver more oxygen.

Anemia is potentially quite serious, so pets with this condition need to be under a veterinarian's care. The first order of business is to treat the underlying problem that is causing red blood cells to decline in number or to work less efficiently. This is usually easy to do. For instance, in pets with parasites, getting rid of the intruders will allow the body's supply of red blood cells to return to healthy levels. In the meantime, your vet may advise supplementing your pet's diet with liver or other foods that are high in iron and B vitamins. These nutrients are essential for boosting the ability of the blood to carry more oxygen.

Arthritis. Joint problems caused by arthritis occur most often in big dogs for the simple reason that the lifelong strain of carrying themselves around puts a lot of wear and tear on the hips, neck, and other joints in the body. But even small dogs (and cats) are prone to this painful problem.

The most common form of arthritis is called osteoarthritis, which occurs when cartilage and bone in joints begin to wear out and break down, says James R. Richards, D.V.M., director of the Cornell Feline Health Center at the College of Veterinary Medicine at Cornell University in Ithaca, New York. Dogs and cats may get other forms of arthritis as well, including rheumatoid arthritis (caused by problems with the immune system), septic arthritis (caused by infection), and Lyme arthritis (caused by a bite from an infected tick), says Jane Shaw, D.V.M., an instructor in the department of anatomy, also at the College of Veterinary Medicine at Cornell University.

Arthritis that is caused by infection, such as Lyme arthritis, can often be cured with medications, especially when the treatment is started early. In most cases, once your pet has arthritis, he has it for life. By controlling the symptoms, however, you can relieve the discomfort and keep the problems from getting worse. (For more information about treating arthritis, see Difficulty Getting Up on page 247.)

Brain tumors. It doesn't happen often, but occasionally dogs and cats will develop a growth, or tumor, on the brain, which can cause a variety of problems, including seizures.

Brain tumors caused by cancer can be extremely serious. But even when the tumor is benign, it may cause problems because it can press on blood vessels or other brain tissues.

Surgery is often the only solution, although in some cases radiation or chemotherapy are used to shrink the tumor, says Dennis O'Brien, D.V.M., Ph.D., a neurologist in the department of veterinary medicine and surgery at the University of Missouri College of Veterinary Medicine in Columbia.

Cancer. We often think of cancer as being simply a tumor, a hard little bundle of unhealthy cells that start growing somewhere in the body. But cancer is more complicated than that. It can affect many parts of the body at once, causing an enormous range of symptoms. As a result, it is not always easy to diagnose right away.

One of the most common symptoms of cancer is the sudden and unexplained weight loss that occurs. Cancer cells are metabolically very active, and as they are growing rapidly, they steal many of the body's nutrients. A pet with cancer can lose weight even when she is eating a lot, says Dr. Shaw.

Cancer also causes pets to be tired and lethargic. Their coats may look dull, and they may have pain in the joints or elsewhere in their bodies.

Since cancer can appear in so many different ways, it is important to call your vet if you begin noticing symptoms that you can't explain. Cancer can sometimes be stopped if you catch it early, before it spreads to other parts of the body.

Your vet will probably need to take a biopsy, samples of cells that will reveal whether malignant cancer cells are present. If they are, your pet may need treatment very quickly. There are many options for treating cancer, including surgery, radiation, and chemotherapy.

Diabetes. We think of diabetes as being a human problem, but it is quite common in dogs and cats. Pets with diabetes are often tired and lethargic because their bodies aren't producing enough of the hormone insulin that is needed to transport sugars from food into their body's cells. Pets will often lose a lot of weight and may need to urinate frequently, the body's attempt to regulate its unbalanced blood-sugar supply.

Dogs and cats, however, are most likely to get a type of diabetes that usually requires insulin injections, says John Saidla, D.V.M., director of continuing education at the College of Veterinary Medicine at Cornell

University. Once your vet shows you how, the shots are easy to give. You will get plenty of practice since they need to be given once (or more) a day.

Even when your pet is taking insulin, you still need to watch her weight and make sure that she gets plenty of exercise. Keeping her fit will help the insulin work more efficiently, which is essential for preventing diabetes from getting worse. In some cases, in fact, pets are able to reduce their need for medications after they have trimmed down, been kept on a healthy diet, and been exercised frequently.

Encephalitis. The brain is very well-protected from hard knocks within its tough, bony shell. But it is not so well protected from viruses, fungi, and other microorganisms. When germs get into the brain or spinal fluid, they can cause a serious infection called encephalitis. This condition irritates brain tissue, which may result in seizures. In some cases, the seizures don't go away even when the infection is cured, says Dr. O'Brien.

Your vet can diagnose encephalitis by doing a spinal tap. Fluid is extracted and then examined for signs of infection. Pets having seizures may also be given an electroencephalogram to test for unusual brain activity.

Pets with bacterial encephalitis will require antibiotics to treat the severe infection. They may need to spend several days at the vet's office as well, says Charles Lowrie, D.V.M., associate professor of neurology and neural surgery at the Veterinary Teaching Hospital at Michigan State University College of Veterinary Medicine.

Epilepsy. The brain is a virtual powerhouse, using electrical currents to send messages throughout the body and to receive signals from nerves, muscles, and organs. Most of the time, these currents are strictly regulated. But in dogs and cats that have epilepsy, the brain's electricity can suddenly go out of control, causing seizures.

Head injuries are a common cause of epilepsy. Poisoning can cause it, as can a brain infection or a brain tumor. But a lot of the time, vets simply don't know the cause, says Dr. O'Brien. So while epilepsy can sometimes be cured by treating the underlying problem, more often, all you can do is help manage the seizures.

Medications usually won't stop seizures completely, Dr. O'Brien says. But with the right drugs, the seizures may occur much less often and with less severity. Most pets that are being treated for epilepsy are able to live fairly normal lives, he says.

Heart block. It is quite rare, but some dogs and cats develop a condition called heart block, in which electrical signals that regulate the heart are periodically interrupted. The heart literally stops beating for a few seconds, halting blood flow. When blood no longer reaches the brain, your dog may suddenly faint and fall over. (Cats with this condition tend to lose weight and have low energy but will rarely faint.) Heart block is especially common in schnauzers.

Heart block is always serious, so if your pet faints even once, it is important to get him to the vet for a checkup, says Andrea Looney, D.V.M., a veterinarian in private practice in Springfield, Massachusetts. Pets with heart block are usually treated with medications at first. In the long run, however, they will usually need a pacemaker to help the heart maintain its proper rhythm.

Hip dysplasia. In big dogs especially, the hip joints don't always fit together the way they should. This condition, called hip dysplasia, causes the hips to wobble, putting a lot of strain on the joints, often resulting in a painful form of arthritis. Hip dysplasia is most common in German shepherds, golden retrievers, and other large breeds. Among cats, Persians and Maine coons have the highest risk of hip problems.

There isn't a cure for hip dysplasia, but there are ways to relieve the discomfort. (To learn more about what you can do to manage this hereditary condition, see Difficulty Getting Up on page 247.)

Hyperthyroidism. The thyroid gland regulates your body's metabolism, keeping your engine running at the proper speed. When the thyroid gland is overactive, however, it is like stepping on the gas. Dogs and cats with a hyperactive condition burn a lot more calories than they are taking in. Weight loss is one of its most common symptoms.

A number of medications can help regulate the amount of hormone that the thyroid gland produces. And vets sometimes remove part of the thyroid gland. Once a piece of the gland is surgically removed, the thyroid produces less hormone, which can bring the body's metabolism back to normal. Another form of treatment, called radioactive iodine therapy, helps shrink the gland and will keep the body running at a normal speed.

Hypoglycemia. Every time your pet empties her food bowl, the chow is converted into glucose, a sugar the body uses for fuel. But blood sugar levels may fall if a pet has a tumor, is experiencing a side effect of medications, or has some other dietary or health problem. The result is a condition called hypoglycemia, which can result in seizures, says Ronald Stone, D.V.M., a veterinarian and clinical assistant professor of surgery at the University of Miami School of Medicine in Florida.

Hypoglycemia can occasionally be treated simply by putting pets on a special diet or by changing medications. More often, your vet will have to treat the underlying problem first. Since hypoglycemia is typically caused by problems with the liver or pancreas, the resulting treatments can be complicated and time-consuming. Once the original problem is taken care of, the blood-sugar problems will go away very quickly.

Hypothyroidism. Just as an overactive thyroid gland causes your pet's engine to run too quickly, one that is underactive can cause it to run sluggish and slow. This condition, called hypothyroidism, occurs when pets don't produce enough thyroid hormone. As their metabolisms run more slowly, energy levels drop. They usually gain a lot of weight as well.

Hypothyroidism is much more common in dogs than cats, with Doberman pinschers, dachshunds, English bulldogs, boxers, Old English sheepdogs, and Great Danes having an unusually high risk. Untreated, hypothyroidism can be quite serious, though once it is diagnosed, it is easy to treat. Giving your pet thyroid supplements will replenish her natural supplies so that her metabolism runs normally again.

Narcolepsy. Pets with a neurological condition called narcolepsy can be playful and running around—and then suddenly collapse into a deep sleep. This mysterious condition usually isn't dangerous, but it is shocking to see for the first time.

The main danger with narcolepsy is that your pet could fall asleep in a dangerous place—by the side of the road or at the top of a flight of stairs. Your vet may recommend medications to control the sleep attacks, but they aren't a cure. The most important thing that you can do is keep your pet in a safe place so that she won't get hurt if she suddenly nods off, says Dr. Saidla.

Condition Index

Underscored page references indicate boxed text. *Italic* references indicate
illustrations.

I

Symptom Index

Italic references indicate illustrations.

T

Tail
chewing of, 78–80
limpness of, 228–29
secretions from oil-producing
glands at base of, 230
Teeth. *See also* Chewing
discoloration of, 310–11
sores on, 313
Temper, 66–68
Testicles, undescended, 231
Thirst, excessive, 40–42
Tilting, of head, 105–6
Tiredness, 402–4
Toes, soreness of, 275–77
Tongue
blue, 286–87
chewing problems and, 288
sores on, 288
spots on, 308–9
Trembling, 413–14

U

Ulcers, decubital, 370–71
Undescended testicles, 231
Urination
crying during, 84–86
difficulty with, 232–34

frequent, 235–36, 398
incontinence and, 109,
218–19
less frequently than usual,
237–38
straining on, 84–86
in wrong place, 109–11
Urine
blood in, 214–15, 420
clear, 237
incontinence of, 218–19
spraying of, 109, 122–23, 235

V

Vision. *See* Eyes
Vomit, blood in, 136–37
Vomiting, 43, 44, 151–52, 420

W

Walking
with arched back, 420–21
in circles, 418–19
Weight
gain, 57, 422–25, *423*
loss, 55, 58, 426–29, 431
Wheezing, 332–34
Whining, 81–83
Wool chewing, 59–60

Subject
Index

Underscored page references indicate boxed text. *Italic* references indicate illustrations.

E